Arthur Hartmann

The diseases of the ear and their treatment

Arthur Hartmann

The diseases of the ear and their treatment

ISBN/EAN: 9783743357372

Manufactured in Europe, USA, Canada, Australia, Japa

Cover: Foto ©ninafisch / pixelio.de

Manufactured and distributed by brebook publishing software (www.brebook.com)

Arthur Hartmann

The diseases of the ear and their treatment

THE DISEASES OF THE EAR

AND THEIR TREATMENT.

BY

ARTHUR HARTMANN, M.D.,

BERLIN.

TRANSLATED FROM THE THIRD GERMAN EDITION BY

JAMES ERSKINE, M.A., M.B.,

SURGEON FOR DISEASES OF THE EAR TO ANDERSON'S COLLEGE DISPENSARY, GLASGOW; LATE ASSISTANT-SURGEON TO THE GLASGOW HOSPITAL AND DISPENSARY FOR DISEASES OF THE EAR.

WITH FORTY-TWO ILLUSTRATIONS.

NEW YORK

G. P. PUTNAM'S SONS

27 AND 29 WEST 23D ST.

1887.

EDINBURGH: PRINTED AT THE UNIVERSITY PRESS FOR YOUNG J. PENTLAND
BY T. AND A. CONSTABLE, PRINTERS TO HER MAJESTY.

THE AUTHOR'S PREFACE TO THE FIRST EDITION.

IN preparing this work I have endeavoured to give a concise account of the Diseases of the Ear and their Treatment, along with an epitome of all that is of value to general practitioners who may undertake the treatment of these diseases. For special study, the text-books of Von Tröltsch, Politzer, Urbantschitsch, and Gruber may be mentioned, to which also reference may be made for the original literature of the subject.

In order to make the book as acceptable as possible I have omitted, or only indicated, whatever is still hypothetical, and not in accordance with the compact and practical character of the work.

I have departed from my original intention of dispensing with Anatomy, and have placed a short anatomical sketch at the beginning of each Chapter, where it appeared necessary, for the purpose of enabling the reader to appreciate the pathological conditions. For the descriptive anatomy and embryology of the Ear reference may be made to the text-books already mentioned, and to works on Anatomy.

My own experience has been the basis of my estimate of the importance of existing views and contributions, and I have given those methods of treatment special prominence which I have found useful, and can therefore recommend.

Dr. ARTHUR HARTMANN.

Berlin, *August* 1881.

THE AUTHOR'S PREFACE TO THE THIRD EDITION.

The concise form and practical character of the First Edition of this Work have obtained for it a much better reception than I anticipated. The rapid sale of the two former editions is evidence that such a book was required.

While the present edition contains many improvements and additions, and all that is new on the subject, care has been taken to preserve the original form of the book. I may therefore venture to hope that the third edition will meet with the same favourable reception as the former two.

Dr. ARTHUR HARTMANN.

Berlin, *September* 1885.

THE TRANSLATOR'S PREFACE.

On account of the increased amount of attention now given to the study and practice of Aural Surgery, this translation has been undertaken with the view of placing in the hands of English practitioners and students a book specially suited to their requirements. Its scientific and practical value is attested by the favourable reception accorded to it in Germany, and by the Author's important and numerous contributions to Otology. The attention which Dr. Hartmann's book deserves has led me to endeavour to make it more widely known.

I have to express my thanks to all who have assisted me, but especially to my esteemed friend Dr. Richard A. D. Robb for his hearty co-operation.

In the Appendix I have placed a list of instruments, and also the therapeutical formulæ in a form for easy reference.

JAMES ERSKINE.

6 Newton Street, Charing Cross,
Glasgow, *January* 1887.

CONTENTS.

	PAGE
HISTORICAL,	1

CHAPTER I.
DIAGNOSTIC.

Inspection without Instruments—Inspection with Speculum and Reflected Light—Examination with Siegle's Speculum—Examination with the Probe—Cleansing the Ear—Testing the Hearing—The Air-douche—The Diagnostic and Therapeutic Application of the Air-douche. 8

CHAPTER II.
SYMPTOMATOLOGY.

Noises in the Ear—Auditory Vertigo—Hyperæsthesia of the Auditory Nerve—Paracusis and Diplacusis—Paracusis Willisii—Autophony, 52

CHAPTER III.

FREQUENCY, ÆTIOLOGY, AND PROPHYLAXIS OF EAR DISEASES, 62

CHAPTER IV.
GENERAL THERAPEUTICS.

Application of Remedies through the External Meatus—Blood-letting—Application of Electricity—Constitutional Treatment—Hearing-tubes, ... 67

CHAPTER V.

DISEASES OF THE AURICLE.

Anatomy—Eczema—Acute Inflammation of the Auricle—Blood-tumour of the Ear—Other Diseases of the Auricle, ... 76

CHAPTER VI.

DISEASES OF THE EXTERNAL MEATUS.

Anatomy — Anomalies of Secretion — Circumscribed Inflammation — Diffuse Inflammation — Desquamative Inflammation — Fungus — Herpes Auricularis—Syphilis—Foreign Bodies—Contraction and Closure—Formation of Blood-cysts—Caries and Necrosis of the Osseous Meatus, ... 82

CHAPTER VII.

DISEASES OF THE MEMBRANA TYMPANI.

Anatomy—Acute Inflammation—Chronic Inflammation—Extravasation of Blood—Rupture—The Artificial Membrana Tympani—Anomalies of Tension, ... 109

CHAPTER VIII.

DISEASES OF THE MIDDLE EAR.

Anatomy—Acute Inflammation—Acute Catarrh—Acute Purulent Inflammation—Contraction and Closure of the Eustachian Tube—Abnormal Patency of the Eustachian Tubes—Neuroses of the Muscles — Foreign Bodies in the Eustachian Tube — Chronic Catarrh—Chronic Purulent Inflammation—Deposits of Exudation Products and Formation of Cholesteatomata—Polypi—Disease of the Osseous Walls—Cerebral Abscess—Meningitis Purulenta—Phlebitis, Thrombosis, Pyæmia—Tuberculosis—Opening the Mastoid Process—Chronic Inflammation of the Middle Ear without Exudation—Nervous Earache—Hæmorrhage into the Tympanum, . 120

CHAPTER IX.

DISEASES OF THE INTERNAL EAR.

PAGE

Anatomy—Physiology—General Remarks—Hyperæmia of the Labyrinth—Anæmia of the Labyrinth—Hæmorrhage into the Labyrinth—Acute Inflammation of the Labyrinth—Chronic Inflammatory Processes—Menière's Complex of Symptoms—Concussion of the Labyrinth—Syphilis of the Labyrinth—Deafness in Leukæmia—Deafness in Cases of Mumps—Diseases of the Auditory Nerve—Other Diseases affecting the Nervous Structures—Deafness in Hysteria—Otitis intermittens—Disease of the Cerebral Tracts of the Auditory Nerve and Centre, ... 207

CHAPTER X.

Traumatic Lesions, Neoplasms, and Malformations, 234

CHAPTER XI.

Deaf-Mutism, 241

Therapeutic Formulæ, . 251

List of Instruments, . . 256

Indexes, . 257

LIST OF ILLUSTRATIONS.

FIG.		PAGE
1.	Ear specula,	9
2.	Mirror attached to head-band,	10
3.	Normal tympanic membrane,	11
4.	Tympanic membrane with perforation,	13
5.	,, ,, calcareous deposit,	13
6.	Indrawn tympanic membrane,	14
7.	Tympanic membrane with large perforation,	15
8.	Bent probe with hook-shaped point,	17
9.	Politzer's bent forceps,	18
10.	Aural syringe with bent nozzle,	18
11.	India-rubber ball syringe,	19
12.	Cotton-holder (Hartmann's),	20
13.–16.	Graphic representations of the results of testing the hearing with tuning-forks,	31, 32
17.	Politzer's inflating bag,	38
18.	Olive-shaped nozzle,	38
19.	Catheter-shaped nose-piece,	38
20.	Antero-posterior vertical section, showing outer wall of right nasal and naso-pharyngeal cavities,	40
21.	Eustachian catheter,	41
22.	Transverse vertical section through the anterior portion of the nasal cavity, showing convexity of the septum,	43
23.	Furuncle knife,	93
24.	Sharp hook for removing soft foreign bodies,	102
25.	Toynbee's artificial tympanic membrane,	116
26.	Hartmann's ,, ,,	118
27.	Section through external auditory meatus, tympanum, and Eustachian tube, showing relation of parts,	121

LIST OF ILLUSTRATIONS.

FIG.		PAGE
28. 29.	} Vertical section through temporal bone, showing variation of sigmoid fossa, ...	124
30. 31.	} Horizontal section through temporal bone, showing similar variation, ...	125
32.	Diagram representing positions assumed by the membranous portion of the Eustachian tube and by the soft palate, . .	127
33.	Instrument for paracentesis, . . .	138
34.	Normal tympanic membrane,	144
35.	Indrawn tympanic membrane, ...	144
36. 37.	} Sagittal sections through the temporal bones of children, three years of age, showing the antrum petrosum and cell-cavities, .	172
38.	Hartmann's metal tympanic tube, .	185
39.	Schwartze's antrum tube, . .	185
40.	Polypus snare, ...	193
41.	Diagram of internal ear, ...	207
42.	Vertical section through one of the windings of the cochlea,	208

DISEASES OF THE EAR

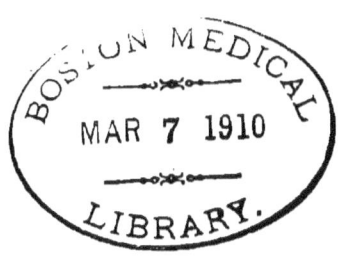

THE DISEASES OF THE EAR.

HISTORICAL.

THE earliest mention of diseases of the ear, according to Professor Brugsch, is to be found in an ancient papyrus scroll preserved in the Egyptian collection of the Berlin Museum. He believes that its date belongs to the reign of Ramses II., who adopted the Jewish lawgiver, Moses, *i.e.* to the fourteenth century B.C. In this scroll, the contents being chiefly of a medical character, two complete prescriptions for ear diseases are to be noticed, one of them a 'remedy for removing a heaviness in the ear,' the other 'for curing eruptions at both ears.' The observation is also notable that 'there are two tubes in the right ear, by which the breath of life enters, and two tubes in the left ear, by which the atmosphere (*sic*) enters.'

Hippocrates (about 460 to 377 B.C.) wrote extensively on the subject of diseases of the organ of hearing. According to his theories of humoral pathology, he considered the mucus and gall as the principal factors in ear diseases. Hippocrates seems to have first recognised the membrana tympani. He described it as a very dry thin skin, like a spider's web in appearance.

For acute inflammation with violent pain, he recommended restricted diet, instillation of oil, and fomentation with sponges dipped in hot water. Otorrhœa was regarded by him as a disease of the head, accompanied by a discharge of mucus.

In the third century B.C., the Empiric *Apollonius* employed a large number of remedies for ear diseases, such as opium for earache, and oil of bitter almonds for fleas and worms in the ear. He removed foreign bodies by means of ear-scoops, pincers, small hooks, and probes; and he even gave directions for softening hardened cerumen, and cleansing the ear with tepid water or oil.

Celsus (about the time of the birth of Christ), in his comprehensive work on medicine, declared that ear diseases are far more dangerous than eye affections, as they sometimes end in insanity and death: 'Ergo ubi primum dolorem aliquis sensit, abstinere et continere se debet.' He distinguished between congenital closure of the external meatus and that caused by ulceration, and held that an operation ought only to be performed when, by the probe, it has been ascertained that the closure is of a membranous character. He directed that a perforation should be made by means of caustics, a red-hot iron, or a knife, and kept open by the insertion of a quill, coated with an ointment to accelerate cicatrisation. Celsus recommended good methods for removing foreign bodies. He directed that fleas which had crept into the ear should be caught by wool saturated with sticky substances, and that inanimate bodies should be removed by vigorous syringing with the ear-syringe (auriculario clystere), or extracted by a probe or a blunt bent hook (specillo auriculario aut hamulo retuso paulum recurvato protrahendum est). The following proceeding is also somewhat ingenious:—The patient was laid on a table, with the ear containing the foreign body directed downwards, and the table being struck with a hammer, whatever was in the ear tumbled out. Torn lobes of the ear, according to Celsus, reunited by means of the blood seam. He also mentioned the plastic operation for replacing loss of substance.

Galen of Pergamum (A.D. 131-210) has, in addition to his anatomical and physiological studies, entered very fully into the subject of ear diseases. He divided them according to the symptoms into five classes:—1. Ὠταλγία, *auris dolor;* 2. Βαρυηκοΐα, *auditus gravitas;* 3. Κωφότης, *surditas;* 4. Παρακοῦσις seu παρακοὴ, *obauditio;* 5. Παρακούσματα, *auditus hallucinationes.* Galen laid down certain principles for the treatment of the various diseases, and protested against the rude empirical methods of some of the surgeons of his time. He condemned the employment of opium, which was then very much in use, and recommended nut-gall and alum as remedies for otorrhœa. He always employed the very mildest remedies at first, and only gradually made use of stronger ones. Galen first gave an exact description of the brain and the cranial nerves, including the auditory nerve.

Alexander of Tralles in Lydia (A.D. 525-605) was the most important surgeon who lived in the period after Galen. He distinguished between external and internal inflammation of the ear, and pointed out the dangers of the latter, as the brain might also become affected. He observed inflammation of the ear with convulsions caused by foreign bodies. For such inflammation he advised first the instillation of oil, and then extraction of the foreign body, which is thereby facilitated after reduction of the inflammation. In his time the greatest variety of hearing-tubes was in use.

Paul of Ægina (seventh century), when the removal of foreign bodies could not be effected in any other way, made a crescent-shaped incision into the meatus behind the auricle, as had been proposed by Hippocrates.

Rhazes, one of the Arabian surgeons (A.D. 850-932), advised the examination of the ear always by sunlight. *Abul Kasem* (died A.D. 1106), who had a great predilection for the actual cautery, used it also for earache, applying it all round the ear in ten different spots previously marked with ink. Adhesions deeply situated in the meatus he also destroyed with the hot iron.

At the close of the Middle Ages, and at the dawn of our own era, ox-gall, human milk, various kinds of urine, and other unapetising fluids were among the chief remedies for diseases of the ear. The urine of male animals was to be applied to male patients, and that of female animals to female patients. *Serapion*, who recommended human milk for otalgia in children, asserted that if the patient be a boy, the milk must be obtained from a woman who suckles a girl. *Gadesden* mentioned a remedy used by a quack for tinnitus:—He put a tube into the meatus, and got some poor person to suck it. This was also done in cases of suppuration. *William of Saliceto* (died A.D. 1277) tied fleshy growths in the meatus with a silk thread or a horse-hair, and burned their roots.

Peter de la Cerlata (died A.D. 1423) first suggested the use of an ear-speculum for examining and dilating the meatus (per inspectionem ad solem trahendo aurem et ampliando cum speculo aut alio instrumento).

While in the Classical and Middle Ages only diseases of the external ear received attention, other affections having been considered as due to the abnormal action of the 'inborn air,' to which *Aristotle* ascribed the power of hearing, we find in the sixteenth century, hand in hand with further progress in anatomy and physiology, a better knowledge also of the organ of hearing and its diseases. The researches of *Fallopius* (1523-1562) were of great importance. He described the labyrinth in detail, and discovered the two fenestræ and the semicircular canals, as also the tympanum, to which he gave its name. He in particular described the canal of the facial nerve, which is named after him.

Eustachius (died 1570) contributed in a very especial manner to the knowledge of the organ of hearing. He discovered the two intrinsic muscles of the ear and the tube connecting the tympanum with the pharynx, which bears his name. Fallopius recommended the use of a mirror for examining the ear. Fleshy growths and polypi were removed by means of a lead tube pushed over them, and the application of a wick dipped in sulphuric acid.

The renowned anatomist, *Andreas Vesalius* (1513-1564), first described the ossicles, but only the malleus and incus. *Ingrassias* (1510-1580) afterwards observed the third ossicle, which he called the stapes.

Hieronymus Capivaccius wrote regarding thickening ulceration, and cicatrisation of the membrana tympani, and pointed out that deafness does not result from defect of the ossicles. He was the first to employ bone-conduction in the differential diagnosis of cases of deafness arising from an affection of the membrana tympani, and from diminished sensibility of the auditory nerve. *Hercules Sassonia* believed that the hearing would be completely destroyed by rupture of the membrane, an opinion which *Willis* afterwards disproved, by experiments on dogs. Beans which had swollen in the ear were reduced in bulk by means of a hot wire, inserted through a tube. *Koyter* first expressed the opinion that sound is transmitted from the membrana tympani to the labyrinth by the ossicula. Otology was considerably enriched by the excellent work of *Du Verney*, 'Traité de l'organe de l'ouïe contenant la structure, les usages et les maladies de toutes les parties de l'oreille,' Paris, 1683. As was formerly exclusively the case, he did not regard tinnitus as an independent disease, but as a symptom of brain-affections, or of various ear diseases. For anatomical reasons, he opposed the opinion prevailing hitherto, that the secretion in otorrhœa had its origin in the brain. According to him, the function of the membrana tympani is to stretch or slacken according to the intensity of the sound. The cochlea, with its nerve structures gradually varying in length from base to apex, he compared to an instrument spanned by many strings, serving to measure the sounds, and to make their variations perceptible. *Le Cat, Boerhaave*, and others were also of opinion that the labyrinth contained a great number of strings which responded to the vibrations produced by every tone. The last-named also asserted, that for high tones the tension of the membrana tympani was greater than for low.

Valsalva rendered a great service to the anatomy and pathology of the ear by his celebrated work 'De aure humana tractatus,' Bologna, 1704, in which, based upon more than one thousand dissections, he gave a most minute description of the external and middle ear, as well as of the labyrinth, and added much to the knowledge of the subject. He declared that hardened cerumen was frequently the unrecognised cause of deafness. In one case, he observed deafness arising from anchylosis of the foot-plate of the stapes with the fenestra vestibuli. As the best method for removing pus from the ear, he recommended forcing air through the Eustachian tube, with the mouth and nose closed. This method was therefore named the 'Valsalvian experiment.' He showed that deafness is frequently caused by obstruction of the Eustachian tube, and mentions the case of a man in whom a nasal polypus extended to the uvula, closing the mouth of the tube, and thereby causing deafness. Although *Schellhammer* had previously (1684) recognised the actual condition of the labyrinth, Valsalva was still of opinion that it was filled with air. *Cotugno* afterwards gave an exact description of the contents of the labyrinth.

In the year 1750, *Cleland*, an Englishman, proposed catheterism of the Eustachian tube by a silver probe-shaped tube inserted through the nose, as a means for injecting air and fluids. He thus gave the first impetus to the rational therapeutics of ear diseases. Some regard *Guyot*, the postmaster of Versailles, as the inventor of catheterism. He introduced through the mouth into the vicinity of the orifice of the Eustachian canal a knee-shaped tube, through which he injected fluids into that region; but it is by no means certain that he succeeded in injecting them into the Eustachian canal itself. The details of catheterism were perfected at a later date, especially by *Deleau*, *Itard*, and *Kramer*.

Treviranus held the view that, without free circulation, the air in the tympanic cavity must soon be changed into nitrogen and carbonic acid gas. *J. L. Petit* first gave a detailed description (1724) of carious processes in the temporal bone, and advocated the operation of trephining the mastoid. In one case he removed with hammer and chisel so much of the bone that the seat of the suppuration was exposed, and a cure effected. Even before his time, *Riolan* (1649) proposed trephining of the mastoid in cases of deafness and tinnitus from obstruction in the Eustachian tube. *Morand* trephined a carious temporal bone in a case of purulent discharge from the ear. After making an opening in the brain-covering below which the pus was lying, he inserted a tube through it, and cured the patient. In Germany, the army-surgeon *Jasser*, in the case of a soldier, successfully trephined both mastoid processes. This operation was afterwards discarded, because a Danish surgeon fell a victim to it through the opening of the cranial cavity. *Cotugno* (1736-1822) first proved conclusively that the labyrinth contained fluid; Aristotle's theory that it was filled with air was hitherto generally accepted. He discovered the two aqueducts, and held that they are designed to let the labyrinthine fluid escape, in order to protect the nerve from too severe concussion. The accidental rupture of the membrana tympani by means of an ear-scoop having resulted in the restoration of a deaf person's hearing, had induced *Riolan* to ask, whether an artificial opening of the membrane ought not to be tried as a remedy for deafness. *Cheselden* desired to perform this operation on a criminal condemned to death, who was to obtain his release on account of it. But as this proposal met with general disfavour, he had to abandon it. The operation was for the first time performed by *Astley Cooper*, in the year 1800; and it soon grew in favour all over Europe, attempts being made everywhere by its means to relieve not only the deaf, but even deaf-mutes.

Anatomical and physiological research with regard to the organ of hearing having thus during the last hundred years made considerable progress, it has been reserved for our own century, by the aid of pathological anatomy, hand in hand with careful clinical observation, to raise the science of otology to that point it has now attained, our diagnosis having obtained well-established foundations on the one hand, and our therapeutics well-defined points of attack on the other. In France, *Itard* and *Deleau;* in England, *Wilde* and *Toynbee;* and in Germany, *Lincke* and *Kramer*, have, during the first half of our century, rendered special service to the advancement of otological science.

In recent times, the publication of periodicals specially devoted to this branch of medicine, in whose pages all the most important contributions are collected, has proved a very important factor in the scientific development of otology. In this way the study of the subject has been facilitated, and encouragement given to renewed research. The 'Archiv für Ohrenheilkunde' is the oldest of these publications, having been started in 1864 by Tröltsch, Politzer, and Schwartze. The 'Zeitschrift für Ohrenheilkunde' was first edited by Knapp and Moos, in 1869, and published as a part of the 'Archiv für Augen- und Ohrenheilkunde,' but subsequently issued separately. It appears now simultaneously in German and English. The 'American Journal of Otology' ceased to appear after existing for four years. In addition to the two publications above mentioned, a number of Journals are published in Germany and other countries, devoted both to laryngology and otology.

CHAPTER I.

DIAGNOSTIC.

INSPECTION WITHOUT INSTRUMENTS.

The inspection of the external meatus may be made in two ways. When the meatus is sufficiently wide, it may be examined in a superficial manner without the use of instruments; but in order to obtain a good view, the ear-speculum and reflected light have to be employed. When the examination is conducted according to the former of these methods, the patient is placed toward a window or a lamp, in such a position that the rays of light fall upon the ear to be examined in the direction of the axis of the external meatus. The auricle is then pulled backward and outward with the one hand, thereby straightening the curve of the meatus; while, with the thumb of the other hand, the tragus is simultaneously pressed forward. Thus the head of the observer does not prevent the light from falling into the ear, and in this manner it is frequently possible, especially in the case of children, to examine the whole meatus and the membrana tympani without the aid of a speculum.

INSPECTION WITH SPECULUM AND REFLECTED LIGHT.

As it is in many cases impossible to inspect the membrana tympani in the manner described above, because the tragus lies in front of the meatus, or hairs at the orifice obstruct the view, instruments which dilate the meatus are required. Formerly, Kramer's bivalve speculum was mostly used for this purpose, but now only the more simple cylindrical cone-shaped specula are employed. They are either formed of vulcanite or metal, generally silver and nickel. Three different sizes of specula are used, according to the width of the meatus, as represented in Fig. 1.

Many aural surgeons still use the conical specula first recommended by Wilde, although even Von Tröltsch, who introduced them into Germany, has long since discarded them for those of the cylindrical cone-shape. The latter cannot be dispensed with in the examination of children, and in cases of stenosis of the external portion of the meatus. It has often been attempted to provide the specula with lenses, in order to obtain a magnified view; but as the method of examination with the simple speculum and reflected light is in all cases sufficient for diagnosis and treatment, such appliances seem to be superfluous. Brunton's speculum, which is so constructed that the speculum and the reflector are connected by a metallic cylinder, is still much used in France and Italy; but as this mirror is only suitable for inspection, and not for the simultaneous introduction of instruments, it can neither be used for thorough investigation nor for rational treatment.

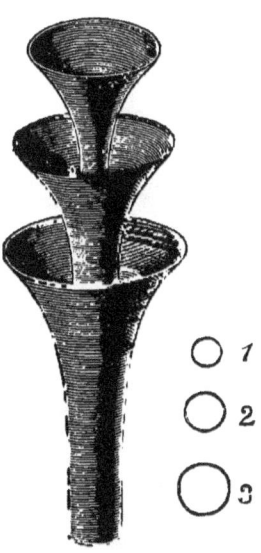

FIG. 1.

The introduction of the speculum ought to be quite painless to the patient, except in cases of inflammation of the external meatus, when great care must be exercised. The examination is performed as follows (right ear):—The auricle being firmly held between the middle and fourth finger of the left hand, and drawn backward and outward, the speculum is inserted with the right hand. The thumb and forefinger of the left hand are then applied to the rim of the speculum, and keep it in position. After illuminating the meatus, the deeper parts can be brought into view, by moving the speculum downward, upward, backward, and forward. By changing the position of the speculum in this way, and not by inserting it deeper, the various parts of the membrana tympani and of the meatus can be inspected. It is to be carefully noted that not only the external rim of the speculum must be moved, but that it is necessary to raise and lower it in its whole length, along with the membranous portion of the external meatus. If these precautions be observed, the patient will never feel any pain from the examination. After introducing the speculum, direct light is generally found to be insufficient to illuminate the meatus; a mirror, with a hole drilled through its centre, is therefore used to reflect the light. Clear daylight, or the light of a good gas or paraffin-oil lamp, supplied with a large burner, is sufficient. The light may be intensified by placing around the flame a metal or earthenware cylinder, with a longitudinal slit in it. During the examination, the ear of the patient is turned away from the source of light, and the rays which fall upon the mirror of the observer are reflected into the ear. The lamp is placed at the right hand of the patient, and on a level with his ear (Fig. 2).

The mirror required for this examination is concave, having a focal distance of 15 to 20 cm., and in its centre a hole about 1 cm. in diameter. It is either furnished with a handle (Hoffman, Von Tröltsch) or it is fixed on the brow of the examiner, generally by means of a head-band. As the left hand is required for holding the speculum, the hand-mirror, if used, must be held in the right hand. But as certain manipulations are frequently necessary in order to make a thorough examination of the membrana tympani, and as one hand must be free for the treatment, the hand-mirror is

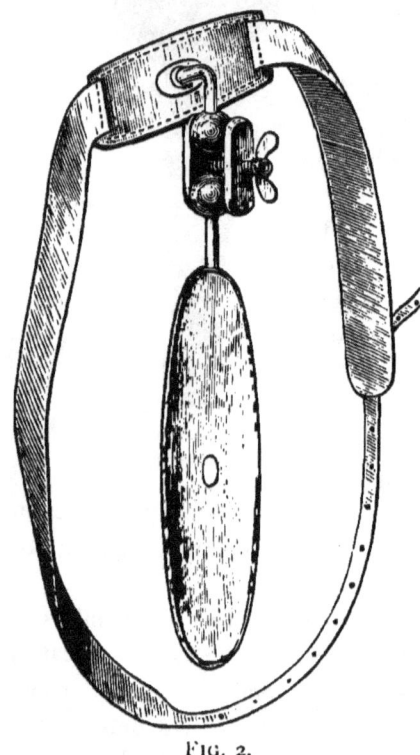

FIG. 2.

rarely used. The mirror can be most simply and efficiently employed when fastened to the head-band (Fig. 2). A mirror of a large size is also suitable for rhinoscopy and laryngoscopy. It is fitted to the head-band in a variety of ways; and as mobility in all directions is of the greatest importance, the manner of fastening it, as represented in the illustration, seems the most suitable. The contrivance consists of a double ball-joint, which allows the mirror to be moved in all directions. The mobility of many head-mirrors is so limited that an examination is rendered very difficult.

Czermak fixed the mirror to a plate which is held between the teeth. This mode of fixture may be recommended most to those who cannot use the head-band. Such a mirror is very handy, as it occupies very little space in the instrument case. The mouth-plate mirror, which the writer employs, is also furnished with a double ball-joint. It can be used very conveniently as a hand-mirror. Semeleder adjusted the mirror to a spectacle frame. Berthold suggested fastening the mirror by means of a ring to a finger of the left hand. When the reflecting mirror is united with the speculum itself, it does not admit of the introduction of instruments during the examination. Sunlight affords the best illumination, and requires a plane mirror; but, unfortunately, sunlight is not always at our disposal, and in summer the heat of the sun is apt to be troublesome.

In examining the external meatus, note should be taken of the presence of hyperæmia, swelling, ulceration, growths, or foreign bodies. In order to obtain a good view, it is often necessary to remove secretion, in the manner to be indicated afterwards. The *membrana tympani* (Fig. 3) appears to the eye as a pearl-grey, transparent membrane, which is inclined towards the long axis of the meatus, and forms with its superior-posterior wall an angle of about 140°. 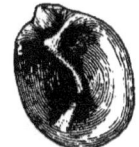

FIG. 3.

The surface of the membrane is conically indrawn. As a landmark in the examination (see Fig. 3, left membrana tympani), the handle of the *malleus*, which first attracts the eye, must be identified. It lies upon the inner surface of the membrane, and appears from the outside like a narrow white ledge, extending from near the anterior-superior boundary towards the centre, commencing with a small white tubercle, the *processus brevis*, and ending with a yellowish spot, the *umbo*. Above the short process of the malleus is situated that portion of the membrane which is called the *membrana flaccida Shrapnelli*. When the convex curve of the anterior wall of the meatus is well marked, the anterior portion of the membrane is sometimes not visible. The normal membrane presents a bright triangular-shaped spot of reflected light, extending forward and downward from the umbo. From its apex at the umbo, it does not quite extend to the margin of the membrane. Politzer has shown that a reflection of light can only appear upon the membrane when the latter is met perpendicularly by the axis of vision. Not unfrequently this cone of reflected light is irregularly formed; it may be divided in the centre, or only a spot-like reflection may appear, either at the umbo or at the margin of the membrane. From such appearances we may infer that the surface of the membrane is not met perpendicularly by the axis of vision, and must therefore either be drawn inward or bulged outward. Another spot of reflected light is frequently to be observed upon Shrapnell's membrane.

In children the membrana tympani is of a dullish white colour, and non-transparent, but it gradually becomes more and more bright, until at the age of 12 to 15 it becomes perfectly transparent and lustrous. Later in life it turns whitish yellow, is less transparent, and loses its lustre.

In order to simplify the description of the different parts of the membrana tympani it is divided, in accordance with its circular form, into four quadrants. The two quadrants of the lower half of the membrane, the anterior-inferior and the posterior-inferior, form each nearly a fourth part of the circle, but the posterior-superior quadrant is larger, and the anterior-superior is smaller than a fourth part, as these two are separated from each other by the handle of the malleus, extending from the anterior-superior boundary towards the centre of the membrane.

Deviations from the Normal Condition of the Membrana Tympani.

1. Its appearance may be changed—

(*a*) By hyperæmia. If the epidermal layer be hyperæmic to a slight degree, the blood-vessels round the short process of the malleus and along the handle are injected, and the vessels radiating from the umbo to the periphery may be distinguished. If the hyperæmia be of a higher degree, extending to the deeper layers of the membrane, a diffused redness is the result, or it may be so great that the whole membrana tympani assumes a scarlet appearance. In cases of hyperæmia of the middle and internal layers of the membrane this diffused redness varies in degree.

Redness confined to the central and posterior portion of a tympanic membrane, whose appearance is otherwise normal, may be occasioned by the hyperæmic mucous membrane of the promontory.

(*b*) By loosening of the epidermal layer under the influence of moist substances. Instillations and secretions destroy the lustre of the surface of the membrane.

(*c*) By inflammatory infiltration, which causes the membrane to be thickened and obscured. The outlines of the malleus are less distinct; the short process is sometimes recognised only as a small projection (see Fig. 4, right membrana tympani with perforation). Degeneration of connective tissue, fatty degeneration, calcification or hypertrophy, produces a whitish or yellowish discoloration of the membrane. Especially as a sequence of purulent inflammation of the middle ear, circumscribed and generally crescentic-shaped calcareous deposits are frequently found (see Fig. 5).

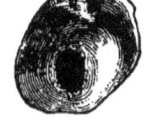

FIG. 4.

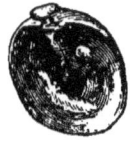

FIG. 5.

(*d*) By opaque mucous fluid in the tympanum, the membrane assuming a darker or bottle-green appearance. When the secretion is purulent and of a yellowish colour, the membrane is correspondingly coloured. Sometimes the line marking the level of the fluid in the tympanic cavity may be observed through the membrane.

(*e*) By chronic secretive inflammation of the external meatus and of the membrana tympani, giving rise to minute red elevations producing a granular appearance of the membrane.

2. Changes in the position of the membrana tympani:—

(*a*) Of the greatest importance is inward curvature of the whole membrane arising from obstruction to the ventilation in the tympanum (see Fig. 6). In such cases the posterior-superior half of the membrane appears diminished in extent, due to the horizontal position which it assumes, while the anterior-inferior half seems enlarged. For the same reason the handle of the malleus appears shortened in perspective. Sometimes the malleus is so much indrawn that the position of the handle is quite horizontal, and is not visible at all. The membrana tympani, by applying itself closer to the malleus, causes the handle to become more prominent, and the short process especially is observed as a strongly projecting tubercle. From this point also extend anteriorly and posteriorly, likewise strongly projecting, the tightly-stretched folds of the membrane. As the peripheric portions are generally more capable of resistance, the central part only is indrawn, causing an indentation of the membrane (Politzer). When the inward curvature is very great, it may lie upon the promontory.

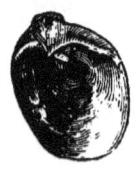

Fig. 6.

(*b*) Cicatrisation produces circumscribed indrawings of the membrana tympani. The cicatrices, in consequence of their thinness, are more transparent, and can easily be distinguished from the surrounding portions of the membrane.

(*c*) These cicatrices bulge outward when air is forced into the tympanic cavity. A bulging of the epidermal layer is observed arising from exudation between it and the membrana propria, with or without communication with the tympanic cavity. We meet with these vesicles or exudation-sacs especially in the posterior-superior quadrant. A uniform bulging of this portion of the membrane is regarded as a characteristic sign of an accumulation of exudation in the tympanic cavity.

(*d*) Visible movements of the membrana tympani occur in the case of unusual patency of the Eustachian tubes, namely, inward curvature during inspiration and outward curvature during expiration. These respiratory movements may be observed in normal as well as in atrophied membranes, and especially in cicatrices. In such cases the author has been able to ascertain, by aid of the manometer, the existence of great patency of the tubes.

3. Losses of substance in the membrana tympani:—

Perforations of the membrane are most frequently found in the anterior-inferior half of the membrane. They vary in extent, being sometimes only punctiform and hardly visible, and in other cases the whole membrane is completely destroyed. In Fig. 4 is represented a medium-sized perforation in the inferior half of the membrane. When the destruction has been very extensive, the superior portion of the membrane, which retains the malleus in position, is generally preserved. In such cases the handle of the malleus is, as a rule, markedly indrawn, and appears shortened, or is invisible. When a large portion of the membrane has been destroyed, the articulation of the *malleus* and *incus* can often be seen in the posterior-superior part of the field of view, the long process of the *incus* along with the *stapes* forming an obtuse angle directed forward and downward (Fig. 7). When both the malleus and incus have been destroyed, the *capitulum of the stapes* is visible as a small projection about the size of a pinhead. Sometimes the *fenestra rotunda* can also be seen as a small depression below the posterior margin of the *sulcus tympanicus* (Fig. 7).

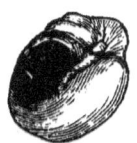

FIG. 7.

Pulsating movements are observed after perforation of the membrana tympani in the course of acute inflammation of the tympanic cavity, and by them the presence of a perforation may be ascertained. These movements show themselves by a reflection of light upon the fluid lying on the floor of the meatus. They are most marked when the perforations are small. The tympanic cavity is filled with fluid, and the blood-vessels, already much dilated, expand with every beat of the pulse, thus exercising a pressure upon the fluid in the tympanum, which extends outward through the perforation, and recedes again when the vessels contract.

Perforations, when small and not closed by secretion, are black in colour. When they are large enough to admit a sufficient quantity of light, the mucous membrane of the inner wall of the tympanum may be seen, which appears more or less thickened, swollen, or reddened. After a cure has been effected the perforation is covered by a firm epidermis of a light grey colour. The surface of the membrane is either smooth or of a granular appearance, due to the formation of small granulations.

Polypi, which in the great majority of cases have their origin in the tympanic cavity, appear of a globular shape more or less reddened, which, if small, project through the perforation; or, if large, occupy the whole extent of the inner part of the meatus.

EXAMINATION WITH SIEGLE'S SPECULUM.

In order to ascertain the mobility of the membrana tympani Siegle constructed his pneumatic ear-speculum. The point of this speculum is covered with an india-rubber tube, which hermetically closes the external meatus. Its outer part consists of a small chamber closed by a glass plate. This chamber, through a lateral aperture, is connected with an india-rubber bag by means of a tube of the same material. By compressing the bag and removing the pressure, condensation and rarefaction of air can be produced in the speculum and in the external meatus. These variations in pressure cause corresponding outward and inward movements of the membrane, which may be observed through the glass plate. We can ascertain either diminished mobility of the membrane (sclerosis) or increased mobility, either of the whole membrane or in circumscribed places (cicatrices or atrophy). It is important to ascertain whether the malleus also moves. Movements of the membrana tympani may be best observed in the posterior-superior quadrant, as also in places where the light is reflected, especially in the anterior-inferior quadrant.

EXAMINATION WITH THE PROBE.

It is sometimes impossible to ascertain the condition of the various parts by inspection only, and in such cases we require the probe (Fig. 8). By no means should it be introduced at random into the ear. Its point must be steadily kept in view while the ear is illuminated by the reflecting mirror. The use of the probe necessitates the greatest caution. It can only be used with safety after practice, as it is difficult to estimate dimensions of depth with one eye. Only very thin knee-shaped probes of silver or steel are in use.

The probe serves to ascertain the presence of growths and foreign bodies in the external meatus. In cases of granulations or polypi we endeavour to find the place of origin by insinuating the point of the probe all round them (Politzer). We can also determine by its means the presence of carious spots, and the hook-shaped point (Fig. 8) serves to ascertain their depth.

Touching the membrana tympani with the probe is disagreeable and painful. In cases of somewhat large perforations we can ascertain the condition of the mucous membrane of the tympanic cavity. Those parts of the tympanum invisible on inspection can be examined by this hook-shaped curved probe. By its means we can discover inspissated secretion, hidden polypi, or carious spots in the tympanum.

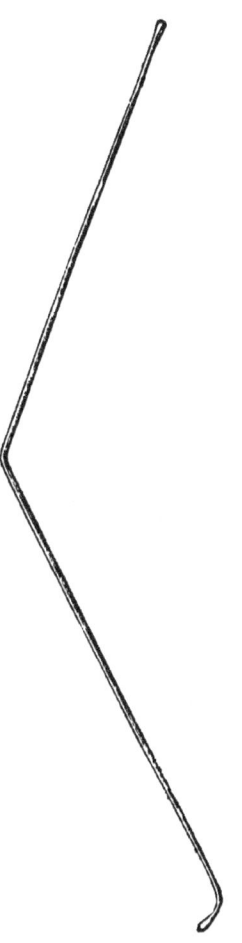

Fig. 8.

CLEANSING THE EAR.

In order to be able to examine the ear, or to apply therapeutic agents, it is first necessary to remove any physiological or pathological products of secretion. Small flakes of epidermis or little pieces of cerumen lying in the way of the speculum can be best removed by the probe or Politzer's bent forceps (Fig. 9).

When the substances are of a larger size, or are situated deeply, they have to be removed by the syringe. In order to remove such masses successfully, it is necessary to produce in the meatus a circulating stream of water by directing the nozzle towards one

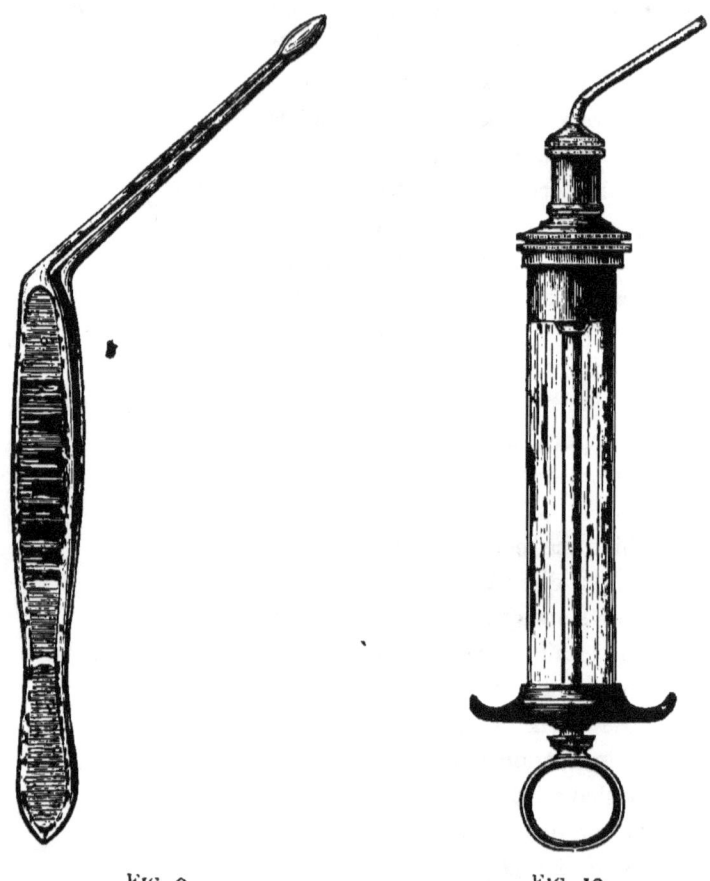

FIG. 9. FIG. 10.

of the walls, along which the fluid will rush to the bottom and, rebounding, make its exit along the opposite wall. To effect this, it is necessary that the nozzle should be thin enough to allow the returning stream a free passage from the ear. A syringe with a thick knobby nozzle is therefore unsuitable. The author uses a syringe whose nozzle consists of a nickel tube, which $2\frac{1}{2}$ cm. from its end is bent at an obtuse angle, so as to prevent it being inserted too far (Fig. 10, half actual size). At the sides of the syringe there are two rings or rests for the index and ring fingers, and one at the end of the piston for the thumb, so that it can be held in position and emptied with one hand.

Little india-rubber balloons, with a tubular point of the same material for a nozzle,[1] are the most suitable for unpractised hands, and for patients who syringe their own ears (Fig. 11, actual size). This little syringe is all in one piece, and the nozzle being soft, the meatus cannot be injured by its introduction. When the secretion is fluid, it may be removed by a single application of this syringe. It is impossible to effect a thorough cleansing with the small tin or glass syringes which are still much used.

In order to straighten the curve of the meatus it is always necessary to draw the auricle backward and outward with the left hand, while the syringing is performed with the right.

A tepid fluid, of the temperature of the body, should always be used for syringing. When it is only necessary to remove small accumulations of secretion from the meatus, water is sufficient; but in affections of the tympanic cavity, a small quantity of common salt, or the following disinfecting substances, may be added, namely, boracic acid, one teaspoonful to 100 grammes of hot water; salicylic acid, 1 to 2 teaspoonfuls of a 10 per cent. alcoholic solution; in cases of fetid otorrhœa, one teaspoonful of 50 per cent. solution of carbolic acid in alcohol, or a 1 per cent. solution of corrosive

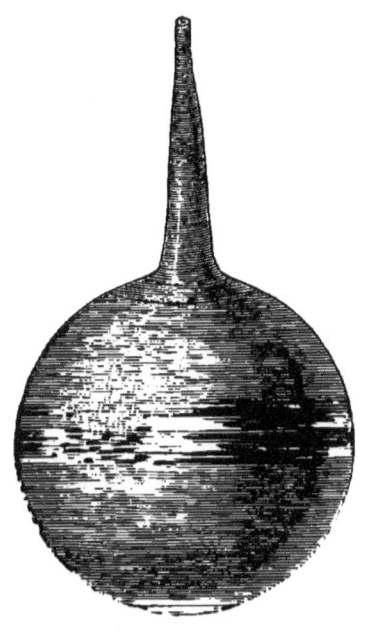

FIG. 11.

---

[1] The air-bubbles to which Von Tröltsch objects can easily be avoided by keeping the balloon constantly filled. Patients must be instructed how to use it.

sublimate to the same quantity of water. In many cases, in order to prevent coagulation of the secretion, Burckhardt-Merian's prescription of a 5 per cent. solution of sulphate of soda proves effective.

Cold fluid will frequently produce giddiness, nausea, and vomiting. These consequences may also ensue if the fluid be injected with too great force. The syringing should always be commenced with a gentle pressure, which should only be increased when the patient bears it well.

The fluid returning from the meatus may be received in any kind of deep vessel, held below the ear. If the patient use the syringe himself, he holds his head over a large basin into which the fluid runs.

After syringing once or twice, the head is inclined sideways, so as to allow the fluid to escape which is still in the meatus, and the orifice is then dried with a cloth. The speculum is then introduced to ascertain whether everything has been removed. If epidermal débris still remain adhering to the walls of the meatus, it may be loosened by the probe and then removed by the syringe or the forceps. Absorbent cotton-wool (not the common kind of cotton-wool) should be used for drying up any fluid which may remain. A small pellet of this cotton, a little larger than a barley-corn, held by the bent forceps, is, under illumination, conducted to the spot which has still to be cleansed. Burckhardt-Merian uses for the same purpose a small metal rod, grooved lengthways, round which the absorbent wool is wrapped. If substances still adhere so firmly to the walls that they cannot be removed by repeated syringing and attempts at loosening them with the probe, they must then be softened by frequent instillations of a salt or soda solution (1 to 2 per cent.) and afterwards removed.

The patient can himself remove liquid secretion by introducing dry pellets of wool deeply into the meatus, either by the bent forceps or Burckhardt-Merian's rod.

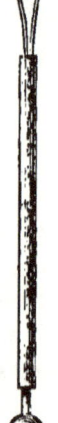

FIG. 12.

The author had a wool-holder made, which is so constructed that the pellet is held fast between its arms by pushing a tube over a portion of them (Fig. 12).

TESTING THE HEARING.

In order to ascertain the perceptive power of the organ of hearing, we have to discover what sound is required in order to excite the auditory nerve, and to make the individual conscious of this excitation.

The waves of sound reach the nerve apparatus leading to the perceptive centre in two ways :—(1) By atmospheric conduction.—The sound-waves travel through the atmosphere to the membrana tympani, and are thence transmitted to the labyrinth by the ossicula. (2) By bone-conduction.—The sound-waves are transmitted by the cranial bones to the labyrinth. Numerous experiments by Politzer and others have shown that by the transmission of sound through these bones the membrana tympani and the ossicula are set in vibration, which is communicated by them to the fluid in the labyrinth. This is called 'cranio-tympanal conduction.' It has not yet been ascertained whether direct conduction of sound can take place, so that the labyrinthine fluid is put into vibration simultaneously with the osseous structures surrounding it.

Normal hearing requires a certain degree of free mobility of the sound-conducting apparatus (membrana tympani, ossicula, and ligamentum annulare of the stapes).

Change in the elasticity or loss of substance of the membrana tympani, anchylosis of the ossicula with each other or with the walls of the tympanic cavity, exudation in the tympanum, or thickening and ossification of the ligamentum annulare,—all such changes which impede freedom of mobility, impair the transmission of sound to the labyrinthine fluid. On the other hand, these same conditions favour bone-conduction; for, the firmer the connection between the cranial bones and the labyrinth, the better will be the transmission of sound.

Bezold[1] explains this by the following experiment :—If we tie a tuning-fork to a small bone tube, and insert the latter into the meatus, when it is struck we will hear its tone very strongly if the string be tightly stretched, and the more we slacken the string the weaker will be the tone, until we cease to hear it altogether.

[1] *Aerztliches Intelligenzblatt*, No. 24, 1885.

It is the same with the transmission through the teeth. Rinne's experiment shows best the prolonged perception by air-conduction over bone-conduction in a healthy ear. A vibrating tuning-fork being placed upon the bones (cranium, incisor teeth, or mastoid process), and kept there until its tone cannot be perceived any longer, when held in front of the open meatus, the tone will still be well heard for a considerable time.

E. H. Weber has pointed out that by covering the ear with the hand, or closing it with the finger, a person hears his own voice, or a tuning-fork placed upon the middle line of the head, louder than with the ear open. Mach's explanation of this is that the sound is prevented from escaping; assuming that, just as the sound penetrates from the outer air by means of the sound-conducting apparatus to the labyrinth, it also escapes again from the labyrinth to the outside by the same means. If this escape be prevented, the sound must be perceived louder. We may, however, assume that under pathological conditions the greater tension of the sound-conducting apparatus plays a more important part in bone-conduction than in the prevention of the escape of sound.

As sound is the less perceived the farther its source is removed, and as it is our object to ascertain the extreme limit at which sound can be heard, we measure the power of perception for air-conduction by the distance at which a certain sound can be perceived. The rule observed in testing the hearing is first to remove the source of sound to such a distance that it cannot be heard at all, and then to bring it gradually nearer to the ear until the sound is distinctly heard. Of course each ear must be tested separately, the ear which is not under examination being closed with the finger. Besides that, and in order to prevent self-deception on the part of the patient, care must be taken that he does not see the source of sound, by placing a hand over his eyes.

As hearing-tests, we employ the watch, speech, specially constructed acoumeters, and tuning-forks.

A. *Testing with the Watch.*

A loudly ticking watch, after it has been ascertained at what distance it can be heard by a normal ear, is gradually brought nearer to the ear of the person examined, until its ticking is distinctly perceived.

Prout and Knapp have proposed to register the hearing-distance by means of a fraction, the numerator representing the distance ascertained, and the denominator the hearing distance of a normal ear for the watch employed. Thus, if we have a watch which is heard by a healthy ear at a distance of 200 cm., and by a patient only at 30 cm., the fraction is $\frac{30}{200}$. If the watch be only heard when applied to the auricle, it is registered as $\frac{i.e.}{200}$ (*in continuo*), or as $\frac{0}{200}$. In order to test the bone-conduction by the watch, it is placed upon the temple or the mastoid process. The hearing-distance for the watch is frequently out of proportion to that for speech. Especially at an advanced age, the watch is badly perceived.

B. *Testing with Speech*.

The most important test is speech. As our hearing has for its chief object the perception of speech, and the deaf desire in the first place to understand speech better, our examination must be conducted so as to ascertain to what extent it is impaired.

The extensive investigations of Oscar Wolf[1] have greatly aided us in forming an opinion from the results obtained by testing with speech. According to Wolf,[1] the vowels possess the greatest volume of sound, *i.e.* they are heard at the greatest distance, while that of consonants is much less. In the same manner, as there is a difference in the intensity of the sound of each letter, they also vary in pitch, our speech comprising eight octaves. The distances at which the different letters were distinctly heard are as follows: *a* as in 'father,' 360 paces (1 pace = 0·7 m.); *o*, 350; *e* as in 'end,' 330; *i* as in 'inch,' 300; *u* as in 'hunt,' 280; *sch*, 200; *m* and *n*, 180; *s*, 175; *g* and *ch* soft, 130; *f*, 67; *k*, 63; *t*, 63; *r*, 41; *b*, 18; *h*, 12.

From the great variation in the perception of the various letters, it of course follows that different words are also heard with varying distinctness. As in loud speech the vowels become very prominent, whispered speech is more suitable for the hearing-test. The

[1] *Sprache und Ohr*, Brunswick, 1871.

louder the speech the worse do very deaf people understand it. Wolf explains this fact thus :—If the voice be raised, only the sound of the vowels is intensified, while the consonants, which cannot be rendered much stronger, are quite drowned. According to the writer's experiments, which on the whole agree with those of others, the average hearing-distance for whispered speech is 20—25 metres, varying somewhat according to the stillness of the surroundings. If a person hear well, the whispering should be very low, if very deaf, it should be strongly accentuated, or loud speech should be used.

Bezold's method of examination is very practical. He only employs the numbers from 1 to 99, and continues to approach the patient until the double numbers, commencing or ending with 7, 5, and 9, whose perception is more difficult, are properly heard. In order to ensure a uniform intensity of sound in whispered speech, he employed the residuum of air left in the lungs after an ordinary expiration.[1]

One who is in the habit of frequently testing the hearing by means of speech, soon discovers which words are well, and which are badly heard. Generally those words are well heard which contain many vowels and hissing sounds or resonants, as, for instance, 'Tisch,' 'Schuh,' 'Mamma,' 'Wasser,' 'Katze,' 'Fenster,' while words in which consonants predominate are heard with much more difficulty.

Testing with speech must always be so contrived that the patient does not see the mouth of the examiner, for many deaf people have acquired a great facility for lip-reading. It is also to be noted that on closing the ear with the finger the hearing power is only diminished, and not altogether abolished, as, by closing the meatus, only direct sound-waves are prevented from entering; while those which are transmitted by bone-conduction are perceived. Lincke mentions the case of a man who heard the watch at a distance of

---

[1] The German recruiting regulations contain a peculiar condition with regard to the intensity of whispered speech. It is to be such that a normal ear can perceive it in the daytime, in the open air, under the most favourable conditions, and for the purpose of repeating it, at a distance not exceeding 2 metres (!). In an enclosed space 8½ metres in width and height, whispered speech is to be understood by a normal ear at a distance of about 23 metres. During the test the ear is to be turned towards the source of sound.

15—20 feet, and who after his ear had been closed with the finger, or with a cotton pellet dipped in wax, still heard it at a distance of 5—6 inches. It is also well known that after closing the meatuses we are still able to understand a loud conversation. This must be specially taken into account in cases of one-sided dulness of hearing or deafness, as during the hearing-test the healthy but closed ear will perceive sound. In order to ascertain by which ear the sound is heard, Dennert[1] proposes also to close the ear which is under examination. If the hearing-distance, previously ascertained, remain the same, it may be assumed that the sound has been heard by the other ear, while a diminution of the hearing-distance proves that it has only been heard by the ear under examination.

C. *Testing with specially constructed Acoumeters.*

A perfect acoumeter must possess the following qualifications. It must have as great a range of tones as possible, which can always be produced with the same intensity; it must be handy and simple, so that it can be employed without difficulty in all ordinary examinations. It must further be so constructed that it can not only be used for testing the air-conduction but also the bone-conduction. Unfortunately we do not yet possess an instrument with all these qualifications, and it is doubtful if its construction is possible in a simple and suitable form. As acoumeters having a large range of tones we employ specially constructed musical boxes (Kessel), and the ordinary musical instruments, especially the pianoforte. By means of the latter we can ascertain whether all or only some of the tones are heard. Most acoumeters give only one kind of sound: they either only make noises or emit a tone of a certain pitch. Wolke and, at a later date, Itard used acoumeters consisting of a sounding body, a board or a ring, struck by a small hammer falling from a certain height. Of the large number of acoumeters, a small instrument designed by Politzer[2] has rapidly come into favour. It consists of a small steel cylinder tuned to the note c^2,

---

[1] *Archiv für Ohrenheilkunde*, vol. x. p. 231.
[2] *Ibid.* vol. xii. p. 104. Manufactured by Gottlieb, instrument-maker in Vienna.

which is struck by a small hammer. This little instrument gives a tinkling sound, whose key-note, c^2, can be easily recognised by a trained musical ear. The degree of sound produced by this instrument renders it better adapted than any of the other instruments for ordinary use in a room, and for testing the various degrees of deafness. But in very slight cases of dulness the watch must be substituted for Politzer's acoumeter, as the rooms in which we make our examinations are generally of small dimensions. The simple construction, handy form, and cheapness of Politzer's instrument render it convenient for general use. On account of its greater intensity of sound, it is more suitable for testing the bone-conduction than the watch. According to the results of the author's examinations of normal ears, Politzer's acoumeter was perceived at a distance averaging 15 metres; but some of the Vienna instruments have a much louder sound.

For producing high tones, in order to test very great deafness, Galton's whistle is used, and for slighter degrees König's steel cylinder—the latter especially to ascertain the extreme limit of the hearing power. After the invention of the telephone, the author endeavoured to obtain an exact gradation of sound by means of electric currents.[1] In the circuit is placed (1) a tuning-fork, by which the current is interrupted at regular intervals, (2) a rheochord, or a sliding induction apparatus, by means of which the intensity of the current can be varied and exactly regulated at will, and (3) a telephone, at which is heard a tone corresponding with that of the vibrating tuning-fork, of more or less intensity according to the strength of the current. Although the hearing-test can be made easily and rapidly by means of such an apparatus, it is unfortunately somewhat too complicated, and as only a small number of tones can be produced, the apparatus has not yet been introduced into practice. The audiometer of Hughes with a microphonic contrivance is arranged on the same principle. The sound produced by this instrument can also be increased or diminished at will.

D. *Testing with Tuning-forks.*

As all the various sounds which reach the ear are composed of

---

[1] Verhandl. der Physiol. Gesellsch. zu Berlin, 11 Jan. 1878.

separate tones, the latter must always form the basis of an exact hearing-test. The ticking of the watch and human speech are merely sounds; while in the tuning-fork we have an instrument by which we can produce tones of sufficient purity for our purpose. In order to ascertain the power of hearing for different tones we employ a variety of tuning-forks. After being smartly struck we ascertain, as with the watch, the distance at which the tuning-fork can be heard. A more exact result is obtained when Conta's[1] plan is followed. The handle of the tuning-fork is covered by an india-rubber tube whose end is introduced into the external meatus. The tuning-fork being struck, the patient hears it for a certain number of seconds, and thus the hearing power is measured. Lucae[2] suggests, after the patient ceases to hear the sound, to hold the tuning-fork to our own normal ear in order to ascertain for what space of time the vibrations still continue. Conta remarks that only a great difference in the strength of the stroke which the tuning-fork receives will make an appreciable alteration in the duration of the vibrations, which, after numerous examinations, the author can confirm. It is therefore not necessary to invent special contrivances in order to secure a uniform strength of stroke. A block of soft wood on which the tuning-fork can conveniently be struck is sufficient.

In order to obtain very pure tones the over-tones which are produced along with the fundamental tone can be diminished, if, as Politzer proposes, clamps are screwed to the prongs of the tuning-fork. The effect of these clamps is however over-estimated. The author has observed tuning-forks with clamps giving very loud overtones. Of more importance than the clamps is the construction of the tuning-fork. The fundamental tone of well-finished tuning-forks predominates so much above the over-tones that the latter soon cease to be heard, and do not become a source of error in our ordinary examinations. Shifting the clamps alters the pitch of the tuning-forks, but it also affects the intensity of the vibrations to such an extent that it serves no practical purpose.

Testing with the tuning-fork can be applied in different ways :—

[1] *Archiv für Ohrenheilkunde*, vol. i. p. 107.
[2] *Ibid.* vol. xv. p. 279.

(a) *Weber's Experiment.*

As already mentioned, when a person with normal hearing puts his hand over the one ear, or closes it with his finger, a tuning-fork placed upon the middle line of the head is heard more loudly in the closed ear. This is also the case when there is an obstruction to sound-conduction in the external meatus or in the tympanic cavity.

When by means of the watch, Politzer's acoumeter, or speech, we have ascertained that only one ear is dull, or that, both being affected, one ear is deafer than the other, we diagnose a disease of the sound-conducting apparatus, if a tuning-fork placed upon the middle line of the head be heard more distinctly by the diseased ear, or, both being affected, by the ear in which the deafness is greater. If we observe the reverse of this, namely, that the better-hearing ear perceives the tone of the tuning-fork, an affection of the nervous apparatus of the other ear may be concluded. The time during which the tuning-fork is heard by the ear may be calculated by seconds. The longer it is heard in comparison with the normal ear, the more certainly may it be inferred that the sound-conducting apparatus is affected.

(b) *Rinne's Experiment.*

Rinne has also shown the usefulness of this experiment in the diagnosis of the part affected, and has pointed out that when it gives a result analogous to that obtained in a normal ear, the auditory nerve and not the sound-conducting apparatus is at fault. If, on the other hand, the patient hear the tone transmitted by bone-conduction as long or longer than that transmitted by air-conduction, disease of the conducting-apparatus may be assumed. Lucae designated the former diagnosis of the ear as a positive, and the latter as a negative, result of the experiment. But it would perhaps be simpler to say, air-conduction, or bone-conduction predominating, $(A+, B+)$.

Lucae confines the application of Rinne's experiment to cases in which whispered speech is heard at a distance of one metre or less. In his opinion, only in such cases the positive or negative result of the experiment can be accepted as proof of an affection of the nerve, or of the sound-conducting apparatus. He, along with Politzer, affirms that in slight cases of deafness the experiment may have a positive result, and that air-conduction may preponderate, even in undoubted affections of the sound-conducting apparatus. The value of Rinne's experiment is also diminished by the fact that it sometimes happens that in the same patient the bone-conduction predominates with high tones and the air-conduction with low tones, and *vice versa*. For this reason alone, in order to form a correct diagnosis of a case of deafness, the examination with a number of different tuning-forks cannot be dispensed with. For Weber's and Rinne's experiments tuning-forks of medium pitch, about c^2 (512 vibrations), are used.

A patient of Bezold's was tested, with the following result:— He heard whispered speech on the right at 6 and on the left at 4 cm., and the tuning-fork upon the vertex continued to be heard about 8 seconds. By Rinne's experiment the right was negative, continuing for 13 seconds, also the left negative, for 12 seconds. On *post-mortem* examination it was found that the foot-plate of the stapes was anchylosed in the fenestra ovalis by extensive calcareous deposition in the ligamentum annulare.

(c) *Testing with Tuning-forks of different Pitch.*

In order to test the hearing power precisely, it is necessary to extend the examination with the tuning-fork over a number of tones, so as to obtain a result from which a diagnosis can be made. This is the more necessary, as Rinne's experiment can only be applied in cases of great deafness, and as its result may be reversed according to the high or low pitch of the tuning-forks with which the patient is examined.

The author, in order to assure himself of the value of testing the hearing with a number of tuning-forks, examined carefully a great many cases of deafness, arising from various diseased conditions. The tuning-forks which he has hitherto employed consist of two of a low pitch, A 106·6, and c^1 256; two of medium pitch, c^2 512, and g^2 768; two of high pitch, c^4 2048, and c^4 3072 vibrations. For each tuning-fork he has ascertained, by experimenting with them on four persons, each with normal hearing, how many seconds the vibrations can be heard, (1) when held before the orifice of the meatus (air-conduction); (2) when placed upon the mastoid process (bone-conduction). In order to arrive at the relative value of the results thus obtained, he has proposed [1] to register them on forms specially printed for the purpose (see Figs. 13 to 16). The averages of the results obtained from examination of the normal ear for air-conduction are entered in the middle, those of the bone-conduction at the bottom. The low A tuning-fork is, for instance, heard for 20 seconds by air-conduction, and for 11 seconds by bone-conduction. When a deaf person is examined, the result obtained (namely, the number of seconds in proportion to a standard duration of perception, which is taken at 100) is entered in a column which is divided into 100 parts. If, for instance, the tuning-fork A, as in Form 1, be heard on the left side for 10 seconds, while it is perceived by a normal ear for 20 seconds, we have the following proportion :—20 : 10 = 100 : x, i.e. $x = 50$. Fifty parts of column A left side are now filled up, either with colour or with oblique strokes as in Figure 13. The results obtained from testing the bone-conduction are not entered in proportion to the normal hearing through the bones, but in proportion to the normal hearing by air-conduction, as in this way a direct comparison of the air- and bone-conduction is better obtained. In the above case the tuning-fork is heard by bone-conduction for 16 seconds, and the proportion is 20 : 16 = 100 : x, i.e. $x = 80$. Therefore in the lower half of the Form 80 parts of column A (left side) are now filled up with oblique strokes. The results obtained with the other tuning-forks are registered in the same manner. Each entry represents the average result of three consecutive tests. For the purpose of understanding the scheme better, the number of seconds has always been given during which a tuning-fork has been heard.

The different diseases of the ear have a variable effect upon the perception of the tones of the tuning-fork. According to the results obtained there are four distinct types :—

---

[1] Die graphische Darstellung der Resultate der Hörprüfung mit Stimmgabeln, *Deutsche medicinische Wochenschrift*, No. 15, 1885.

Type I. Approximately uniform diminution of the duration of perception by air-conduction. Good hearing by bone-conduction. This type is to be met with in acute and chronic processes in the middle ear. Figure 13 is the record of a patient who had suffered from purulent inflammation of the middle ear on both sides. The left membrana tympani was totally destroyed; in the anterior part of the right membrane, a milk-white opacity was present, of the size of a hemp-seed, as also a cicatricial adhesion to the promontory.

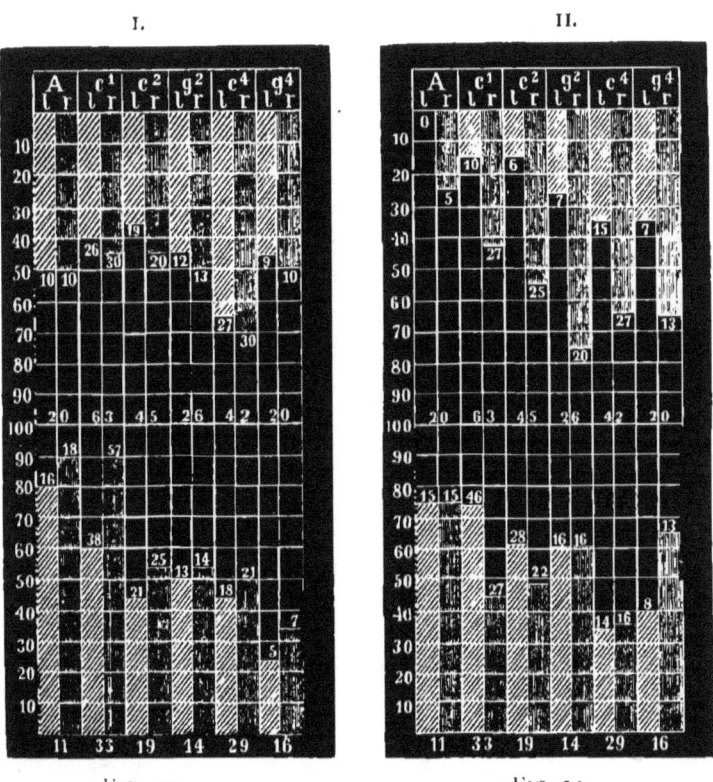

FIG. 13. FIG. 14.

Type II. The low tones heard badly, but as the tones become higher the perception improves. Hearing better by bone-conduction than by air-conduction, especially low tones. This condition is due to pathological processes, which lead us to suspect an anchylosis of the stapes in the fenestra ovalis, the result of purulent inflammation of the middle ear, and of sclerosis.

Figure 14 represents the hearing power of a female patient who had suffered, years previously, from purulent inflammation of the middle ear as a sequela of scarlet fever. The perception through the cranial bones being good, it may be assumed that the nerve was not affected by the disease.

Type III. Good perception of the low tones, and diminished perception as the tones rise in pitch. Bone-conduction diminished, especially as regards high tones. This kind of perception we find in boilermakers, artillerymen, and in diseased conditions of the nervous apparatus.

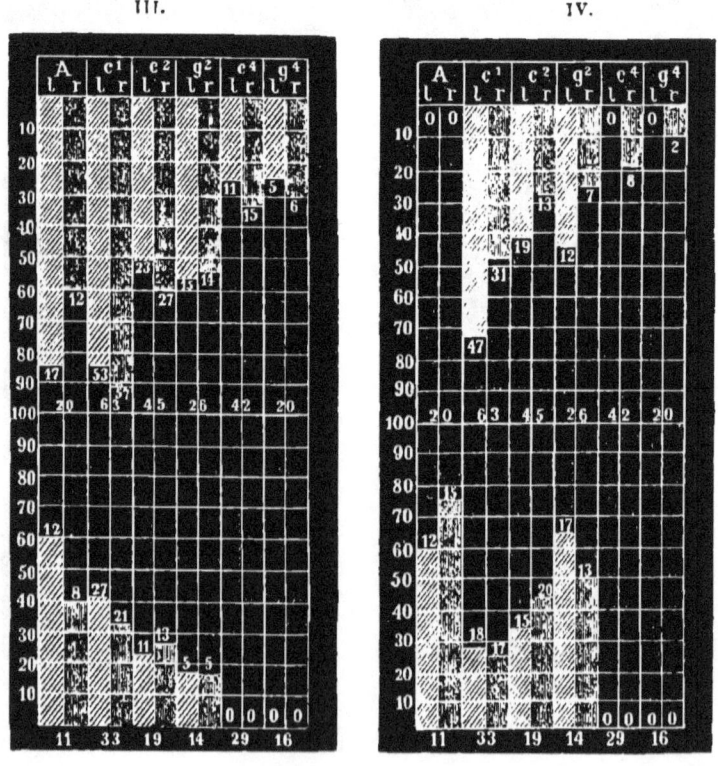

FIG. 15.   FIG. 16.

Figure 15 concerns a boilermaker who had been at that trade since 1867, and who was for five years what is called a 'holder-on,' sitting inside the boiler. The bone-conduction is considerably diminished, the two highest tones not being perceived at all. This shows that the injurious action of the noise in boiler-shops is chiefly expended upon those portions of the sound-perceiving apparatus, which serve for the perception of the higher tones.

Type IV. Irregular perception of the varying pitch, by air-conduction as well as by bone-conduction. This manifests itself in various forms, the high and low tones being heard badly, while those of medium pitch are heard well, or the middle tones being perceived indistinctly, while the higher and lower are heard well, etc. Sometimes the bone-conduction is increased for certain tones; sometimes it is decreased, or is entirely abolished. This irregular perception takes place in diseases of the nervous apparatus, when it is partially affected. There is also frequently a simultaneous affection of the sound-conducting apparatus. A reliable diagnosis of a labyrinthine affection can be made, if there be gaps in the range of the tones perceived.

Figure 16 represents the case of a patient with chronic progressive deafness without objective proof of changes in the sound-conducting apparatus. By air-conduction the A is not heard, nor the c^4 and g^4 on the left side, and only badly on the right, while c^1 and c^2 are heard comparatively well. The low A being heard well by bone-conduction points to the participation of the sound-conducting apparatus in the disease. When testing the hearing with several tuning-forks, it must be borne in mind that if not of the same make they may have a different quality of sound, so that by using such, varying results may be obtained. But practical experience proves that these differences are not so considerable as to lessen the value of the results obtained by the examination. The general application of the hearing-test with tuning-forks of different pitch is rendered impracticable by the fact that the whole examination, especially if both ears be affected, occupies much time. However, when an exact diagnosis is desired, it is essential that the perception of a large number of single tones be ascertained, and this mode of procedure, although it takes up much time, cannot be dispensed with.

Instead of the tuning-forks already mentioned, the author now uses the following, namely, c, c^1, c^2, c^3, c^4, g^4, manufactured by

Mr. Wesselhöft, instrument-maker in Halle on the Saale. As a rule, tuning-forks which can be heard by a normal ear for 25 to 50 seconds are the most suitable for this method of examination. A longer duration of the vibrations, causing the examination to be much protracted, is not required.

In testing the bone-conduction with a tuning-fork of high pitch, we meet with the difficulty, that when placed upon the bones its tone is heard just as long, sometimes even longer, by air-conduction as by bone-conduction. In order to avoid this as much as possible, the writer has had tuning-forks made with long handles. In doubtful cases it is necessary first to ascertain how many seconds the tuning-fork is heard when placed upon the bones. At the next test the tuning-fork is lifted a little from the bone before the number of seconds, already ascertained, has been reached, and the patient is asked whether he still hears the sound, and if so, it may be assumed that he hears by air-conduction, but if not, by bone-conduction. As our methods of examination become more perfect, the value of the pathologico-anatomical results will also increase. Unfortunately, *post-mortem* examinations of cases carefully observed during life are still very rare. In a very interesting case which was examined by Moos and Steinbrügge where the high tones were not perceived and speech not understood, the histological examination showed atrophy of the nerve-fibres of the first turn of the cochlea, bearing out Helmholtz's theory, according to which this turn is the recipient of the higher, while the upper turns receive the lower tones.

Moos first observed that for understanding speech the perception of the higher tones is of more importance than that of the lower. The power of perceiving low tones may be perfectly normal while the higher are heard indistinctly or not at all. Speech in these cases is likewise understood badly or is not heard at all. When the power of hearing speech is completely lost, disease of the nervous apparatus must be assumed.

E. *Testing the Hearing in suspected Malingering.*

When it is suspected that dulness of hearing or deafness is simulated, both ears must in the first instance be carefully examined, as information may be thus obtained as to the degree of deafness from pathological. changes which perhaps actually exists. In testing the hearing in such cases, we must note whether dulness or complete deafness on one or both sides is simulated, and when only the former, its degree must be exactly ascertained, while the eyes of the suspected malingerer are covered. As repeated tests made in this way, in the case of truthful patients, must always give an unvarying result, important indications may thus be obtained which will lead to the detection of simulation.

When deafness on both sides is pretended, it should be contrived, by careful watching or by a sudden surprise, to detect the malingerer while he thinks he is unobserved. For the purpose of distinguishing simulated deafness from great dulness of hearing in one ear, the writer has repeatedly found the following plan to succeed very well. The person to be examined is placed in such a position that the healthy ear is turned away from the examiner, thus making him believe that only the alleged deaf ear, which is turned towards the examiner, is being examined. The malingerer will pretend that he hears nothing, although he must hear with the healthy ear. In this way the deception is discovered. In a similar manner Voltolini[1] recommends the application of a large hearing-trumpet to the ear alleged to be deaf, and then closing the healthy ear with a perforated plug. Moos closes the healthy ear with a lint plug and places a vibrating tuning-fork upon the middle line of the head. If the person examined pretend that he does not hear the tuning-fork at all, not even with the healthy ear, he is unquestionably malingering. Teuber introduces an india-rubber tube into each ear of the person examined, who is then asked to repeat words rapidly spoken through the tubes. When the words are repeated which are spoken into the tube leading to the ear alleged to be deaf, the deception is discovered.

THE AIR-DOUCHE.

For diagnostic and therapeutic purposes air is propelled through the Eustachian tube into the tympanic cavity by various methods.

---

[1] *Monatsschrift für Ohrenheilkunde*, No. 9, 1882.

This procedure is called the air-douche. The merit of first recognising its great importance in the treatment of ear diseases belongs to Deleau, who in consequence of the astonishing results which he obtained by it, recommended its application so strongly that Itard was led to say, 'God alone could give hearing to man by a mere breath.' The methods employed are the following :—

1. *The Valsalvian Experiment.*—After a deep inspiration the mouth and nose are closed, and by a strong expiration the air is driven into the tympanic cavity.

2. *Politzer's Method.*—During the act of swallowing, which shuts off the upper from the lower part of the pharynx, in consequence of the soft palate applying itself to the posterior pharyngeal wall, and which also causes the simultaneous opening of the Eustachian tubes, the air in the naso-pharynx is compressed by forcing more air into it by means of an india-rubber bag, or by special compression contrivances producing a graduated pressure.

3. *Catheterism.*—Air, condensed either by means of an india-rubber bag or other compression apparatus, is forced directly into the tympanic cavity through a catheter introduced into the orifice of the Eustachian tube.

1. *The Valsalvian Experiment.*

The expiratory pressure which can be exerted varies very much in different individuals, according to age, sex, bodily strength, and especially according to the condition of the lungs, and ranges from 70 to 220 mm. of the mercury column. According to the author's examinations, the entrance of air into the tympanic cavity, when the Valsalvian experiment is performed under normal conditions, takes place at a pressure of 20—60 mm. mercury, in exceptional cases with a minimum of pressure. In cases of naso-pharyngeal catarrh, with swelling of the mucous membrane of the Eustachian tube, greater pressure is required, or the expiratory pressure increased to its fullest extent may be altogether insufficient to force air into the tympanic cavity, although there is no defect of hearing. If therefore an expiratory pressure of upwards of 60 mm. mercury do not force any air into the tympanum, only obstruction in the tubes may be inferred, and not defective ventilation of the tympanic cavity.

The entrance of air into the tympanic cavity is ascertained by a crackling sound, which is perceived by the patient, and also by the surgeon with the aid of an auscultation-tube. Outward curvature of the membrana tympani from the entrance of air may be also observed. Performing the act of swallowing while the nose is closed is called 'the negative Valsalvian experiment.' It produces rarefaction of air in the naso-pharynx and the simultaneous opening of the Eustachian tubes. An inward curvature of the membrana tympani is caused thereby, along with a crackling sound. When both the positive and negative Valsalvian experiments are successful, a normal condition of the Eustachian tubes may be concluded. The Valsalvian experiment can only rarely be employed in treatment, as a slight obstruction in the Eustachian tube will prevent the air from entering into the tympanum. If an entrance be effected, the force of the currenti s so slight that this kind of air-douche proves insufficient in most cases. Where the membrana tympani is perforated, the Valsalvian experiment may be employed to remove secretion from the tympanic cavity. In doing so the expiratory pressure must be rapidly increased, and a continuous pressure must be avoided, as it occasions venous congestion, which in many cases, especially in acute inflammation, may produce most unfavourable consequences. A patient recommended to employ Valsalva's method requires to be cautioned against doing so too frequently.

2. *Politzer's Method.*

The india-rubber bag [1] (Fig. 17) is, for this method, the most suitable appliance. To the nozzle is attached an india-rubber tube about 3 cm. long, which is introduced into the posterior part of one nostril. The alæ nasi are compressed over it with the thumb and forefinger of the left hand. When the words 'now,' or 'one, two, three' are said, the patient swallows water, while with the right hand the india-rubber bag, which is held between the palm and thumb, is rapidly and firmly compressed. It is a matter of practice to hit upon the moment correctly at which the patient swallows.

[1] Inflation with the mouth, as is sometimes practised, is distasteful to patients.

The bag is kept compressed until the india-rubber tube is withdrawn from the nose, to prevent secretion being sucked into the tube or bag. In order to guard against infection by pathological products, each patient receives a small tube for his own special use. As an improvement upon this, Politzer recommended a vulcanite tube (Fig. 19), flexibly connected with the bag by an india-rubber tube. Beginners using this apparatus are apt to allow the india-

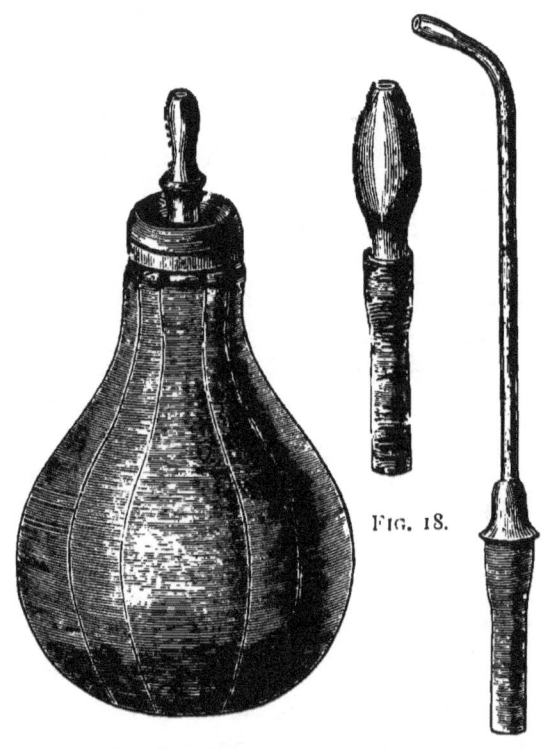

FIG. 17.   FIG. 18.   FIG. 19.

rubber tube to get doubled up during the compression of the bag, thereby obstructing the passage of the air. As children very frequently resist the introduction of such an apparatus into the nose, it is best to employ for their treatment an olive-shaped nozzle (Fig. 18) which occupies the whole nostril, and closes it. This nose-piece may be either connected with the bag by an india-rubber tube or firmly and directly inserted into it. During inflation the other nostril must be closed with the finger.

The pressure applied to the naso-pharynx by Politzer's method amounts to half an atmosphere. It depends upon the rapidity and force with which the bag is compressed, also upon the capacity of the nasal cavity and the naso-pharynx, and upon the power of resistance of the soft palate. In cases of slightly defective function, as well as in acute affections of the tympanic cavity, Politzerisation must be performed with gentle pressure; while in other conditions, especially in chronic cases, great pressure must be exerted. If air cannot be forced into the tympanum by this method, or only to a small extent, catheterism must be resorted to. In Politzerisation, as air is always driven simultaneously into both tympanic cavities, it must be performed with great care, and with slight pressure in cases in which only one ear is diseased. The healthy ear may also be protected by pressing the finger into the external meatus. Especially in the case of children, pain in the region of the stomach is often complained of after inflation, when the compression is made either too late or too early. This results from air entering the stomach and suddenly distending it. In such cases the writer lets the patient drink a little water, after which the air escapes by eructation, and the pain subsides. In children Politzerisation can often be performed even without swallowing, as contraction of the muscles of the soft palate is caused by the inflation itself. It can also be done while the child is crying.

Lucae[1] and Gruber[2] have recommended, for the purpose of effecting the closure of the soft palate, the phonation of vowels or of words with k (hick) instead of swallowing. According to the author's manometrical records, the power of resistance of the soft palate in pronouncing vowel sounds is so slight that sufficient pressure cannot be obtained in the naso-pharynx. The resistance is more considerable when 'k' or 'hick' is pronounced. But, at any rate, Politzer's original method is to be preferred to these modifications, as being more effectual. It should, however, be pointed out that there are cases in which, during the act of

---

[1] Virchow's *Archiv*, vol. lxiv., 1875.
[2] *Monatsschrift für Ohrenheilkunde*, 1875.

swallowing, air does not pass into the tympanic cavity, while it enters during phonation.

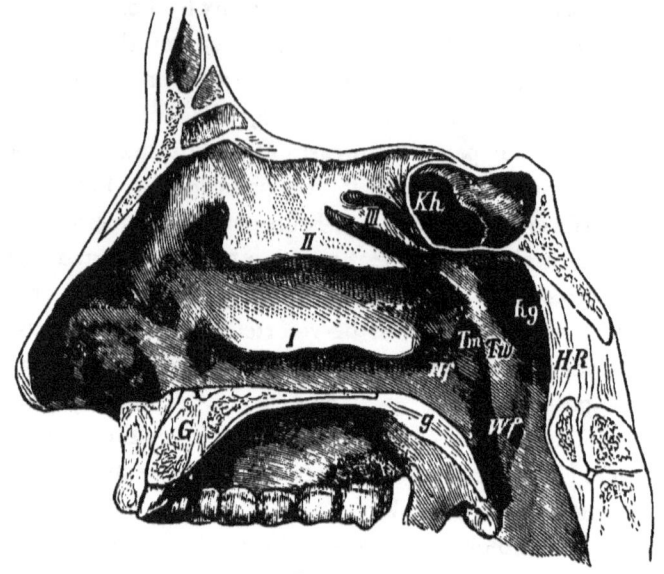

FIG. 20.

Tm. Mouth of Eustachian tube. *Tw.* Eustachian prominence. *Wf.* Salpingo-pharyngeal fold. *Hf.* Salpingo-palatine fold. *Rg.* Rosenmüller's fossa. *I.* Lower turbinated body. *II.* Middle turbinated body. *III.* Upper turbinated body. *G.* Hard palate. *g.* Soft palate. *HR.* Posterior wall of pharynx. *Kh.* Sphenoidal sinus.

The great advantage of Politzerisation over Catheterism lies in the fact that it avoids the disagreeable feeling arising from the introduction of the catheter, which sometimes renders its employment impossible, especially in the case of children. Besides, it is frequently possible to force a greater volume and a stronger current of air into the tympanic cavity by Politzer's method than by the catheter.

3. *Catheterism.*

The pharyngeal orifice of the Eustachian tube is situated (see Fig. 20) on the lateral wall of the pharynx, on a level with the lower turbinated body, 1 cm. above the floor of the nasal cavity, at an average distance of $7\frac{1}{2}$ cm. from the border of the anterior nares, $1\frac{1}{2}$—2 cm. from the posterior pharyngeal wall, and 2—$2\frac{1}{2}$ cm. from the septum narium. The pharyngeal opening of the tube is directed forward, being bounded above and behind by the hook-shaped cartilaginous portion, the central cartilaginous plate projecting posteriorly toward the middle line as the Eustachian prominence. The long axis of the Eustachian tube lies at an angle of 40° to the horizontal plane.

Catheters (Fig. 21) are either made of metal, silver being preferable, or of vulcanite; the latter are not affected by medicaments, and are more agreeable to the patient. They should however be manufactured from well-hardened material, so that they do not lose their shape by cleansing in hot water. They are 14—15 cm. in length, including the beak, which is 2—2½ cm. long, and has a curvature of 145°. The thickness is 2—3 mm. Different sizes must be used according to the width of the nasal cavities. The length of the beak must also vary according to the capacity of the naso-pharynx. At one end the catheter is widened like a funnel, into which the nozzle of the india-rubber air-bag can be fitted. At this end a ring is fastened to it, which serves to indicate the direction of the beak when introduced into the mouth of the Eustachian tube. Any secretion in the nose should first be removed, either by blowing or syringing.

Catheterism consists of three acts. In the first act the catheter is introduced into the naso-pharynx; in the second, the point of the beak is inserted into the mouth of the Eustachian tube, and the catheter fixed in its position; and in the third act, air is driven through it by means of the india-rubber bag or an air-compressing apparatus.

Act I. The thumb of the operator's left hand is placed upon the point of the patient's nose, the other fingers upon the bridge of the nose and the fore-

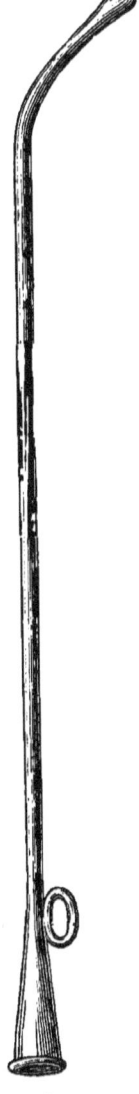

FIG. 21.

head, and the point of the nose is tilted upward. The catheter is held between the thumb and forefinger of the right hand like a pen, and its beak is pointed downward. The beak is introduced into the nostril in such a manner that its point rests upon the floor of the nasal cavity; next, the outer end being raised, the catheter is slowly and carefully pushed forward in a horizontal direction until the point of the beak reaches the posterior wall of the pharynx. Any obstacle at the soft palate can be overcome by slightly lowering the outer end of the catheter, or by the relaxation of the muscles of the soft palate produced by the patient breathing through the nose or swallowing.

The introduction of the catheter is most frequently obstructed by malformations of the septum of the nose. They are as a rule met with in its inferior portion, and somewhat diminish the space between the lower turbinated body and the septum. Figure 22 represents a transverse section through the anterior portion of the nasal cavity, showing a convexity of the septum to the left side (Vk). This obstacle can generally be overcome by directing the point of the catheter downward and outward, and then pushing it forward in the direction indicated by the arrow. The beak, after passing the constricted part, should then be raised perpendicularly and pushed forward. The tube of the catheter then generally glides through the narrowed portion in the inferior nasal meatus, or this only takes place when the beak is in the naso-pharynx, and after making attempts to pass it by turning it in different directions. If it be found impossible to pass the beak of the catheter beyond the place of constriction in this manner, its point, instead of being brought again toward the perpendicular, should be turned still more outward. If the beak be short and the lower nasal meatus wide, its convex surface will then slide across the convexity of the septum down into the lower meatus, where it will now lie. It can then be pushed forward, the beak again being raised perpendicularly by lowering the outer end of the catheter, or it is even better to push the beak forward in a horizontal direction into the posterior portion of the nasal cavity, and then to turn it upward behind the posterior border of the lower turbinated bone. After the beak with its point directed upward has been introduced into the naso-pharynx, it receives another turn through an angle of 180°, which will again give it a downward direction. It is advisable to employ in such cases thin catheters with a short beak. In cases of obstruction the introduction of the catheter may be much facilitated by a

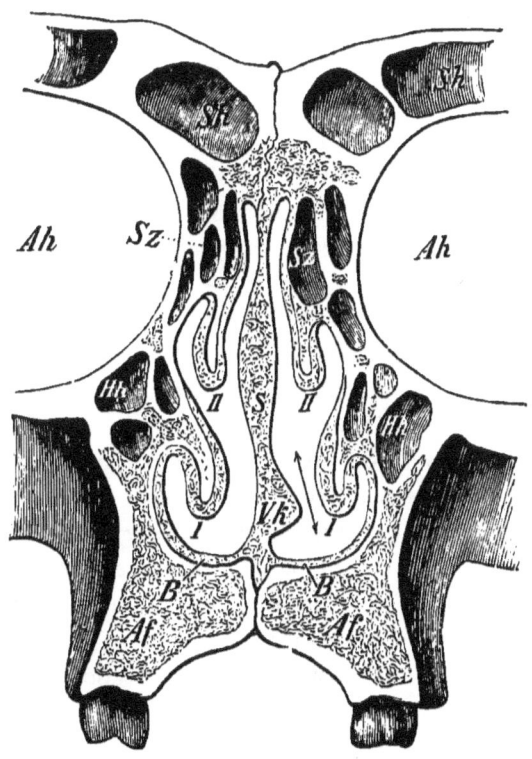

FIG. 22.

S. Septum.   *Vk.* Convexity.   *I.* Inferior meatus.   *II.* Middle meatus.   *B.* Floor of nasal cavity.   *Af.* Alveolar process.   *Hh.* Anterior extremity of Antrum of Highmore.   *Sh.* Frontal air-sinus.   *Sz.* Ethmoid cells.   *Ah.* Orbit.

careful preliminary inspection of the nasal cavity, and by ascertaining the nature of the obstruction. If the catheter lie in the middle meatus, the second act of catheterism, namely, turning the beak in the naso-pharynx, and inserting its point into the orifice of the Eustachian tube, will be very difficult, or impossible. If the one nostril will not admit of the passage of the catheter, an attempt should be made to introduce one with a long beak through the other nostril, and thence to insert it into the opposite Eustachian tube.

Act II. After the point of the beak has reached the posterior pharyngeal wall, the catheter is held between the thumb and forefinger of the left hand in order to support it easily; its introduction into the orifice of the tube can then be accomplished by one of three methods :—

1. Withdrawing the catheter $1\frac{1}{2}$—2 cm., and giving its beak one-eighth of a turn outward, so that while touching the outer wall of the pharynx, the cartilaginous Eustachian prominence is felt, after passing over which the catheter receives another quarter of a turn (Politzer's Method).

2. Withdrawing the catheter 1—2 cm. with the point of the beak directed downward until the resistance offered by the soft palate is felt. If the point be now turned outward and upward, it will enter the mouth of the tube (Kramer's Method).

3. The third method, which the writer finds described for the first time in Frank's book (p. 101), consists in turning the beak toward the middle line, and in withdrawing it until its concave surface meets the nasal septum. It then receives an outward turn of 180°, which causes the point to enter the orifice of the tube.

The first of these three methods is most in use, but many employ the second. The successful introduction of the catheter by either method is simply a matter of practice. If both the first and second methods fail, the third will frequently succeed.

Under the following conditions the introduction of the catheter into the Eustachian tube will not be successful :—(a) If the catheter do not lie on the floor of the nasal cavity, but be elevated at its inner end, so that the point of the beak is situated above the orifice of the tube. (b) If it be not withdrawn far enough, and its point lodge in Rosenmüller's fossa. (c) If it be withdrawn too far, its point getting into the nose, and being held fast by the inferior turbinated body. (d) If the soft palate contract spasmodically, the operator should wait till it is relaxed, which can be effected by speaking or breathing through the nose.

The most important sign that the catheter is in proper position is obtained by auscultation while air is being passed through it. It may also be assumed that the point of the catheter is properly inserted when resistance is felt on moving the catheter backward and forward, and also on attempting to turn its point upward. After the catheter has been inserted by one of the three methods into the orifice of the tube, the middle, ring, and little fingers of the left hand are placed upon the forehead and bridge of the nose of the patient, and the catheter is firmly held between the thumb and forefinger close in front of the nostrils.

Act III. The catheter being fixed in this manner in the mouth of the Eustachian tube, air is forced through it by means of the india-rubber bag (Fig. 17, p. 38) furnished with a conical or rounded nozzle fitting into the outer end of the catheter. The bag, held laterally in the right hand, is placed in the longitudinal axis of the catheter and rapidly compressed. When compressing the bag, care has to be taken that the nozzle changes its position as little as possible, as such movements cause considerable pain. After the bag has been compressed, it is withdrawn while in that condition, to prevent mucous material entering the catheter. It is then allowed to expand and is again compressed in this way a number of times. If the catheter be well fixed, and no unnecessary movement made during compression of the bag, the air-douche is quite painless. When compressing the bag, care should be taken not to press the beak of the catheter against the posterior wall of the Eustachian tube.

For thorough disinfection of the catheter, a 5 per cent. solution of carbolic acid at boiling heat is most highly recommended. Patients who require to be catheterised frequently, ought, if possible, to have catheters of their own. This is particularly required in the case of syphilitic patients. Burow (*Monatsschrift für Ohrenheilkunde*, No. 5, 1885) reported six cases, in each of which the same practitioner inoculated syphilis by means of the catheter. According to Köbner and Burow, cases of syphilitic infection from the pharynx are specially characterised by high fever, early appearance of well-marked skin eruption, and above all, by distinct swelling of the cervical glands.

Instead of the single india-rubber bag, a double bag may be used (Lucae), by which means a continuous but much weaker current of air can be furnished. Lincke used a pair of bellows. The author employs a large india-rubber bag which can be compressed with the foot. Heidenreich, and afterwards Erhard, obtained compressed air at any desired pressure by means of cylinders submerged in water upon which weights were laid. It is rare that so great pressure is necessary that force-pumps, such as have been constructed by Politzer and Von Tröltsch, have to be employed. The older aurists attempted to exhaust the tympanic cavity of air by means of the catheter. Pomeroy and Kessel have advised catheterism from the mouth with specially shaped catheters. Fixing the catheter after insertion into the tube with nose-clamps, such as have been designed by Kramer, Bonnafont, and Delstanche, is not required in the methods now in use.

In the normal condition it only requires an exceedingly slight pressure to force air through the catheter into the tympanic cavity, but in cases of swelling in the Eustachian tube, a high degree of pressure may be required, and sometimes it is only possible while the patient swallows as the air is injected.

Alarming and even dangerous accidents may be caused by the catheter injuring the mucous membrane and inflating the subjacent and surrounding tissues with air. This happens most frequently after passing bougies into the Eustachian tube. The emphysema produced in this manner extends to the lateral wall of the pharynx, the soft palate, the uvula, and even to the glottis, sometimes extending also externally down the neck even to the chest. Its symptoms are a feeling as of a foreign body in the throat, pain, difficulty in swallowing, and, in very severe cases, a choking sensation. In the throat the little swellings have the appearance of transparent bullæ, yellowish-white in colour. On the side of the neck externally, the emphysema can easily be recognised by palpation. It subsides without treatment in a few days. A gargle of iced water may be used for the pain. In order to remove this condition rapidly, incisions should be made. Blowing the nose is to be avoided. Alarming symptoms sometimes happen after catheterism. Fainting occasionally occurs. Hinton observed, in an otherwise healthy man, giddiness, unconsciousness, and epileptiform convulsions. Two fatal cases are on record, both of which occurred while the force-pump was applied. A third unexplained case of death, which happened in a town in Silesia, was related to the writer verbally. Death seems to have been caused by emphysema of the mucous membrane of the glottis. Baginsky's experiments on animals give another explanation. He found that injections into the external auditory meatus, made under great pressure, could bring about the death of animals by rupture of the membrana tympani and of the membrane of the fenestra rotunda, along with penetration of fluid into the cranial cavity through the aquæductus cochleæ.

THE DIAGNOSTIC AND THERAPEUTIC APPLICATION OF THE AIR-DOUCHE.

In a diagnostic aspect the air-douche is chiefly important on account of the sounds which may be heard by means of the auscultation-tube when air is injected into the tympanic cavity by means of Catheterism or by Politzerisation. The auscultation-tube or otoscope (Toynbee) consists of an india-rubber tube, about one metre long, one end of which is put into the ear of the patient and the other into that of the surgeon. The one end is generally furnished with an olive-shaped nozzle for the patient's ear, while the other end has no nozzle.

When the Eustachian tube is in a normal state, a sound, produced by the current of air striking against the walls of the tympanic cavity and the membrana tympani, is heard. The sound varies according to the force of the air-current, the patency of the Eustachian tube, and the lumen of the catheter. It commences more or less sharply, and changes into a blowing noise, giving the impression that a full current of dry air is entering the tympanic cavity. When the passage of air is obstructed by pathological changes in the Eustachian tube, and only a weak current enters the tympanum, we do not hear the sound made by the air striking against its walls, but merely a slight short blowing noise, which sometimes has a hissing or whistling sound of high pitch.

In some instances the sound may be interrupted, and a brief pause may occur during which no air enters.

When secretion is present we perceive rattling noises, either a fine crackling râle or a loud bubbling sound, which may arise from the secretion in the Eustachian tube being propelled into the tympanic cavity, or from the formation of air-bubbles in the secretion in the tympanum. The character of the râle varies according to the quantity and consistency of the secretion.

When the membrana tympani is perforated, the air is driven into the tympanic cavity, and passes into the auscultation-tube, giving the observer the impression that air is being blown directly into his own ear,—the characteristic sound produced by a perforation. In the absence of secretion, the sound is full and loud, and varies according to the calibre of the tube and size of the perforation, assuming a blowing, breathing, or hissing character. Secretion being present, a loud râle can easily be heard even without the auscultation-tube.

All these auscultation sounds not only can be heard during catheterism, but also in Politzerisation, and when air enters the tympanic cavity by the Valsalvian experiment. During catheterism, however, when a stronger and more continuous current of air is produced, the sounds are most pronounced and most easily distinguished.

During auscultation, sounds are also heard, although the air does not enter the tympanum, but rushes back along the catheter from the Eustachian tube into the naso-pharynx, and when the point of the catheter is not in the tube at all, but in Rosenmüller's fossa. These sounds are, however, much weaker, and appear more distant than the sounds caused by the entrance of air into the tympanic cavity, which give the impression that they are produced close to the ear of the observer.

When under a minimum of pressure, the air passes freely into the tympanum through the catheter, while a greater pressure is required for Politzer's method, it may be inferred that the constriction has its seat at the mouth of the tube.

The air-douche can further be employed diagnostically and prognostically to ascertain the nature and condition of the pathological processes in the sound-conducting apparatus. An abnormal position and tension of the membrana tympani and of the ossicula, resulting from diseases of the Eustachian tube or the formation of adhesions, may be remedied by the pressure effected by the air-douche upon the inner surface of the membrane. The excessive tension of the sound-conducting apparatus accompanying inward curvature of the membrane is removed when the latter returns to its normal position. If the hearing be quite restored after the air-douche, the cause of the deafness must have been purely mechanical, resulting from the impaired function of the Eustachian tube; if only an improvement be effected, the dulness of hearing must arise from exudation or from new growth and swelling within the limits of the sound-conducting apparatus. The greater the improvement, the more insignificant will be the nature of the obstruction, and the easier removed. Although the air-douche produce little or no improvement, the prognosis is still favourable, if, on further examination, the presence of secretion be detected; otherwise, the prognosis is unfavourable. In giving a prognosis it is also important to observe the duration of the improvement after the air-douche; the more rapidly the hearing becomes worse, the more unfavourable the prognosis.

Therapeutically, the air-douche is chiefly valuable in effecting the restoration of the normal position and tension of the sound-conducting apparatus. By means of Politzer's method, exudation may be most readily removed from the tympanic cavity by inclining the head forward and downward to the side opposite the diseased ear, which will cause the secretion to be brought to the orifice of the Eustachian tube. When the membrana tympani is perforated, the secretion is driven into the external meatus, and removed by means of the syringe. Frequent repetition of the air-douche also promotes the reduction of hyperæmic swelling and cessation of the secretion.

Not only air, but various solutions and vapours are injected into the tympanum by means of the catheter. Vapours especially have been formerly much employed, most frequently steam, which was led through the catheter into the middle ear from a bottle containing boiling water, a method which even now is sometimes employed with good results. The use of sal-ammoniac vapour, which was formerly so much practised, has now become obsolete. The vapour of chloroform, ether, or oil-of-turpentine may be injected by means of the india-rubber bag, to which it is supplied from a spray-bottle having a stopper penetrated by two glass tubes.

An insufflation capsule is very useful, made like Zaufal's disinfection capsule. It is made of vulcanite, and consists of a globe which can be unscrewed in the middle. At its two poles there are nozzles, one of which is inserted into the india-rubber bag, and the other into the catheter. Each half of the globe contains a perforated plate. Between these two plates is placed a piece of cotton wadding, which has first been saturated with the evaporating fluid. At the side of the globe is a perforation fitted with a valve, opening inward. Another valve, opening outward, is placed in the nozzle which is intended for the catheter. The whole apparatus can be attached to any bag. The air entering the capsule by the lateral opening is by compression of the bag forced through the layer of wadding into the catheter.

To apply medicated fluids to the mucous membrane of the tympanic cavity, Pravaz's syringe is employed, furnished with a long conical nozzle, or with a simple drop-counter, a few drops of the fluid being injected into the catheter, which has first been placed in its proper position and then driven into the tympanum by a current of air from the air-bag. In order to convey the fluid direct into the tympanum, the tympanic tube (Paukenröhrchen) may be employed.

Ph. H. Wolf[1] first recommended the insertion of a thin flexible tube (Paukenröhrchen) into the osseous portion of the Eustachian tube through the catheter. Wolf employed for this purpose a silver tube, and Frank a more flexible leaden one, and recently Weber-Liel a tube made of a soft bougie material. The injections through these small tubes are made in the same manner as through the catheter. In order to convey larger quantities of fluid into the tympanum, which is chiefly desirable in cases of secretion with perforation of the membrana tympani, a catheter with a beak as thick and as long as practicable must be introduced as far as

---

[1] S. Frank, *Handb. der prakt. Ohrenheilk.*, p. 102.

possible into the Eustachian tube, and the injection then made with a large syringe.

Fluid can be injected into the tympanic cavity without a catheter by Politzer's method, if the bag be filled with fluid instead of air, and discharged during an act of swallowing (Saemann). It can also be done by first conveying the fluid into the nasal cavity and then Politzerising. As in each of these methods the fluid enters into both tympanic cavities, they can only be employed when both ears are affected.

When it is impossible to remove a constriction of the Eustachian tube by injections or by treatment of the naso-pharyngeal mucous membrane, bougies may be used. They are $\frac{2}{3}$—$\frac{4}{3}$ mm. in thickness. Kramer recommended catgut as the most suitable material for them; whalebone sounds were afterwards employed, and now the so-called English bougies, prepared with wax, are in use. Laminaria bougies, which Schwartze formerly recommended, have not proved suitable, as it repeatedly happened that they broke in the Eustachian tube. When introducing the bougies, it is to be borne in mind that, on the average, the Eustachian tube is 36 mm. long, but that this length is subject to considerable variation. One-third of it is formed by the osseous portion, and two-thirds by the cartilaginous and membranous portion. The bougie will, therefore, be in the osseous portion when its point is more than 24 mm. distant from the curved beak of the catheter. The measurements may be marked at the external end of the bougie.

In order to cauterise the mucous membrane of the Eustachian tube, the older aural surgeons employed metal sounds, upon which nitrate of silver had been fused. These were passed into the tube through the catheter. Saissy first recommended an instrument for dilating the Eustachian tube by bleeding.

CHAPTER II.

SYMPTOMATOLOGY.

NOISES IN THE EAR. (SYNONYM: *Tinnitus aurium.*)

NOISES in the ear form one of the most frequent symptoms in ear diseases. They differ very much in their origin, character, and intensity. Sometimes they are so weak that they can only be perceived with the closest attention; sometimes they are so intense that they become a source of great trouble to the patient, robbing him of sleep, and, in the most extreme cases, driving him to suicide in order to escape from their torture.

We distinguish three kinds of noises—namely, (a) *nervous*, also called *subjective;* (b) *entotic;* (c) *objective.* We assume that the first mentioned are caused by irritation of the nervous apparatus, either in the labyrinth or in the brain, arising from alteration in the blood-supply, or some other influence, such as inflammation. The entotic noises have their origin in the middle ear or its neighbourhood, and are transmitted to the internal ear. They arise either in the blood-vessels (*carotis, arteria auditiva interna, vena jugularis, sinus transversus*), from contraction of the muscles (*tensor tympani, stapedius*), from movements of the membrana tympani or of the walls of the Eustachian tube, and from mucous collections in the tympanum. The perception of these noises is favoured (1) by all factors increasing resonance in the ear, (2) by hyperæsthesia of the auditory nerve (Brunner). Sometimes these entotic noises are so loud that they are also heard by others, in which case they are named 'objectively perceivable.' In many cases it cannot be decided whether the sounds are subjective or entotic.

We distinguish the character of noises in the ear as follows:—

1. *Tinnitus of a high pitch*, with which we class what is described as singing, hissing, and chirping. Such a sound occurs spontaneously even in healthy ears, and can also be produced by the application of the constant current, when it occurs at the closure of the cathodes and the opening of the anodes. According to Brenner,[1] it corresponds with c^1 (256 vibrations) or g^1 (348 vibrations), and, according to Hagen,[2] with a^3 (1705·6 vibrations). When the membrana tympani is destroyed it may be produced by touching the stapes. Brunner observed that a loud, clear sound occurred every time he touched a granulation on the promontory. The sound sometimes heard on closing the eyelids Brunner calls 'reflected tinnitus.' A sound of a very high pitch, which may continue for weeks and months, results from hearing a sudden loud report. In one case Wolf found after such a detonation, not only tinnitus, but defective perception of sound, which was confined to the second treble octave (German, *zweigestrichene*, double-lined). One of the author's patients, a professional musician, who suffered from catarrh of the middle ear, with implication of the labyrinth, had transitorily a very troublesome tinnitus corresponding in tone with d^3 (1152 vibrations). While this tinnitus lasted, the corresponding tone of the pianoforte could only be heard when it was very loudly sounded. Most frequently tinnitus occurs in active or passive hyperæmia of the organ of hearing, in acute or chronic catarrh, and especially in implication of the labyrinth.

These noises are best explained by the theory of stimulation of individual nerve filaments, or groups of filaments, in the labyrinth, just as we have ocular phenomena resulting from hyperæmia or pressure on the eyeball.

Kiesselbach[3] found, in the case of himself, that the sound produced by the constant current corresponded in tone exactly with that of the resonance in his ears, which was b^4 (German, h^4, 3840 vibrations) on the right side, and a^4 (3411·2 vibrations) on the left. According to him, the vascular sounds were intensified, being perceived when the nervous structures were in a high state of stimulation induced by the current.

[1] *Elektro-Otiatrik*, p. 110.   [2] *Prakt. Beiträge zur Ohrenheilk.*, vol. vi. p. 18.
[3] Pflüger's *Arch. f. ges. Physiol.* vol. xxxi.

2. *Tinnitus of a low pitch*, as rushing and humming.

Many cases of tinnitus must be considered as nervous, especially such as occur with cerebral tumours, with diseases confined to the labyrinth, and with affections in the middle ear, causing increased pressure in the labyrinth, by forcing the stapes inward. But a great number of these sounds must be classed as entotic, arising in the neighbouring blood-vessels or muscles, and perceived under various conditions. The venous sounds are continuous; the arterial, pulsating; both can, as a rule, be affected by pressure upon the vessels in the neck. The muscular sounds have a correspondingly low tone, of a humming character. Most frequently noises of this kind seem to be perceived when the conditions of resonance in the ear are especially favourable, as when the external meatus is closed by plugs of cerumen or by polypi, or when accumulations of secretion have formed in the meatus or in the tympanic cavity. Vascular and muscular sounds are also perceived in cases of hyperæsthesia of the auditory nerve, especially the former, if they have been previously well marked. Moos was able to trace, in one case, the cause of tinnitus to the dilatation of the sinus of the internal jugular vein. Tinnitus in anæmic and chlorotic persons may be considered as autoperception of the so-called nun-like or bellows-like sound, caused by the blood flowing from the lateral sinus into the sinus of the internal jugular vein. Patients as well as observers have frequently noticed, synchronous with the pulse, a noise of a blowing character in cases of aneurism, either transmitted from the aorta and the carotids, or as an accompanying sign of cerebral aneurism.

Gottstein observed a rustling noise in the ear, which occurred spasmodically and simultaneously with blepharospasm. The rustling disappeared when the spasm of the eyelid ceased. Gottstein believes that it was caused by a spasm of the stapedius muscle. A female patient described to the author the noises occurring simultaneously with facial spasms as the slow rattling of a mill, which afterwards changed into a low hum. Habermann removed, by tenotomy of the stapedius muscle, a hollow droning noise which occurred four or five times at every closure of the eyelid.

3. Various entotic noises are caused by movements of exudation in the middle ear, or by changes in the position of the moveable parts of the middle ear. The sounds of scraping, crackling, gurgling, rattling, and bubble-bursting may be explained as arising from movements of exudation, and they vary according to its consistence. If it be of a serous character, bubbles are formed by air passing through the Eustachian tubes, causing noises both when forming and bursting. A loud report in the ear is caused by the bursting of the membrana tympani in acute inflammation, also by the Eustachian tube becoming suddenly permeable after closure for some time.

Many persons are able to produce at will in their ears a snapping or crackling noise simultaneously with the contraction of the muscles of the soft palate. According to Joh. Müller, this noise is caused by the contraction of the tensor tympani; according to Politzer, by the detachment from each other of the walls of the Eustachian tube previously in apposition by means of secretion. The author can produce this noise in his ears, and is convinced that it arises in the middle ear, either by a change in the tension of the membrana tympani itself, or by an alteration in the position of the ossicula in consequence of the contraction of the tensor tympani. The tensor veli, along with the tensor tympani, is supplied by the motor portion of the trigeminus. An observer can also perceive this noise objectively by auscultation, which sometimes is so loud that it can be heard at a distance of several feet. A patient of Bremer's could produce this noise 100—150 times per minute, by spasmodic contraction of the tensor tympani. Boeck and Holmes observed this noise in cases of clonic spasms of the extrinsic muscles of the larynx and of the soft palate. An entotic sound should be mentioned here which takes place synchronously with inspiration and expiration, and which the author observed in two patients, to whom it occasioned great annoyance. It is caused by in- and out-going currents of air through abnormally wide Eustachian tubes.

4. *Hearing full melodies* is of much rarer occurrence than that of the noises which have hitherto been discussed. It can hardly be otherwise assumed but that it arises from a state of excitation

of the cerebrum, and must be regarded as a kind of hallucination, although no other psychical phenomena are observed. Not only well-known but even unknown melodies are heard. With such perception of musical sounds may be classed the hearing of human voices, the croaking of frogs, and suchlike. Brunner observed a case of hearing of melodies in a patient who had taken large doses of quinine, and also in an apoplectic patient. A musically trained lady, who was under treatment by the author for nervous dulness of hearing in a very advanced stage, heard for a long time the most beautiful melodies, mostly well known to her. But subsequently she unfortunately heard them jumbled together, so that discordant sounds were created.

In many cases an alteration or a temporary or lasting diminution or cessation of the noises can be produced by external influences, as by pressure upon the mastoid process, or upon the first cervical vertebra (Türck); also, according to Weil, by blowing upon the walls of the meatus with the india-rubber bag, by the action of electric currents, and by external sound. Lucae[1] attaches the greatest importance to the influence of the latter, and even divides subjective sounds into those which increase in intensity by the influence of external sound, and those which decrease. In the treatment of the former, the patient is kept away from all noise; in the latter, the 'tone-treatment' is resorted to. Lucae employs the influence of a low tone for whistling and hissing of a high pitch, and that of a high tone for low-pitched whistling and humming.

The prognosis of cases in which the noises remain un altered and continuous is unfavourable; while in the case of those of varying intensity, and especially if they temporarily cease altogether, there is some ground for hope. An alteration in the noise after the air-douche may be regarded as a favourable sign in the prognosis of the case. If the noise alter in consequence of rarefaction of air in the external meatus, an abnormal state of tension may be inferred, admitting of treatment.

According to Von Tröltsch, Schwartze, and Köppe, noises produced by peripheric affections may occasion psychical disorders,

---

[1] *Zur Entstehung und Behandlung der subjektiven Gehörsempfindungen*, Berlin, 1884.

hallucinations of hearing, melancholy, and even reflex-psychosis. L. Meyer observed the case of a patient suffering from melancholia, with continuous hallucinations of hearing, who was cured by the removal of a plug of cerumen. Psychosis may be produced by various ear diseases, especially in persons predisposed to psychical affections. When the ear disease is removed, the psychosis will also disappear.

AUDITORY VERTIGO.

Giddiness and disturbance of equilibration may occur in a variety of ear diseases. As a rule, these symptoms are accompanied by hissing or ringing sounds in the ears, and by nausea or vomiting.

For the proper recognition of these symptoms of vertigo, various observations on the organ of hearing in health and disease are of importance :—

1. According to experiments by Schmidekam and Hensen, a column of cold water lying upon the membrana tympani will produce giddiness, nausea, and vomiting, symptoms which do not occur when warm water is used or under the influence of air-pressure. As already pointed out, giddiness is also occasioned when the water used for syringing is even only of a slightly too low temperature.

2. Giddiness may be caused by foreign bodies or ceruminal plugs lying upon the membrana tympani, or upon the walls of the tympanic cavity. Urbantschitsch mentions a case in which a tendency to fall and giddiness were produced by touching polypous growths lightly with the probe, which were situated near the fenestra ovalis.

3. Schmidekam first observed that giddiness, nausea, and singing in the ear were caused by the loud tones of the syren, and also by the action of other sounds—for instance, a gun report.

4. Numerous experiments, made after the manner of Flourens, regarding the function of the semicircular canals, have shown that a section through these canals in animals produces disturbances of equilibration, especially in cases of deafness. Various movements of the head were observed according to the canal through which

the section was made; likewise, nystagmus of both eyes occurs. These phenomena do not appear by exposing the osseous canals only, without opening the membranous canals. Goltz draws the conclusion from these experiments that in the internal ear there must exist the terminal ramification of a nerve which by conducting the stimulation to the brain produces vertigo.

5. The most strongly marked symptoms of vertigo and disturbance of equilibration in man are caused by injuries of the labyrinth. The author had the opportunity of observing such an injury which had taken place without any further complication. A girl had with great force driven the point of a knitting-needle in the direction of the fenestra ovalis at the posterior-superior border of the membrana tympani. She fell at once, had to be put to bed, and every movement was accompanied by the most extreme vertigo, along with uncontrollable vomiting and loud subjective noises, in addition to a moderate degree of deafness. These symptoms lasted in their full intensity for about two days, when a gradual improvement began to take place.

As in man the centre of the power of equilibration has its seat in the cerebellum, we must, on the ground of the above experiences, assume, with Goltz, that in the ear, especially in the labyrinth, there are nerve-structures, the stimulation of which produces in a reflex manner disturbance of equilibration and giddiness, as also nausea and vomiting; and for the sake of simplicity we therefore designate such vertigo and its accompanying symptoms as 'reflex vertigo.' From experiments upon animals Baginsky regards 'reflex vertigo' as the result of direct irritation of the brain, produced by pressure upon the labyrinthine fluid and penetration of the latter into the cranial cavity through the aquæductus cochleæ.

HYPERÆSTHESIA OF THE AUDITORY NERVE.

By this term we designate a peculiar sensitiveness of the organ of hearing with regard to sound-impressions, which are either perceived better than by a normal ear (hyperacusis) or accompanied by the sensation of pain. This symptom must for the most part be considered as cerebral, and is frequently accompanied by an increased sensitiveness with regard to the other senses. Abnormally acute hearing is sometimes met with in cases of hysteria, or in weakened conditions of the nervous system. Lucae observed abnormally acute hearing of all musical tones, especially of low ones, in some forms of facial paralysis. This is explained by paralysis of the stapedius and the predominating action of the tensor tympani. Hearing accompanied with pain may be limited only to single tones and certain noises, or it may extend to every sound. Even with a high degree of deafness this symptom may exist. Brenner regards as 'hyperæsthesia acustica' the stimulation of the auditory nerve produced by a weak action of the galvanic current.

PARACUSIS AND DIPLACUSIS.

By paracusis we understand the false perception of a tone, the impression made upon the ear not corresponding with the actual tone. While the tone is heard correctly by the healthy ear, its pitch appears to be either higher or lower in the diseased ear. The person thereby receives the impression as if he heard double, which is called diplacusis. The difference is either insignificant, or it may include several tones. This condition is not unfrequently met with, but as a rule it can only be exactly ascertained in patients with a musical ear. Most frequently paracusis is a consequence of acute inflammation of the middle ear, and is also caused by other tympanic and labyrinthine affections. We must assume that paracusis is caused by altered tension of some of the cochlear nerve fibres. A particular kind of paracusis may result from changes in the sound-conducting apparatus producing abnormal tension, according to which tones are transmitted to the perceiving apparatus with more or less intensity. In such cases paracusis does not exist when sound is transmitted by bone-conduction.

PARACUSIS WILLISII.

A considerable number of patients suffering from dulness of hearing exhibit the striking peculiarity of 'hearing better during a loud noise.' While travelling by rail, or in a carriage amid a great noise in the street, during the roll of drums, or while a vibrating tuning-fork is placed upon the cranial bones, some patients hear speech, and the sound of the instruments employed in testing the hearing, better than they would do without the influence of such loud sounds. The case related by Willis himself, of a man who could only converse with his wife when a drum was beaten, is well known. Willis first described this peculiar condition of hearing, and it was called after him 'Paracusis Willisii.' In the objective examination of patients with this symptom, frequently no changes from the normal state are found, and it has not yet been ascertained whether chronic disease of the middle ear or an affection of the labyrinth is the cause. Löwenberg points out that many cases of paracusis are accompanied by cerebral symptoms. It has been already observed by Frank that this may also occur in cases of destructive changes in the tympanic cavity in consequence of purulent inflammation of the middle ear. The prognosis of these cases is exceedingly unfavourable, as no improvement in the hearing can be effected by treatment. Johannes Müller was of opinion that this peculiar symptom was produced by torpor of the hearing-nerve, which requires to be stimulated in order to rouse it into activity. Politzer, however, thinks that by vigorous shaking, the ossicular chain is released from the fixed position it has assumed, and becomes thereby better adapted for the transmission of sound.

AUTOPHONY.

To the category of symptoms which are rarely observed belongs autophony, or tympanophony, namely, hearing one's own voice with extreme loudness, which seems to enter directly into the ear with great intensity. It is occasioned by abnormal patency of the Eustachian tube, so that the sound of the voice straightway reaches the tympanic cavity and causes the membrana tympani to vibrate very strongly. One's own voice is heard extremely loud, and has a pealing sound; it is most unpleasant to the patient, and he requires to take care not to speak loud. At the same time the passage of air to and from the tympanum during respiration causes a very disagreeable feeling. Autophony is especially well marked when the consonants *m*, *n*, *ng* are pronounced. Brunner in his treatise on autophony describes two such cases, and the author had an opportunity of observing one. Such cases are due to the fact that in the articulation of these sounds no closure by the soft palate takes place, so that the sound vibrations reach the orifices of the tubes unobstructed. By auscultation of the ear the entrance of the sound of the voice can be easily perceived. While in most cases the abnormal patency of the Eustachian tube can be easily and positively ascertained by examination with the manometer, some cases of autophony are difficult to explain, as they sometimes occur in acute or subacute inflammation of the middle ear with naso-pharyngeal catarrh. In such cases, according to our experience, obstruction of the tubes should be assumed. As in the normal ear the mucous covering of the Eustachian tube forms only a very loose, valve-like closure, Brunner's [1] theory appears rather probable that in a fresh catarrh of the middle ear, due to inflammatory swelling, the soft lining of the tube is less fitted to produce this valve-like closure.

[1] *Zeitschrift für Ohrenheilkunde*, vol. xii. p. 268.

CHAPTER III.

FREQUENCY, ÆTIOLOGY, AND PROPHYLAXIS OF EAR DISEASES.

EAR DISEASE is of very frequent occurrence. Von Tröltsch holds that in middle age, that is, from 20 to 50 years, on an average one out of three persons does not hear normally and well, at least in one ear. We possess exact statistics of the frequency of deafness in childhood. Reichard,[1] who only examined with the watch, which is unsuitable for this purpose, found among 1055 children 22·2 per cent. dull of hearing. The most extensive examinations were made by Weil[2] in Stuttgart with 5905 children. He found ceruminal plugs in 11 per cent. of the boys, and in 15·1 per cent. of the girls; prominence of the posterior fold of the membrana tympani (in-drawing of the membrane) in 8·2 per cent. of the boys, and in 6·0 of the girls; suppuration of the ears in 1·9 per cent. of the boys, and 2·3 per cent. of the girls; calcareous deposit in 1·5 per cent. of the boys, and 0·9 per cent. of the girls. More than 30 per cent. of all the children were dull of hearing. In the schools attended by the children of the wealthier classes the hearing is on the whole better than amongst the poorer children. In Munich, Bezold[3] found, by examining the 3836 ears of 1918 school children, that 79·25 per cent. of these children had normal hearing, and in 20·75 per cent. the hearing was imperfect. The latter heard whispered speech at a distance of 8 metres or less, *i.e.* at one-third the normal distance or less. Although Weil's examinations showed that affections of hearing increase during school years, Bezold

---

[1] *Petersburger med. Wochenschrift*, No. 29, 1878.
[2] *Zeitschrift für Ohrenheilkunde*, vol. xi. p. 106.
[3] *Ibid.* vol. xiv. p. 253.

could not confirm this. The dulness of hearing is mostly unknown to the children themselves and to their relatives, as well as to their teachers, so that Weil justly demands of the school authorities that the ears of all children who seem inattentive should be examined.

When Bezold applied the statistics which he had collected with regard to the frequency of dulness of hearing in the different classes to the rate of progress of the school-children, the following extremely important fact was noticed, namely, 'that not only had it an influence on the progress of the children, but that even a gradual increase of this influence could be proved, corresponding with the degree of the existing deafness.'

According to the statistical reports of aural surgeons [1] the male sex suffers more from ear disease than the female, the ratio being 3 to 2. Of all the various diseases of the ear, 25 per cent. belong to the external ear (eczema, 2 per cent.; otitis externa circumscripta, 3·5 per cent.; otitis externa diffusa, 5 per cent.; aspergillus, 0·1 per cent.; ceruminal accumulation, 14 per cent.; myringitis acuta, 1 per cent.); to the middle ear, 67 per cent. (acute inflammation, 17 per cent.; chronic catarrh and sclerosis without perforation, 25 per cent.; chronic purulent inflammation, 20 per cent.); to the nerve apparatus, 8 per cent.

Colds, according to the laity, play the most important part in the origin of ear disease; indeed, it cannot be denied that in a number of cases they furnish the real cause. Immediately after the influence of cold, as a draught, or the entrance of cold water, we observe acute inflammation of the membrana tympani, or of the tympanic cavity, and exacerbation of chronic processes. More frequently than by direct influence ear diseases arise, especially in children, from extension of catarrhal inflammation of the mucous membrane of the nose and naso-pharynx to that of the Eustachian tube and of the tympanic cavity. Cases of total deafness also occur suddenly after a severe cold, as from sleeping in the open air, which must be considered as labyrinthine.

According to Bezold's investigations more than one half of all the cases of disease of the Eustachian tube occur in children.

---

[1] Bürkner, 'Beiträge zur Statistik der Ohrenkrankheiten,' *Archiv für Ohrenheilkunde*, vol. xx. p. 81.

Nervous dulness of hearing is found in 6·9 per cent. of children, and 93·1 per cent. of adults. The percentage of chronic non-perforative disease of the middle ear is similarly low in children.

Under ordinary conditions the healthy ear does not need to be protected from cold; only during extreme cold or stormy and rainy weather ought cotton-wool to be inserted, into children's ears especially. The same precaution must be taken in the case of every ear predisposed to inflammation. All persons whose membranæ are perforated ought to protect their ears with cotton-wool. The entrance of cold fluids into any ear must always be prevented, and so, while bathing or diving, the ear ought to be plugged. Patients with perforations of the membrane should be very careful in this respect, as violent inflammation may be caused by the entrance of cold water.

Persons subject to catching cold should wear woollen under-clothing. Hardiness of constitution may be acquired by cold baths and vigorous rubbing, exercise in the open air, and active employment. In cases of catarrh, or a catarrhal disposition, smoking, the use of alcoholic liquors, and residence in a damp or dusty atmosphere, should be prohibited.

A continuous or sudden loud sound, as an explosion, may cause rupture of the membrana tympani, or lesion of the nervous structures, with temporary or permanent dulness of hearing or deafness. Very many cases of this sort are found among artillerymen. Workmen who are exposed to the continuous action of loud sounds, such as boilermakers, millers, etc., suffer from sclerotic processes with greater or less dulness of hearing. Artillerymen should endeavour to protect their ears somewhat by firmly inserting into the external meatus plugs of cotton wadding. The increase of deafness caused by the particular occupation can only be prevented by a change of employment.

The dulness of hearing which develops in drivers and stokers of locomotives has deservedly received special attention (Moos [1]), because by their inability to hear signals or verbal orders, serious accidents may be occasioned.

Not unfrequently the ears of children are more or less injured

---

[1] *Zeitschrift für Ohrenheilkunde*, vol. ix. p. 370.

by blows; therefore parents and teachers should never lose sight of the fact that the ear is not a proper place for inflicting chastisement.

Sometimes inflammation is caused, or foreign bodies get into the ears, by injudicious application of remedies for toothache—chloroform, eau-de-Cologne, ether, and other fluids being instilled, or pills, onions, and other nostrums inserted into the ears. Patients should be warned against such folly.

It is sometimes necessary to cleanse the orifice of the meatus of an accumulation of cerumen. In the case of children this should only be done if the deposits can be seen from the outside, when they may be removed with the corner of a handkerchief or with an ear-scoop. To enter deeper into the meatus is not advisable. In the case of adults, inspissated cerumen can best be removed by means of the ordinary ear-scoop, or by the aid of the author's wadding-holder (Fig. 12). By the use of sharp or pointed instruments, injuries of the tympanic membrane or of the walls of the external meatus may be caused. Unnecessary syringing may produce loosening and desquamation of the epidermis, as well as inflammation, so that its injudicious employment should be avoided, as also the instillation of oil and the introduction of steam.

A great many cases of ear disease are caused and maintained by affections of the nose and naso-pharynx. Catarrhs and diphtheritic processes extend from these parts to the mucous membrane of the Eustachian tube, and the tympanic cavity, or the swelling in the tube obstructs the ventilation.

Next to scrofula, the exanthemata play the most important part in giving rise to ear affections, namely, scarlet and typhoid fever, measles, and small-pox. Tuberculosis and syphilis may likewise localise themselves in the ear, and all diseases connected with disorders of the circulation may have an unfavourable influence upon the ear (heart disease, plethora, emphysema, goitre, aneurism), either producing disease in it or preventing the cure of existing affections.

As the ear receives branches from the trigeminus and the sympathetic, it is thereby placed in communication with distant organs. Decayed teeth may, in a reflex manner, produce inflammation of the ear and nervous otalgia. Sometimes ear affections occur during pregnancy, which become aggravated at every return of that condition. Menstruation also has sometimes an unfavourable influence upon the ear.

From the close connection between the labyrinth and the cranial cavity, through the sheath of the auditory nerve and the aqueducts, the labyrinth and brain are often both affected. Moreover, the auditory nerve, at its origin or in its course, may be affected in sympathy with various diseases of the brain.

A hereditary predisposition to chronic disease of the tympanic cavity, as well as of the labyrinth, is met with in many families, a large number of the members being afflicted with dulness of hearing earlier or later in life. Bezold points out that hereditary deafness can be proved, especially in such forms in which, from the negative appearance of the membrana tympani, from the ineffectiveness of the air-douche, and from a predominance of bone-conduction, we conclude that the affection results from loss of mobility of the structures at the labyrinthine fenestræ.

A most important part of the prophylaxis of ear diseases consists in preventing acute affections from assuming a chronic character. Although we must confess that a number of ear diseases cannot be arrested in spite of all treatment, we are nevertheless able in the majority of cases, by early treatment, to effect a cure or to arrest further development. We must urge especially that acute purulent inflammation of the middle ear should not be neglected, as it involves the patient in great danger, because it mostly assumes a chronic form, which may lead to a high degree of dulness of hearing, even total deafness, and to other complications so often associated with chronic suppuration. The neglect of catarrhal affections also leads in most cases to irreparable defects.

CHAPTER IV.

GENERAL THERAPEUTICS.

APPLICATION OF REMEDIES THROUGH THE EXTERNAL MEATUS.

REMEDIES applied through the external meatus will only be effectual when that portion of the ear to be acted upon is free from the products of secretion, so that a most careful cleansing must take place before every application. Medicated fluids may either be employed in syringing the ear, thus reaching the desired spot, or, if only small quantities are to be used, they may be applied, previously warmed (10—20 drops), instilled either direct from a medicine-glass, or by means of a drop-counter, a small spoon, or small syringe. In order to allow the fluid to reach the bottom of the meatus, and especially if, in case of destruction of the membrana tympani, the fluid be intended for the tympanic cavity, the meatus should be straightened during the instillation, and the head being inclined toward the opposite side, the tragus should repeatedly be pressed into the meatus, in order to drive the fluid by compression into the tympanum. The entrance of the fluid into the tympanic cavity can be facilitated by the act of swallowing, with the mouth and nose closed, whereby the air is drawn from the tympanum towards the pharynx.

In order to localise the action of the fluid to certain parts of the meatus or of the tympanic cavity, as in using the liquor ferri perchloridi or sulphuric acid, it is most convenient to dip a probe into the fluid and to apply the drop at its point to the part. In such cases it is advisable to wrap a little cotton wadding round the point of the probe. Special care must be taken with strongly corrosive applications; the external meatus should be protected by an ear-speculum or by covering its walls with an ointment.

Ointments are applied by means of a small brush or cotton wadding.

Powders may be introduced through the speculum, the head being inclined toward the opposite side and the meatus straightened. This is still better effected by using a powder-blower, consisting of a tube made of vulcanite or glass, with a lateral opening through which it can be filled. The opening is closed with the finger or with a special contrivance, while the powder is blown into the ear. The insufflation can best be done with the mouth and an india-rubber tube. Politzer constructed a powder-blower with a special compartment for holding the powder. For the application of boracic acid, the insect powder-blowers are quite suitable.

Of solid substances, nitrate of silver is chiefly used; it is either introduced by a special holder, or in the simplest manner by a silver probe, upon the point of which the caustic is melted. The probe is heated over any suitable kind of flame, and the desired quantity of caustic is melted upon it. When chromic acid is used, its crystals are generally in such a moist condition that they adhere to the point of the probe, and are then melted upon it by heating over a flame, and afterwards introduced into the ear.

BLOOD-LETTING.

Blood-letting is often employed with very favourable results in acute inflammation of the different parts of the organ of hearing, or in acute exacerbations of chronic inflammation, accompanied by great hyperæmia and violent pain. In purely chronic hyperæmia also, although only in rare cases, energetic blood-letting is useful. Usually leeches are employed, 3—6 for adults, 1—2 for children. As the blood-vessels of the external and middle ear are partly drained into the venous ramifications in the neighbourhood of the maxillary joint, blood-letting at this point proves very effective, the leeches being applied close in front of the tragus. On the other hand, when the inflammation is deep-seated in the tympanic cavity or in the mastoid process, blood-letting on the surface of the latter is of advantage. In any case it should be employed when the mastoid process itself is painful. In acute inflammation of the middle ear, leeches are placed round the external ear, on the mastoid process, the retro-maxillary fossa, and in front of the tragus. In order to prevent the leeches from creeping into the external meatus, it must be stopped with cotton.

Besides leeches, Heurteloup's artificial leech is in use. As is well known, any desired quantity of blood can be extracted by its means in a very short time, and therefore its application is highly to be recommended if it be desirable to withdraw a large quantity of blood. The artificial leech is placed, according to the seat of the disease, either in front of the tragus or behind the ear, but in the latter situation its application is somewhat difficult on account of the surface of the mastoid process being so irregular. Frequently it is only possible to fix the instrument close behind the mastoid process. Blood-letting at this place chiefly proves effectual when the patient is suffering from congestion of the labyrinth or from cerebral symptoms.

General blood-letting is not employed in the treatment of ear diseases.

APPLICATION OF ELECTRICITY.

Both the induced faradic current and the constant galvanic current are employed. According to the author's experience, the former is the most advantageous in cases in which vaso-motor defects are suspected, also in the later stages of acute inflammation of the middle ear, and in chronic inflammatory processes, when simultaneously a feeling of pressure and pain in the head or neck is present on the diseased side. The one electrode is placed upon the mastoid process, or upon the neck, behind the angle of the lower jaw, so as to act upon the sympathetic nerve. The second electrode is placed upon a more distant part of the body.

The constant current is employed most frequently and with most success. To Brenner[1] belongs the merit of establishing a rational basis for its application and proving its practical value. Brenner's statements have been confirmed by Hagen, Erb, and others, but have long been doubted by many aural surgeons, so that the galvanic treatment has been little employed. Only re-

---

[1] *Untersuchungen und Beobachtungen auf dem Gebiete der Elektrotherapie*, Leipzig, 1868.

cently reports of the favourable result achieved by means of the constant current have been increasing in number, especially as regards the treatment of tinnitus, when all other methods have failed.

For the galvanic treatment of the ear a good battery is necessary, which must be supplied with a commutator and a rheostat. Although Brenner himself inserted the ear-electrode into the external meatus after it had been filled with salt water, which is called the internal application of the electrode, the external application, recommended by Erb, is now generally in use. By this method, the ear-electrode of medium size is placed directly in front of the ear so as to cover the tragus. The second electrode is placed upon the sternum, the neck, or the hand of the opposite side.

Brenner was successful in showing that, by the action of the constant current, the auditory nerve reacts in a manner corresponding to the law of contraction of the motor nerves. With a current of medium strength, the cathode on closure of the circuit (KaS) produces the sensation of sound, which gradually decreases while the closure lasts (KaD). The cathode, on opening the circuit (KaO), and the anode on closure (AS), and during closure (AD), produces no result; while the anode on opening (AO) reproduces a weak sound. Brenner's formula [1] for normal hearing is therefore as follows:—

KaS—K (sound), KaD—K > (decreasing),
KaO—(no sound), AS—, AD—, AO—k (weak sound).

In most cases it is easier to produce a reaction of the auditory nerve in persons with ear disease than those with normal hearing, *i.e.* a weaker current will suffice to produce sensations of sound. Brenner designates this condition as 'simple galvanic hyperæsthesia' of the auditory nerve. This form of reaction is observed in the greatest variety of ear diseases, in purulent inflammation of the middle ear, in chronic catarrh, in sclerosis of the tympanic cavity, and also in affections of the nervous structures. The accompanying tinnitus is lessened or removed by the action of the current. On closure of the circuit, and during closure, the anode (AS and AD) effects diminution or cessation of the tinnitus, while the cathode, on

---

[1] Ka = Cathode (the negative pole). A = Anode (the positive pole). O = Oeffnung, opening. S = Schliessung, closing. D = Dauer, duration. K = Klang, sound. k = weak sound.

closure, and during closure (KaS and KaD), increases it. The cathode on opening (KaO) may produce a temporary decrease. Sometimes it happens that the reaction is reversed, namely, a decrease in the tinnitus during the action of the cathode and an increase during that of the anode. According to Erb, the general principle of the treatment consists in continuing that form of stimulus which lessens or removes the tinnitus as powerfully and as long as possible, while those which increase the tinnitus should be managed as cautiously as possible. When therefore the tinnitus is lessened during the action of the anode (AD), a strong closure is made, and the current is allowed to act for several minutes, and then decreased by means of the rheostat or by lessening the number of elements, which must however involve no opening reaction.

The galvano-cautery is of very limited application to the ear. Middeldorpf has used the galvano-caustic snare for the removal of polypi, but as the ordinary snares have been found much simpler, the galvano-cautery has proved superfluous for this purpose. Most frequently it is employed for the destruction of the remains of polypi, as well as for the removal of fibrous tumours in the external meatus, and for artificial perforation of the membrane. The extent of the action of the cauterisation cannot always be exactly reckoned. In all cases where the bone lies immediately beneath the diseased tissue, and especially in the tympanic cavity, the galvano-cautery must be applied with the greatest care. Thin wire and the finest platinum points are used.

CONSTITUTIONAL TREATMENT.

As a large number of the pathological processes in the organ of hearing owe their origin or their delay in healing to diseases of other parts of the body, we must not confine ourselves to the local treatment of the ear, but we must also have regard to the general state of health. It is of the greatest importance in cases of anomalies in the constitution, mal-nutrition, and the scrofulous and phthisical diatheses, to promote a more healthy condition by suitable treatment. By regular living, a rational diet, by preparations of iodine, iron, and quinine, cod-liver oil, and other constitutional remedies, beneficial results may be obtained.

Of special importance in the treatment of ear diseases are baths, which are employed in all chronic diseases in order to promote absorption, to invigorate the nervous system, and to improve the constitution generally. Cold baths are only suitable for strong, well-nourished persons, and warm baths for weakened systems requiring careful treatment. Baths of 25°—29° R. (88°—97° F.) are soothing; baths of a higher temperature than the blood are stimulating in their effect. The mineral elements and the carbonic acid gas act as an additional stimulant upon the skin.

Saline baths are most frequently prescribed in the treatment of ear diseases, and especially in all cases of a tendency to recurrent catarrh with profuse secretion and a protracted course, and where the affection may be traced to the scrofulous diathesis. The baths should be taken warm, 26°—27° R. (90°—93° F), each bath lasting 15—30 minutes, and the whole course of treatment 4—6 weeks. In choosing a saline bathing-place, it is important to consider, on the one hand, the proportion of salts, and, on the other, that of carbonic acid gas, existing in the waters; as also the situation, climate, and arrangements for patients. The greater the proportion of saline ingredients the better will be the effect. It should be noted that generally those waters which are rich in carbonic acid are more stimulating than those containing little of it. For highly sensitive, excitable, and otherwise nervous patients, or for those with dry chronic inflammation of the middle ear or labyrinth, accompanied by great tinnitus and congestion, the weaker waters should be chosen, such as Ragatz, Pfäffers, and Gastein, as well as Wiesbaden, Baden-Baden, Soden, and others. Weak saline waters contain 2—4 per cent. of salt; the strong waters 6—8 per cent. Those of Kösen, containing 5 per cent., and of Harzburg, containing 6½ per cent., may be used undiluted; while the concentrated saline waters of Reichenhall, Kreuznach, Ischl, and Salzungen can be diluted at discretion.

The waters containing salts and carbonic acid in large proportion are to be recommended chiefly in the case of patients of an apathetic nature, with the so-called 'pasty' form of scrofula, also in otorrhœa and catarrh with exudation. In cases of recent aural deposits of small extent in persons of good general health, the thermal saline waters of Nauheim and Rehme, which contain much carbonic acid, are to be recommended; while, for deposits of older date and larger extent, Kreuznach and similar watering-places are indicated as preferable. For sulphur baths Cauterets stands especially high in reputation in the cure of ear diseases.

The absorption effected by these baths is assisted by simultaneously drinking natural mineral waters, especially saline waters containing iodine and bromine, such as Kreuznach, Adelheidsquelle in Heilbrunn near Tölz, and Hall in Upper Austria. In anæmic conditions benefit is obtained from taking waters especially containing iron, along with saline baths. In cases of digestive derangement, or in plethoric conditions, Marienbad, Karlsbad, Kissingen, Friedrichshall, and similar wells, should be resorted to.

HEARING-TUBES.

In many cases of great dulness of hearing, conversation may be facilitated by instruments which either conduct sound to the ear or cause a greater volume of sound to act upon it.

As in passing through tubes the intensity of sound is not diminished, speech, conducted to the ear by means of a tube, is heard just as well as if uttered close to it. If the tube have a conical shape, the sound is at the same time collected, intensified, and reflected into that portion of it which is inserted into the meatus.

The number of ear-tubes in use is exceedingly large, and they differ in form as well as in material. When choosing one, the degree of the dulness of hearing, as well as the affection causing it, require to be taken into consideration. Generally it may be assumed that the smaller the instrument, the slighter will be its effect. In cases of dulness produced by slow processes, resulting in sclerosis of the mucous membrane of the tympanic cavity, or in an affection of the labyrinth, those of soft material should be employed. When tinnitus is present, and is increased by the use of the instrument, it must not be employed, or at least as seldom as possible. If pathological processes long since exhausted, suppuration, or previous injuries, have produced great dulness, instruments made of tin are to be preferred. Frequently only after prolonged experience will the patient himself discover which kind of hearing-tube is the most suitable.

The hearing-tubes most in use are the following :—

1. Dunker's hearing-tube, about a metre in length, made of a soft substance surrounded with wire, having a conical ear-nozzle and at the other end a funnel-shaped horn for speaking into. As it is troublesome for the patient to hold the short ear-nozzle for a length of time in his ear, it is more convenient to substitute for it a firm tube, by which the instrument can be held.

2. Funnel-shaped instruments of vulcanite or soft material, soft leather being very suitable. These can be folded up and put into the pocket, and assume their conical shape again as soon as they are relieved from pressure.

3. Tin hearing-tubes :—

(*a*) Adapted for fastening to the head. Small semicircular curved tubes are so placed around the ear that their aperture is directed outward. Ladies especially prefer them, as they can for the most part be covered by the hair, but they are of little use.

(*b*) Conical tin tubes of very reduced size, which are either straight, with an external funnel-shaped sound-receiver, or bent double, so that they become very short and can be held in the hollow of the hand. Politzer constructed a very small instrument for the deaf, based upon his experience that sound is heard much louder when the surface of the tragus is increased in a backward direction, by applying to it a small solid plate, because a greater number of the waves of sound which are reflected by the concha enter the meatus. It is made of vulcanite, and consists of a small tube bent at a right angle, whose narrower inner end is inserted into the external meatus, while its external broader end lies in the auricle. This instrument is said to be especially advantageous when the face of the deaf person is turned towards the source of sound, as is indeed usually the case. Politzer claims for it as a special advantage that it may be worn in the ear unobserved. Leiter, surgical instrument-maker in Vienna, has recently constructed a useful hearing-trumpet, consisting of a somewhat flattened vulcanite funnel and a bent tube. The instrument while in use is placed in the breast-pocket. Among the instruments which are employed for the improvement of hearing are also the small tubes, designed by Abraham, to keep open the lumen of the meatus in case of collapse of its walls.

Sometimes an improvement is effected by the so-called otophones, which, being placed behind the auricle, force the latter outward and forward. Rhodes of Chicago recently patented an instrument, called the audiphone, by whose aid persons very dull of hearing and deaf-mutes are said to hear. The audiphone consists chiefly of a thin plate of vulcanite, a convexity of its surface being produced by means of cords. The edge of this plate is placed against the upper teeth and the sound of the voice is directed towards it. Colladon employs with similar results a piece of thin-pressed cardboard, which at three of its sides is cut straight, and the fourth is semicircular (30 cm. broad and 40 cm. long). It is bent into a curve by pressing it against the upper teeth. Another instrument, the dentaphone, also an American invention, is arranged in such a way that the sound of the voice is received by a thin metal plate, which, similar to the telephone, is situated at the bottom of a wooden cone. From the centre of this plate extends a wire, at whose end is a wooden plate which the deaf person takes between his teeth. From the plate in the dentaphone the waves of sound are transmitted by means of the wire to the wooden plate, and then by the teeth and bone-conduction to the labyrinth.

After the most varied experiments with the audiphone and the dentaphone, it may be said that sometimes really an improvement in the hearing is effected by these instruments, but their effect does not exceed that of the ear-trumpets, which are much more convenient for daily use. When the dulness of hearing is very great, and speech is not even understood by the aid of ear-trumpets, lip-reading should be acquired.

CHAPTER V.

DISEASES OF THE AURICLE.

ANATOMICAL.

The auricle is formed of reticulated cartilage, which is covered by a very firmly adhering perichondrium. Its skin is thin, and contains no layer of fat. The part leading into the external meatus has the shape of a shell (*concha auris*), and is bordered by two ridges, the *helix* and the *antihelix*, between which lies the *fossa navicularis*. Below the commencement of the helix lies in front the *tragus*, partly covering the orifice of the meatus; behind and opposite the tragus, at the termination of the antihelix, is another small projection called the *antitragus*. Between these two points lies the *incisura intertragica*.

Below is situated the appendage of the integument, called the *lobule*. The auricle extends conically into the external meatus, the boundary between the two being formed by a ridgelike projection.

ECZEMA.

Acute eczema of the auricle occurs mostly along with that affection of the surrounding skin; more rarely is this disease confined to the ear alone. Its onset is generally very suddenly followed by great swelling and redness of the skin of the whole auricle, which assumes a very unsightly, bulky appearance. A feeling of tension, pain, and heat is associated with it. The extension of the swelling to the adjoining skin causes the auricle to project from the head. When the orifice of the meatus has also been implicated, a narrowing or closure takes place. When the affection is only slight, the superficial layers of epidermis peel off in the form of scales without exudation (*eczema squamosum*). In inflammation of a high degree, so frequently met with, serous exudation occurs, separating the epidermis by the formation of isolated vesicles, or extending over a larger area (*eczema rubrum*). It then presents a very moist, reddened surface, which after becoming dry forms a crust (*eczema impetiginosum*). The exudation is often very copious, a continuous dripping of the fluid sometimes taking place as if squeezed out of a sponge. With suitable treatment it becomes less after a few days, the swelling and redness subside, and the epidermic layer forms again. For some time the redness remains, and a pityriasis-like desquamation ensues, after which a complete cure soon follows. Relapses frequently occur during recovery, caused by renewed inflammation; in other cases the disease takes a protracted course and resolves itself into chronic eczema. The secretion becomes purulent, the crusts become larger, and form a thick scab, and the corium or true skin is implicated in the disease. Sometimes *rhagades* (fissures) are formed, which cause great pain, especially when the ear is touched. In protracted or frequently recurring cases of the disease a thickening of the cutis sets in, which remains even after cure, and gives the ear a deformed appearance. Sometimes this thickening is so considerable that the lumen of the meatus is occluded. This closure sometimes becomes complete by growth of tissue uniting the opposed surfaces.

In many cases chronic eczema consists only in great swelling and redness, with a moderate degree of desquamation, associated with a feeling of burning and itching.

If the eczema be only confined to particular places, it appears either as a fissure in the line of junction of the auricle with the head, or some other parts of the auricle are affected. It frequently attacks the lobule after it has been pierced, an operation which parents in the various grades of society cause to be performed on their children, partly from superstition, 'in order to prevent disease,' partly for wearing ear-rings. Not infrequently the wearing of such articles of jewellery produces circumscribed inflammation, which may cause the perforation to enlarge, and gradually to extend downward through the lobule.

In children especially, in consequence of discharge from the tympanic cavity and the external meatus, excoriations and crusts form at the orifice and on the inner surface of the auricle.

Treatment.—In the first stage of acute eczema it is most advisable to apply as mild treatment as possible. When tension, itching, or pain is felt, it is best to employ, as a mild soothing remedy, a 1—2 per cent. solution of carbolic or salicylic acid in olive oil, either applying it with a brush or on linen. The oil forms the best protection against external influences, alleviates the pain, and loosens the crusts. For very moist eczema, powders are used, especially starch mixed with an equal quantity of oxide of zinc. To this mixture salicylic acid or alum (1—2 per cent.) may be added. The rest of the treatment consists in protecting the parts from irritation. Watery applications generally cannot be endured, as water increases the tension and swelling of the skin. Any scab which forms must be carefully removed by softening it with oil. In chronic eczema, after the exudation upon the surface has ceased, the application of salicylic acid with vaseline (1 : 20—50), or of Hebra's ointment (Rp. Emplastr. litharg. spl., Vaselini $\bar{a}\bar{a}$, leni igne misce) is recommended. The ointments are spread upon thin linen and placed upon the parts affected. The application of these remedies should be preceded by the careful removal of all exudation products. A cure will only be effected when the substances are applied direct to the diseased surface. In the treatment of great infiltration of the skin, spirit of soap or soap ointment may be used. For dry desquamation, preparations of tar are very effective, *e.g.* ol. picis liquidæ, with oil or alcohol in equal parts, applied twice daily with a brush. Fissures are treated with nitrate of silver, either solid or in solution. In particularly obstinate cases the daily administration of 2—6 drops of Fowler's solution (Liquor potassæ arsenitis) may be necessary. In addition, the constitution of the patient must be taken into consideration.

ACUTE INFLAMMATION OF THE AURICLE.

(SYNONYM : *Perichondritis auriculæ.*)

Acute inflammation of the perichondrium, one of the rarer diseases of the auricle, is described in old text-books as a tumour of the auricle or as a cystic formation. It seems that many cases described as othæmatoma are included with it. The swelling forms upon the anterior aspect of the auricle, and presents a smooth dark-red surface. It increases rapidly, may occupy the whole of the front of the auricle, and grow larger than a pigeon's egg. The orifice of the meatus is then completely closed. The swelling is painful, hot, and fluctuant. If incised, a cavity is found which is mostly filled with yellowish viscid fluid, more rarely with pus or blood. On examining it with the probe, it will be found that the perichondrium has been detached from the cartilage, the soft parts surrounding and covering it have become densely swollen, and even after the removal of the fluid show little tendency to return to their original state. This produces for a long time, or even permanently, thickening and disfigurement. Without incision the cystic formation may exist for months, and its reduction is very slow. In one case the author found the whole cartilage of the external ear affected by perichondritis. The cure took a long time, as repeated attacks occurred in various parts of the cartilage. He once observed perichondritis after a burn, in which case recovery took place after incision and drainage, leaving however atrophy of the auricle. Sometimes serous cysts develop in the auricle, unaccompanied by any symptoms. In a case recently observed by the author, the cyst almost filled the concha. After incision, and insertion of a lead drainage tube, a cure was effected in eight days without any deformity.

Treatment.—During the first stage of the inflammation the treatment of perichondritis is antiphlogistic. Such cases are generally only observed when fluid has accumulated. The soft tissues must be freely incised, and drainage of the fluid which continues to form must be provided for by the insertion of tubes or tents of cotton wadding. If the exit of the fluid be obstructed, it will again accumulate, and a second incision will be necessary. When granulations form, they must be removed with a sharp scoop.

BLOOD-TUMOUR OF THE EAR.

(SYNONYM: *Othæmatoma.*)

Hæmatoma has given rise to much discussion in connection with the pathology of the auricle, its determining causes especially having been the subject of frequent controversy. Having been frequently observed in persons suffering from mental disorders, it was assumed that hæmatoma was connected with pathological processes in the cranial cavity, especially with *pachymeningitis hæmorrhagica*. Gudden and others, however, are of opinion that it is chiefly produced by injury. The extravasation of blood only occurs in such cases from a predisposition arising from degeneration of the cartilaginous tissue, a fact which was especially demonstrated by L. Meyer. In many cases the actual cause cannot be traced. The extravasation of blood takes place between the perichondrium and the cartilage, or between the layers of cartilage, almost exclusively on the anterior surface of the auricle. The skin exhibits a bluish discoloration, and bulges more or less according to the quantity of the effusion, and is rarely inflamed. As a rule, it is accompanied by pain and a feeling of tension and burning. According to the length of time that the effusion has existed, it consists either of fresh blood, of sanguineo-serous fluid, or of coagulated fibrin, which may be converted either into connective tissue or fibro-cartilage. In cases of extensive effusion, with subsequent new growth of tissue and contraction, the auricle assumes an unsightly appearance. Very rarely does the exudation become purulent.

Othæmatoma is distinguished from perichondritis auriculæ by the absence of inflammation and by the contents of the tumour.

Treatment.—The treatment consists in drawing off the extravasated blood. In cases in which the contents were fresh blood the author obtained a rapid cure by withdrawing it by means of Pravaz's syringe, and by subsequently compressing the swelling. In other cases the tumour refilled. When the exudation has existed for some time, it is necessary to incise the tumour in order to remove the coagulated blood.

Meyer[1] of Copenhagen in two such cases promoted absorption

[1] *Archiv für Ohrenheilkunde*, vol. xvi. p. 161.

in a short time by massage,—kneading and rubbing the tumour for a quarter of an hour several times a day.

OTHER DISEASES OF THE AURICLE.

Besides the diseases described, the auricle may be affected by the most varied pathological processes such as also appear in other parts of the body. Not infrequently the external ear is affected by *erysipelas*, which appears and runs its course as in other situations. Various *neoplasms* form on the auricle, namely, encysted tumours, fibrous tumours, especially on the lobule, cavernous tumours, aneurismal dilatation of the arteries, and malignant growths.

In gouty patients deposits of salts of uric acid (*tophi*) are frequently found in the auricle, appearing as yellowish-white spots on the anterior surface of its upper portion.

Frost-bite in varying degree not unfrequently affects the auricle, and may be either confined to the external margin or extend throughout the whole of it. Only a bluish-red discoloration may appear, caused by temporary or permanent dilatation of the capillaries. Sometimes a more or less extensive *gangrene* sets in. The author observed a circumscribed gangrene in a cachectic patient at the external margin of each auricle, without being able to trace it to the action of cold. The gangrene was of the same extent on both sides, and was quite symmetrical in form.

Wounds of the auricle unite readily on suturing the edges together. Several cases have been observed in which parts that had been severed from the auricle reunited.

CHAPTER VI.

DISEASES OF THE EXTERNAL MEATUS.

ANATOMICAL.

THE external meatus, closed at its inner end by the membrana tympani, consists of a tube 24 mm. long. It is divided into two portions—the cartilaginous, forming one-third, and the osseous, two-thirds of its length, meeting at an angle open forward and downward. It is therefore necessary in making an examination to straighten the meatus by drawing backward and upward the cartilaginous portion, which is composed of a tubular channel, incomplete posteriorly and superiorly. This gap is occupied by fibrous tissue, by which it is firmly adherent to the squamous portion of the temporal bone. Situated also in the cartilaginous portion are two transverse fissures of fibrous tissue, the *incisuræ Santorini*, which tend to make the canal more mobile. The inferior wall of the osseous meatus has a convex curvature upward (Fig 27). Near the membrana tympani it forms a depression, which frequently is the receptacle of foreign bodies. The lumen of the meatus is subject to great variation. On the average it is 8 mm. high and 5 mm. wide in the cartilaginous portion, and 10 mm. high and 6 mm. wide in the osseous portion (Luschka). The cutis covering the cartilaginous portion contains numerous convoluted glands, the *glandulæ ceruminales*. In this part it is 1½ mm. thick, and only 0·1 mm. in the osseous part. In this latter situation the cutis is inseparably connected with the periosteum. The superior wall of the meatus is separated from the middle cranial fossa by a plate of bone, varying in thickness, and containing cellular spaces. Between the posterior wall of the meatus and the mastoid antrum is compact bone 3—4 mm. thick.

In the newly-born child the osseous meatus is absent, and only develops during the first years of childhood from the *annulus tympanicus*.

The blood-supply of the external meatus is chiefly furnished by the *ramus auricularis profundus* of the *maxillaris interna ;* to a lesser degree, by branches of the *auricularis posterior* and the *arteria temporalis superficialis*.

The nerves of the meatus consist of the *ramus meat. audit. externi* of the *trigeminus*, and a small branch of the *vagus*. By irritation of that portion of the skin which is supplied by the latter, coughing and vomiting may be caused.

ANOMALIES OF SECRETION.

The numerous ceruminal glands of convoluted structure in the external meatus—which, according to Kölliker, are to be considered as sweat-glands, exhibit even in their normal condition great variation with regard to their secretion. In some individuals the surface of the epidermis is very dry and free from cerumen; in others its frequent removal is necessary in order to prevent accumulation. The quantity of the secretion corresponds with the activity of the glands of the skin of the rest of the body. While in former times it was held that the secretion of cerumen exerted great influence on the diseases of the ear, and although as recently as within the first half of this century Buchanan considered his instructions for the removal of accumulations of cerumen to be an advance in aural treatment such as had not been made for centuries, yet, according to our present views, it cannot be assumed that any material relationship exists between the two.

(a) *Diminished Secretion of Cerumen.*

The dryness of the walls of the external meatus, caused by insufficient secretion of cerumen, produces an unpleasant feeling of tension and itching, which induces scratching. Sometimes this is accompanied by a pityriasis-like desquamation of the epidermis. This abnormal dryness is frequently met with after inflammation of the external meatus, as well as simultaneously with chronic diseases and sclerosis of the middle ear.

Treatment.—The treatment is chiefly that of the symptoms. By moistening the surface of the external meatus, or applying to it substances which do not evaporate, we are able to abolish the unpleasant sensations. Painting the meatus with glycerine or vaseline is most effective. Patients who have been treated with the constant electric current frequently assert that it has been the means of restoring the natural moist condition.

(b) *Increased Secretion of Cerumen.*

(SYNONYM: *Thrombus sebaceus.*)

While normally the wall of the meatus is only coated with a thin layer of cerumen, a greater accumulation may take place by increased activity of the glands and insufficient removal of the secretion. From the ceruminal glands new secretion is being continually poured out upon the walls of the auditory canal; the older layers of cerumen are thereby approximated, and so the lumen of the meatus becomes more and more narrowed, till at last it is completely filled up by a so-called ceruminal plug or *thrombus sebaceus*. The character of this plug differs according to the composition of the secretion. If mainly composed of fatty matter, it is very soft, while it is much harder when its ingredients are chiefly solid. In the latter case the surface of the thrombus will be found to be opaque, yellowish green, and uneven, while in the former it is lustrous, smooth, and of a dark or black colour. The size of such a ceruminal plug may be such that it either occupies only a portion of the meatus or may fill it completely. If it extend to the membrana tympani, the inner end of the plug after removal may bear an exact impression of the membrane. The growth of the plug is, as a rule, very slow. Years may elapse before the accumulated secretion comes under notice, while, on the other hand, a thrombus may form again in half a year or a year after removal. The narrower the meatus, the more readily does obstruction occur. If such a plug remain in the ear for a long time, atrophy of the soft or osseous walls of the meatus may take place. The thrombus, by lying upon the membrana tympani, may produce atrophy or inflammation, and even a dangerous inflammation of the middle ear may be caused thereby.

The ceruminal plug is most frequently found in people of middle age, and rarely in children. Sometimes it is accompanied by other ear diseases, and it is principally met with after inflammation. Toynbee found that only in 36 per cent. of his patients was the hearing quite normal after the removal of the thrombus. In Wendt's experience, on the other hand, 68 per cent., and in Schwartze's 81 per cent., of the cases were completely cured. This affection occurs in all classes of the population, both in those well situated in life, observing careful cleanliness, as well as in the poorer classes who live amongst dust and dirt.

The symptoms which are chiefly observed when the meatus has been occluded are a feeling of fulness, dulness of hearing, tinnitus, pain, and giddiness. If the closure be only confined to the outer portion, the former two symptoms predominate; if, however, the thrombus press upon the membrana tympani, great tinnitus, giddiness, pain in the ear and in the head will be added. In many cases vomiting and a feeling of faintness also occur—symptoms which may be mistaken for Menière's disease or a cerebral affection. The symptoms sometimes appear slowly, and may begin with tinnitus, accompanied by dulness of hearing. Sometimes they appear at once, a sudden shaking or manipulation of the ear causing the plug to change its position and enter the deepest part of the meatus. Frequently the sudden occurrence of these symptoms results from the entrance of fluid into the meatus, especially while bathing or washing, causing the mass to swell and close the meatus.

Treatment.—Our treatment is confined to the removal of the thrombus, which in cases of soft plugs can be done simply with the syringe and tepid water. If the accumulation be more solid, a number of injections may require to be made, which as a rule will be successful. The better the current of water is made to circulate along the walls of the meatus, after the manner described at p. 18, the more rapidly and safely the removal will be achieved. If the syringe be unsuccessful, the probe and forceps may be used; but care must be taken not to push the plug inward and thereby aggravate the symptoms. The abandonment of instruments in such cases the author considers unjustifiable, and always resorts to the probe if the thrombus cannot be removed by repeated syringing.

When the plug firmly adheres to the walls of the meatus, the fluid cannot be made to circulate. In such a case its detachment by means of the probe will sometimes be sufficient to give more effect to the syringe. The surface of the thrombus being rough and uneven, or if successfully detached from the walls of the meatus, the whole plug can be removed at once by the forceps, or by the other instruments (see p. 102) employed for the removal of foreign bodies. It is scarcely necessary to mention that instruments should only be used when the meatus is illuminated, and that nothing should be done at random.

If the removal of the thrombus be attended with difficulty, or if giddiness and symptoms of fainting should occur during the syringing, further treatment should be postponed, and the thrombus first softened. For this purpose we generally employ repeated instillations of tepid water, to which soda may be added, or of soap and water. After softening, the accumulation can easily be removed by syringing. Last century extensive experiments were made with regard to the varying solubility of cerumen. Haygarth, for instance, after experimenting with water, lime-water, brandy, oil, and other fluids, found that it dissolved most readily in tepid water. Wedel arrived at the same conclusion in his *Dissertatio de Cerumine*, 1705.

After the thrombus has been removed, care must be taken to protect the meatus and the membrana tympani against external influences by means of cotton-wool. Frequently dulness of hearing remains after the removal of the obstructing plug, caused either by inflammatory processes in the tympanic cavity, or by an inward curvature of the membrana tympani in consequence of the pressure exerted upon it. In the latter case the dulness of hearing is removed when the membrane is restored to its proper position by propelling air into the tympanum.

INFLAMMATION OF THE EXTERNAL MEATUS. OTITIS EXTERNA.

(a) *Circumscribed Inflammation.*

(SYNONYMS : *Furunculosis ; Otitis externa circumscripta.*)

Furunculosis of the external meatus is a very painful and torturing affection. Like furunculosis appearing in other parts of the skin, a reddened elevation, painful from the beginning, and especially when touched, may arise at any part of the surface of the external meatus. It either subsides at this stage, or a purulent degeneration of the inflamed tissues takes place; a yellow point forms on the swelling, from which, for three to six days, pus is discharged, and finally a core of diseased tissue, after which healing sets in. It may be assumed that the inflammation has its origin in one of the glands, which are so numerous in the cutis of the external meatus, and that by reactive inflammation of the surrounding tissues suppuration of the gland is produced.

The extent of the swelling and inflammation varies very much. It may be very slight, or so great that the lumen of the external meatus becomes closed. The whole meatus takes part in the inflammation, and not unfrequently an inflammatory swelling of the tragus, as well as of the cutis and of the glands in the neighbourhood of the ear, occurs. Furuncles form mostly in the cartilaginous portion of the meatus. In most cases not only one furuncle appears, but several, either simultaneously or one after the other, so that the process which subsides in a few days without this multiple formation, may extend over several weeks. The cause of the inflammation cannot generally be ascertained. Löwenberg maintains, along with Pasteur, that he has invariably found a copious formation of *micrococci* in the pus of the furuncle in the ear, as in furunculosis of other parts; and he draws from his experiments the conclusion that each furuncle is caused by an invasion of a special kind of microbe, which penetrates from the atmosphere, under certain conditions which are as yet unknown, into a gland-follicle, grows exuberantly there, and produces inflammation. The relapses are supposed to be caused by extension of the pus containing the *micrococci* to the neighbourhood of the furuncle, whence a further invasion into the gland-follicles takes place. This view of Löwenberg's is confirmed by later investigations regarding the formation of furuncles, according to which furunculosis may be produced by rubbing the sound skin with *staphylococci*. Kirchner recognised in furunculosis of the ear the *staphylococcus pyogenes albus*. Besides furunculosis proper, dependent on the formation of *staphylococci*, a circumscribed inflammation of the external meatus may also be caused by mechanical irritation, by foreign bodies, or by manipulations in the ear. Not unfrequently it is caused during the treatment of other ear diseases by applications which act as irritants upon the cutis.

Furunculosis seldom occurs in children; among adults it attacks anæmic and delicate persons, especially females, more frequently than strong well-nourished individuals. Many patients are peculiarly predisposed to this disease, and at varying intervals they are affected by it. The pain is usually very great, causes sleeplessness, and has a very depressing influence upon the patient. It is especially severe in the evening and during the night. In the morning it generally decreases, or it may cease altogether, only to set in again in the evening with its former severity. The pain radiates into the surrounding parts, extending entirely over the same side of the head as the ear affected, and frequently toothache is simultaneously complained of. It is increased particularly by movement of the lower jaw, and in such cases eating of solid food must be dispensed with. The accompanying fever produces constitutional disturbance. The dulness of hearing is very marked when the external meatus is closed by the swelling, or by accumulation of exudation products in the deeper parts of the meatus. After the inflammation has subsided granulations frequently appear at the spot where the furuncle had its seat. They either disappear or develop into polypi, which must be removed in the usual manner.

(b) *Diffuse Inflammation.*

(SYNONYM: *Otitis externa diffusa.*)

Diffuse inflammation of the external meatus cannot be discussed separately from the circumscribed, as the former is very frequently connected with the latter, and as the diffuse inflammation is also frequently followed by the formation of abscess. In most cases acute otitis externa diffusa forms one of the symptoms of an acute inflammation of the middle ear, as will be shown when we come to the investigation of its diseases. If it occur independently its cause is generally local irritation of a chemical, heat-producing, or mechanical nature, such as the entrance of cold water, the instillation of eau-de-Cologne or alcohol, and unskilful attempts at extraction of foreign bodies. These cases are frequently complicated by congestion and inflammation in the middle ear.

This disease is generally only unilateral, and is observed oftener in children than in adults.

As the soft covering of the external meatus is in immediate connection with the periosteum, the latter is always more or less affected; and this explains why the inflammation is so very painful. The bone itself often becomes diseased, resulting in exfoliation of a sequestrum, or caries. Some cases have been under observation in which the disease extended into the middle cranial fossa, or through the cells of the mastoid process into the lateral sinus, thereby proving fatal. On the other hand, an accumulation of pus in the mastoid process may make its way into the external meatus, and simulate otitis externa. Suppuration of the neighbouring parotid gland may make its appearance in the external meatus, passing as a rule between the cartilaginous and the osseous portions of the meatus. By collateral hyperæmia symptoms of cerebral irritation may develop.

Diffuse inflammation of the external ear begins with a feeling of tension and itching in the ear, accompanied by heat, pulsation, and subjective noises. Pain, which is rarely present from the first, sets in soon after, with fever and constitutional disturbance. The pain rapidly becomes more severe and unbearable, radiating from the ear all over the same side of the head, and is increased especially by movements of the jaw, so that patients are sometimes scarcely able to open the mouth. Generally in the course of a few days after the disease has passed its worst stage, all the symptoms subside and a complete recovery quickly takes place.

At first the cutaneous covering of the meatus is greatly hypertrophied, and of a livid-red appearance. The swelling may become so great that the walls touch each other. The more the meatus is contracted and obstructed by the products of secretion, the greater is the dulness of hearing, which may also be the result of a simultaneous affection of the middle ear. The membrana tympani, which is only visible at the beginning, appears greatly congested, swollen, and excoriated. During the first few days a serous exudation takes place. This fluid is frequently at first of a yellowish-green colour, due to the secretion of the ceruminal glands, but sometimes contains an admixture of blood; afterwards the discharge becomes viscid and muco-purulent. In milder cases a cure takes place rapidly after a short serous exudation, while in others muco-pus forms, with a continuance of the inflammatory symptoms.

In severe cases swelling of the region in front of the ear occurs, or the mastoid becomes inflamed, so that it is painful on pressure. In children we find considerable swelling of the glands behind the ramus of the jaw. In many cases, and especially in those accompanied by most violent pain, granulations form in consequence of superficial necrosis of the bone (Wolf). As a rule, these granulations disappear in the course of the healing process, as in furunculosis, or they develop into polypi, and afterwards require to be removed. It frequently happens that during the course of the inflammation, perforation of the membrana tympani occurs, and then the mucous membrane of the tympanic cavity is also implicated. Shedding of the epidermis of the meatus often happens in the first stage of the disease, thin white patches of it being formed, which are either thrown out with the discharge or remain attached by their lower surface. The latter occurs chiefly in the advanced stages of the disease, when the acute symptoms and the exudation have decreased. When the inflammation subsides the secretion also becomes less, and disappears altogether in a short time. In other cases the process develops into chronic inflammation. A muco-purulent discharge persists, which may either be derived from the cutis remaining inflamed, or from the middle ear in the case of perforation of the membrana tympani.

Chronic inflammation of the external meatus may also occur without a previous acute attack. It sets in with or without swelling and secretion in the meatus, but these symptoms may continue for some time in a greater or less degree.

Diphtheritic inflammation of the external meatus is caused either by extension of pharyngeal diphtheria to the tympanic cavity and the meatus, or it is idiopathic, being confined to the external meatus only. Cases of the latter kind have been described by Wreden, Moos, Bezold, and Blau.

Treatment.—During the treatment of acute inflammation of the external meatus, circumscribed as well as diffuse, care must be taken, in the first instance, to protect the ear from all hurtful influences. Everything that might cause congestion of the head or of the diseased organ must be avoided, such as bodily exertion, stimulating food or liquids, especially alcohol, changes of temperature, and mechanical irritation, such as indelicate examination and syringing of the meatus, neither of which should be done in the first stage of the disease. In order to reduce congestion, purgatives and local blood-letting may be resorted to. Patients will feel as a rule very much relieved by the application of 4—6 leeches in front of the tragus.

The application of heat and cold plays an important part in the treatment. Hippocrates endeavoured to remove inflammation by fomenting the parts with sponges compressed after being dipped in hot water. According to Von Tröltsch, nothing alleviates the pain so much as ear-baths, *i.e.* frequently repeated instillation of tepid water into the external meatus. Poultices, which were formerly employed almost without exception, are now contraindicated, because their continued application induces an increased supply of blood to the entire ear. Patients who have for some time been poulticed are frequently grateful to the surgeon when he abandons them and applies cold instead. During the first days of the inflammation, the author is in the habit of using ear-baths of hot salt-water or oil, or of placing for a short time upon the orifice of the external meatus small sponges dipped in hot water, as warm as can be borne. When the inflammation is very violent, cold compresses or bags of ice may be placed upon the region of the ear from the beginning. The author confines the action of cold to the maxillary and retro-maxillary region as well as the side of the neck. For the removal of the pain, ear-baths and hot sponges may be employed simultaneously. By a combined application of cold and heat the author in many cases has observed that the symptoms rapidly abated. By cold the total supply of blood to the parts is lessened, and by warmth the severity of local symptoms is reduced. During the time when no fomentations are applied, especially before bed-time, the author advises the embrocation of the region of the ear with blue mercurial ointment, generally mixed with an equal quantity of vaseline. In order to reduce the tension and swelling of the skin, and thereby allay the pain, weak ointments or olive oil with carbolic acid (1—2 per cent.) may be used. The well-known popular remedy of inserting a small piece of bacon into the meatus is of good service.

Especially in the case of furunculosis, thorough disinfection must be aimed at, which can be effected by early incision and cleansing with a solution of corrosive sublimate of the strength of one in a thousand. Absolute alcohol, first recommended by Weber-Liel, proves in many cases to be very useful. Whether suppuration exist or not, the meatus is kept filled with the alcohol for five minutes, then dried, and a compress laid upon it. The application of this remedy may be repeated every hour or half-hour. In diffuse inflammation it may be of advantage to insert a firm tent of cotton wadding into the meatus in order to exert gentle pressure on its walls.

There is a diversity of opinion as to whether and when the furuncle should be incised. Kramer especially held the view that an artificial opening was never necessary, while Von Tröltsch recommends an early incision. Others, again, only incise after suppuration has set in. When certain parts of the meatus are markedly bulging, and are more painful when touched with the probe than the surrounding parts, an incision should be made. An early incision is painful, but if extensive enough, it will lessen the suffering, but will not remove it altogether. If, on the other hand, the incision be made after suppuration has already set in, the pain will at once completely cease. But the whole contents of the furuncle must be evacuated after the incision, which is effected by pressure upon it laterally with the probe.

For the incision the author employs, instead of the ordinary bistoury, a small furuncle-knife, with a straight back and a two-edged sharp point (Fig. 23). The knife is inserted through the base of the bulging point, the edge of the blade being directed towards the centre of the lumen of the meatus. In this way a cut is made through the whole swelling from base to surface. Thus a thorough opening of the furuncle is effected safely and quickly and with little pain. Löwenberg, in conformity with his views regarding bacteria, recommends an early incision, with subsequent antiseptic treatment.

After the acute symptoms have passed away, the removal of the exudation which remains, and of the detached epidermis, must be attended to. The regular removal of the former, especially by the dry method, with tents of cotton-wool, should bring about its cessation. The meatus must also be dried after syringing. When granulations are present, showing no tendency to disappear spontaneously, they must be removed by means of the snare.

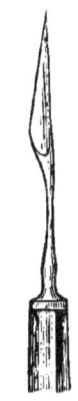

FIG. 23.

If the discharge continue long, as it always does in cases of chronic otitis externa, the employment of boracic acid, which was introduced into aural surgery by Bezold, is most efficient. It is used in the same way as in chronic suppuration of the middle ear, which will be described afterwards. Sometimes a discharge from the external meatus which has lasted a month, or even a year, will be successfully stopped by a single application. In most cases, however, it must be frequently repeated.

Granular swellings, which are often the cause of chronic otitis externa, disappear on touching them with nitrate of silver or with chromic acid.

DESQUAMATIVE INFLAMMATION OF THE EXTERNAL MEATUS.

(SYNONYM: *Otitis externa desquamativa.*)

In 1874 Wreden[1] first described twelve cases of obstruction of the external meatus which differs in many ways from that caused by ceruminal accumulation. In a purely practical respect, the difference between the two accumulations consists in the fact that the ceruminal plugs can be easily removed by syringing, perhaps preceded by instillation of a soda-solution, while the obstructing masses described by Wreden firmly adhere to the walls of the meatus, and can only very slowly and with difficulty be softened

[1] *Arch. für Augen- und Ohrenheilkunde*, vol. iii. 2, p. 91.

and removed. They consist of a whitish, somewhat solid substance, composed of a large number of layers of epidermis arranged concentrically, which, on microscopic examination, prove to be constructed of epidermic cells. The pathological process, which Wreden calls *Keratosis obturans*, is therefore to be considered as a copious desquamation of the epidermic layers of the external meatus. It appears that the disease may arise spontaneously or in consequence of inflammatory processes. As a rule, the more internal parts of the external meatus, with the membrana tympani, are affected by this disease, in many cases almost exclusively the latter, when it is called *Myringitis desquamativa*. The symptoms which are caused by the epidermic plug are the same as those produced by the ceruminal accumulation, namely, dulness of hearing and tinnitus. As these accumulations occur at the bottom of the meatus, and lie upon the membrana tympani, the symptoms set in even when they are small in bulk. Wreden only observed the unilateral formation of these epidermic plugs. The author has seen one case in which they were present in both ears. In a boy, twelve years of age, the obstruction of both ears recurred annually for five years, and had repeatedly led to perforation of the membrana tympani and acute inflammation of the middle ear. That this disease may also appear in an acute form is evident from a case communicated by Gottstein,[1] which he called *myringitis desquamativa acuta*, and which may be classed under this head. Accompanied by severe pain and fever, greyish-white membranes formed at the deepest part of both meatuses, which on removal exhibited a perfect impression of the membrana tympani. On microscopic examination the epidermal character of the membranes was proved.

Treatment.—According to Wreden, the treatment consists in the preliminary use of softening alkaline lotions, followed by the removal of the softened epidermic masses by injections of water. He then advises the application of solutions of corrosive sublimate or iodide of potassium, in order to restore the covering of the external meatus to its normal condition. As already remarked, the removal presents great difficulties, as the membranous formations firmly adhere to the walls of the meatus and to the membrana

---

[1] Paper read at the second International Congress in Milan.

tympani. Large pieces cannot be removed with the forceps, as the loose fragments that are seized are easily torn. Sometimes they can be removed by loosening the plug by means of the probe or small spatula from the walls of the meatus, along with repeated syringing. The author has obtained but little success with alkaline lotions, such as soda-solution and lime-water, but instillations of a 2 per cent. solution of salicylic acid in oil proved most useful, followed by syringing with alkaline solutions, if the former alone did not prove effectual. After the removal of the masses, the cure is completed by instillation of a corrosive sublimate solution (0·1 : 30—50 water). In a case which was complicated by granulations in the outer part of the meatus, the author was obliged to remove the masses with a small sharp spoon after administering chloroform.

FUNGUS IN THE EXTERNAL MEATUS.

(SYNONYM: *Otomycosis aspergillina.*)

Mayer,[1] in the year 1844, described cases of fungus-growth in the external meatus, but Wreden[2] first gave a complete description of the disease and its symptoms, based upon a large number of cases which he had observed. More recently the significance of fungus-growth in the ear was made clear by the experimental work of Siebenmann.[3]

The fungi found in the ear are mould fungi, *Aspergillus niger, flavus et fumigatus.* Viewed macroscopically, they are found to consist of a felt-like structure, composed of fine filaments, varying in colour according to the species of aspergillus. Under the microscope we see the thallus, consisting of thin filaments (mycelia) with septa (hyphæ), from which extend the fruit filaments, either perpendicularly or at an acute angle. These terminate in a rounded bladder-shaped capsule, the fruit-head or sporangium. On its surface it is covered with radially arranged globular cells, the fungus-spores or conidia. Although these spores are almost always present in the atmosphere of our dwellings, the normal walls of the

[1] Müller's *Arch. f. Physiol.* 1844, No. 12.
[2] *Arch. f. Ohrenheilkunde*, vol. iii. p. 1, and *Arch. f. Augen- und Ohrenheilkunde*, vol. iii. 2, p. 56.
[3] *Die Fadenpilze*, etc. Wiesbaden, 1883.

external meatus offer no favourable soil for their development. When cerumen, or even pus, is present, the formation of fungi does not take place. According to Siebenmann, serum is most favourable for the development of fungi; we therefore find otomycosis only in eczema of the external meatus, or when purulent otorrhœa has become serous in its character, with scanty secretion. Attempts to inoculate healthy ears with fungous material have failed.

Otomycosis chiefly affects the membrana tympani and the innermost portion of the external meatus. It may, however, extend over the whole meatus, and lead to obstruction, in cases of prolific growth. The fungous membranes lie upon the surface of the Malpighian layer or of the corium, more rarely upon the epidermis. The mycelia do not penetrate into the tissue, but single filaments may be found surrounded by the cells of the Malpighian layer. In the absence of exudation, only single whitish or blackish spots, or a complete layer, is found lying upon the membrana tympani, or upon the walls of the meatus. When exudation is present the fungous membranes in the meatus are black-spotted, resembling wet newspaper.

In many cases the fungous formation gives rise to no symptoms. In most cases, however, the patient complains of itching in the ear, a slight degree of dulness of hearing, and tinnitus, resulting from obstruction in the meatus. Sometimes pain and a slight serous exudation are the first symptoms of the affection, being due to the dermatitis with which it is accompanied. Perforation of the membrana tympani and inflammation of the middle ear are rarely produced by otomycosis.

Instillations of glycerine and of solutions of zinc, alum, and tannin, as well as of oil, favour the development of otomycosis, as also mechanical injuries to the walls of the meatus producing dermatitis.

Treatment.—The treatment consists in the removal and destruction of the fungus. The eczema or otorrhœa originally favouring its development must also be treated. It is rarely possible by means of the syringe to remove the fungous membranes, so firmly are they attached. They must first be loosened, which can be done by using the probe. If this cannot be easily accomplished, agents for destroying the fungus are employed. Antiseptic remedies, dry or in solution, are somewhat ineffective. The instillation of pure alcohol is most certain in its effect; and, as proposed by Bezold and Burckhardt-Merian, 2—4 per cent. of salicylic acid may be added. Alcohol not only effects the destruction of the fungi, but it also reduces the exudation. The removal of the fungous masses alone is not sufficient, as they form anew after a few days. According to experiments made by Walb, boracic acid has no influence upon fungous formations.

HERPES AURICULARIS.

This is especially a disease of the external ear, and occurs either in the auricle or in the outer portion of the meatus. It sets in with a feeling of great tension and itching, soon followed by intense pain, such as already described under acute diseases of the external meatus. On examination, the wall of the meatus is found to be markedly reddened and swollen. On its surface appear little vesicles containing serous fluid, which, after a few days, on the decline of the symptoms, dry up, and form brownish crusts. Sometimes an exudation of a mucous fluid also occurs. This disease is met with either idiopathically or accompanied by acute inflammation of the external meatus and of the tympanic cavity. Adults mostly suffer from it. Ladreit de Lacharière's opinion, that it is always a result of gastric disturbance, has not proved correct. As a rule, it is of very brief duration, a cure usually taking place after a few days.

Treatment.—The treatment is confined to soothing the pain by the application of ointments, which lessen the tension in the first stage of the disease, *e.g.* the extract of belladonna with vaseline in the proportion of 1 to 10. Of narcotics, hydrate of chloral proves most effective.

SYPHILIS OF THE EXTERNAL MEATUS.

Sometimes general syphilitic disease manifests itself in the external meatus by the development of *condylomata*, which make their appearance as secondary symptoms. Broad red papules form, which at first have a dry and afterwards a moist surface. They become gradually larger, and when they form on all the walls of the meatus they may produce complete closure. On examination a very characteristic condition is found. The lumen is filled up with ulcerated, slightly bleeding swellings, and there is generally a considerable amount of sero-purulent discharge.

The disease is either confined to the external portion of the meatus or extends downward, invading and perforating the membrana tympani. The hearing is affected according to the degree of swelling. No pain is usually felt, except when fissures form. A cure may take place spontaneously, but by treatment healing can be effected in a shorter time.

Treatment.—During the first stages of the disease the treatment is the same as that applied to condylomata on other parts of the integument, namely, application of precipitate ointment, painting with a solution of corrosive sublimate, and powdering with calomel. The author has observed very rapid cures occurring in cases of deeply ulcerated patches by thorough cauterisation without any simultaneous general treatment. Healing is promoted by carefully cleansing the meatus with disinfecting fluids. When the local treatment is not effectual, and constitutional symptoms appear, treatment by inunction should be resorted to.

FOREIGN BODIES IN THE EXTERNAL MEATUS.

The greatest variety of foreign bodies may get into the ear. Sometimes they are hard, such as small stones, cherry-stones, glass beads, etc., sometimes soft, as pellets of cotton-wool, corn-seeds, and other vegetable substances. Many of them, such as corn-seeds, swell, and thereby occupy more space. Further, especially during sleep, insects enter the ear, such as flies, bugs, fleas, and the so-called ear-wig (*Forficula auricularis*). In the ears of patients with a discharge of matter, worm-like larvæ develop from the eggs of flies (*Musca domestica et sarcophaga*). Generally these larvæ appear in large numbers, show great activity, and, when the membrana tympani is perforated, easily creep into crevices in the tympanic cavity.

Foreign bodies usually get into the ear by accident; but sometimes they are intentionally introduced for therapeutic purposes, *e.g.* onions and other substances as remedies in toothache, pieces of bacon in inflammation, and plugs of cotton for protection.

Most frequently foreign bodies are found in the ears of children, who have a peculiar inclination to insert small articles into their various orifices.

Foreign bodies remain in the outer portion of the meatus, or they are pushed further inward, and, especially when small, are lodged in the depression formed by the lower wall of the meatus immediately in front of the membrana tympani, so that they are partially hidden from view on examination. In other cases the membrana tympani may be injured either by driving the object inward or by manipulation in the ear, and the foreign body may even get out of the meatus into the tympanic cavity. It is well known that foreign bodies may long remain in the external meatus without causing the slightest inflammation. A carious molar tooth remained in the meatus for forty years (Rein). Politzer removed a piece of lead (pencil) an inch long and several lines thick, which had lain in the meatus for twenty-two years, without causing the slightest trouble. Brown found both meatuses of an imbecile boy filled with a large number of stones, which had been there for seven years without causing inflammation.

The symptoms of the presence of foreign bodies are the same as those of the thrombus sebaceus. A feeling of obstruction and dulness of hearing are complained of when the whole meatus is filled, or the foreign body lies in its outer portion. Tinnitus, giddiness, pain, and sometimes vomiting, are observed when the foreign body is in contact with the membrana tympani. Most intolerable noises are occasioned by insects reaching the innermost part of the meatus, and producing movements of the membrana tympani. The symptoms accompanying the presence of the larvæ of flies are, on the other hand, of little account.

Foreign bodies are a source of great danger when unpractised hands attempt their extraction by means of instruments, especially when the manipulations are conducted without illuminating the ear, and the forceps are introduced at random. The meatus is injured thereby, the foreign body being pushed inward, and, after rupturing the membrana tympani, enters the tympanic cavity. By lesion of the surrounding parts, or by consequent inflammation, death may result. One fatal case is communicated by Wendt. A carob- or locust-seed, by rough attempts at extraction, was driven into the innermost part of the meatus, and after a consequent violent inflammation was removed under chloroform; but with symptoms of meningitis the case proved fatal. Sabatier reports a case resulting in death, which was caused by the unskilful attempts at extraction of a pellet of cotton-wool. Levi quotes the case of a soldier, who, in order to obtain exemption from military service, had put a pebble into his ear. After extraction, a large perforation was found in the membrana tympani, followed next day by facial paralysis, otitis media, and death from meningitis. E. Fränkel describes an analogous case, in which also a pebble, by attempts at extraction, had been pushed into the tympanic cavity, destroying the ossicula, and even causing a lesion in the wall of the labyrinth. Death was caused by purulent meningitis of the convexity of the brain. Moos tells of a man into whose ear a splinter of stone had entered. Without illumination, several of his companions made attempts at extracting it with pincers, which led to hæmorrhage and to twitching of the same side of the face, followed by repeated copious bleeding, rigors, delirium, and death. Post-mortem examination revealed destruction of the floor of the tympanic cavity and of the ossicula, opening of the jugular vein, and of the canal of the facial nerve, metastatic deposits being found in the lungs and muscles. Pilcher relates a case in which the surgeons of a London hospital looked in vain for a nail supposed to have entered the ear. They extracted the 'hammer,' and the patient died in two days. At the post-mortem examination no foreign body at all was found.

The nervous symptoms, which, however, are only seldom occasioned by the presence of foreign bodies, are very interesting. They consist of coughing, obstinate vomiting, hemicrania, dysphagia, paralysis, atrophy, epilepsy, and general marasmus. Frank remarks in his Manual that after the prolonged presence of a foreign body even the opposite and healthy ear is sympathetically affected with dulness of hearing.

Treatment.—When the presence of a foreign body has been ascertained, and is found to consist of a solid object, especially a glass bead, or a small round stone, it can be made to roll out of the ear by simply inclining the head to the corresponding side, and then suddenly shaking the head by a moderately strong blow. In all other cases the sovereign remedy is the syringe and tepid water. But although Kramer states that it has been proved by experience that any foreign body can be removed from any part of the ear by means of the syringe, yet that cannot be held as absolutely correct. There are many cases in which foreign bodies, either from swelling or from irregularity of surface, get squeezed in between the walls of the meatus, and cannot be moved out of their position by a stream of water. In such cases we must use instruments for the purpose of extraction.

During syringing, as well as the employment of instruments, the oval shape of the external meatus must be taken into consideration. In the case of round foreign bodies, a free space exists above and below, through which the stream of water or the instruments may be passed. Syringing is most effectual when the current is directed along a wall of the meatus. When it has been ascertained by examination where the lumen of the meatus is open, the stream must be directed toward that side. The injected fluid then passes behind the foreign body, and forces it from the inside outward. Its expulsion is favoured by inclining the head towards the corresponding side during syringing. It is sometimes possible to increase the effect of the water by moving the foreign body from the wall of the meatus by means of a small flat spatula.

Zaufal recommends syringing with oil in order to prevent vegetable substances swelling. According to him, swollen foreign bodies can be made to shrink by means of glycerine. When using the syringe, and especially when using instruments, great care must always be taken not to push the foreign body inward. If a high degree of inflammation have already set in, causing great swelling of the walls of the meatus, external to the foreign body, it is most advisable to delay its extraction until the inflammation has subsided.

The choice of an instrument for extraction depends upon the

shape, character, and situation of the foreign body. The following are in use:—1. The hook-shaped probe. The common thin silver probe is bent hook-like, and passed behind the foreign body, which is thus extracted. It is necessary, of course, in such a case that the lumen of the meatus be not entirely occupied. Any kind of foreign body can, under such circumstances, be removed in this manner. Instead of a silver probe, a hair-pin, as suggested by Deleau, may be used, bent in the same manner, and fixed into a piece of cork for a handle. Flat spatula-shaped instruments similarly bent may also be employed. The author has repeatedly used the small sharp scoop.

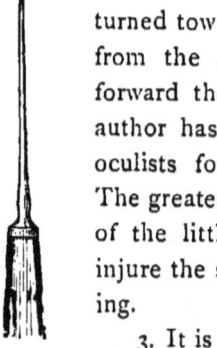

Fig. 24.

2. The small sharp hook (Fig. 24) is chiefly used for the removal of soft foreign bodies. This instrument is laid flat against the wall of the meatus and pushed in between it and the foreign body. The point is then turned towards the object, and is firmly pressed into it from the side. By moving it slowly backward and forward the foreign body can now be pulled out. The author has frequently used the Iris-hook employed by oculists for extracting foreign bodies from the eye. The greatest care must be observed in the introduction of the little hook, so that its sharp point does not injure the skin of the meatus and cause pain and bleeding.

3. It is very dangerous to use pincers or forceps, as they are liable to drive the foreign body inward. They should not be employed at all for extracting round hard objects with smooth surfaces. Only when the foreign body projects externally, and is sufficiently soft to be easily and safely seized with these instruments, is their employment advisable.

4. Boring instruments may be employed with advantage for the extraction of soft objects, especially corn-seeds. Those with sharp points and double spirals are the best. The instrument is inserted through a tube and long speculum, and then firmly screwed into the foreign body. These instruments must, however, only be employed when, by previous examination with the probe, it has been ascertained that the foreign body cannot be pushed further inward. In

many cases the sharp points of the drill penetrate so easily into the object, and hold it so firmly, that, even when tightly wedged in, it can be extracted with ease.

5. In the case of the foreign body being driven into the innermost part of the meatus, or into the tympanic cavity, it may be necessary, by reason of the development of symptoms threatening immediate danger, arising from purulent inflammation of the tympanic cavity and of the mastoid process, to remove it by the operation of detachment of the auricle; and, if required, by chiselling an opening in the posterior wall of the external meatus. According to Moldenhauer, the detachment of the auricle is effected by an incision down to the periosteum along the line of attachment of the auricle. The cartilaginous part of the meatus is then separated by means of the handle of the scalpel, and its inner end laid open. For loosening the foreign body, Moldenhauer[1] recommends small levers bent at an obtuse angle and grooved on their inner surface.

When the membrana tympani is destroyed, an attempt may be made to remove the foreign body by acting upon it from the Eustachian tube either by Politzerising or by injecting water. Deleau describes a case in which he removed a stone from the tympanic cavity in this manner.

The annoying sensations produced by the entrance of insects into the ear may at once be allayed by filling the meatus with fluid. Their removal can be effected by syringing, but in many cases they must be killed first. This is done by instillation of water, oil, or alcohol. In the case of the larvæ of flies, Politzer recommends the addition of a few drops of petroleum or turpentine to the oil. 'A few minutes after the instillation, the larvæ leave their hiding-places, and creep out of the external meatus.'

Among other methods may be mentioned the extraction of a foreign body by suction effected through a small tube, which was recommended by Alexander of Tralles. The agglutinative method is also to be noted. Hocker first described a case in which a stone was removed from the ear adhering to a plug of cotton-wool dipped in a solution of shellac. Löwenberg recently recommended glue.

[1] *Archiv für Ohrenheilkunde*, vol. xvi. p. 59.

The older aural surgeons suggested a red-hot wire for the destruction of a soft foreign body. Voltolini proposed the galvano-cautery for the same purpose. The author tried it in one case; but although the speculum was deeply inserted (under illumination), and the point of the cautery was placed immediately upon the foreign body, it caused such violent pain that he had at once to desist. Gruber, acting upon Voltolini's recommendation, had a similar experience; such violent inflammation set in that he had to refrain from making further attempts. Zaufal reports a case in which attempts at destruction of a foreign body by the galvano-cautery were followed by meningitis and a fatal termination.

CONTRACTION AND CLOSURE OF THE EXTERNAL MEATUS.

Contraction of the orifice of the meatus is sometimes met with in women, whose auricles, through oft-repeated pressure to the head by bonnet-bands, have assumed an abnormal position. As the inner portion of the auricle, the concha proper, has the form of a section of a globe, its anterior margin, *i.e.* the posterior boundary of the orifice of the meatus, is driven forward when pressure is exerted upon the outer margin of the auricle. When this pressure is repeated very frequently or continuously, the auricle remains in this position, and contraction or closure takes place. When the auricle is drawn outward, the meatus is opened.

Narrowing and displacement of the external meatus may also be caused by loosening of the posterior wall, which often occurs in patients who have frequently suffered from inflammation, and especially from furunculosis. The swelling which occurs in these affections, causing the soft covering to become raised and loosened from its attachment, may produce complete closure of the meatus. This condition can be recognised by the fact that when the meatus is examined, its relaxed walls can be easily pressed back with the speculum or with the probe, allowing a free view of the deeper parts.

Treatment.—In order to improve the defective hearing, small tubular instruments may be fitted into the meatus to keep the lumen open.

Narrowing and closure may also be produced by chronic inflammatory processes, especially eczematous conditions, which lead to thickening of the skin. Sometimes the orifice is completely closed. When the case is only one of great contraction, the orifice itself should be dilated with laminaria or with sponge tents. When the closure is complete, an operation should be performed by making a crucial incision and removing the flaps. In one case the author dilated the orifice by excising the whole margin with a blunt-pointed knife. The subsequent treatment requires the greatest care. It has been recommended, in order to prevent the margins re-uniting, to keep the meatus open by continued insertion of materials capable of expansion. The author has not found this mode of treatment successful, as the laminaria tents could not be tolerated. He has effected a cure with leaden tubes coated with ointment and worn in the ear for several weeks until cicatrisation had taken place. Any one can prepare these leaden tubes for himself by rounding with a knife one end of a small piece of tube, while the other end is dilated into the shape of a funnel by slitting it in halves and bending them asunder.

EXOSTOSIS forms in the osseous portion of the external meatus. It makes its appearance either without any traceable cause, probably through hereditary disposition, or as a consequence of inflammatory processes. In the former case its growth is very slow, and the osseous tumour formed is exceedingly hard (*ivory exostosis*). If exostoses form after inflammation, well-marked tumours may develop in a short time. There appears either only a single swelling, sessile or pedunculated, generally situated upon the superior-posterior wall of the meatus, or several osseous growths are formed which constrict the lumen. In very rare cases a uniform occlusion of the meatus is observed from concentric formation of new bone. The osseous growths which arise from inflammatory processes are not so hard as the ivory exostoses.

The symptoms of exostoses vary. While the smaller growths remain unnoticed, the larger cause dulness of hearing of a high degree. This may arise from exudation, or epidermis filling up the small existing chink in the canal. In such cases, the hearing can be temporarily restored by removal of the obstructing material.

In cases of suppuration, the life of the patient may be endangered by retention of pus.

Moos saw a case of neuralgia of the trigeminus caused by exostosis of the external meatus, which was cured by operation.

Treatment of Exostosis.—This is limited to removal of obstructing matter, so long as the contraction is not very great, and the dulness of hearing is only caused by temporary obstruction of the space which exists. When it is not possible to clear the passage by syringing or by loosening the obstructing material with the probe, the 'thin tympanic tube' (Paukenröhrchen) may be used with advantage. This is passed behind the place of constriction and a current of water injected through it. As a rule, the exostosis should be removed as early as possible, especially if still growing, as the operation is more easily performed the less the meatus is occluded. When these osseous growths are pedunculated and project markedly, they may be removed with one stroke of the chisel.

Operation upon large hard exostoses is associated with greater difficulty. The narrow space in which operations can only be performed under illumination, and the troublesome hæmorrhage which obstructs the view of the parts, combine in forming this difficulty. The operation associated with the least danger is most certainly that in which the chisel is used. After inducing chloroform narcosis, a hollow ground chisel, without regard to the thin soft covering, is driven along that wall of the meatus from which the exostosis projects, and a piece or the whole of it is chiselled off. In this way the author has succeeded in removing at one operation an ivory exostosis occupying the whole lumen of the meatus. It was 14 mm. long, 7 wide, and 5 thick. If it cannot be removed all at once, the exostosis should be reduced bit by bit. Operation with the drill is more dangerous and tedious and less certain than that with the chisel. The number of operations hitherto performed is yet small. Heinicke and Lucae operated with the chisel, and also Knorre and Bremer, after they had been unsuccessful with the drill. Field repeatedly employed the dentaldrill, and it took about an hour to pierce an exostosis when using a narrow drill. In one of his cases the drill slipped into the tympanic cavity, producing facial paralysis, which, however, was subsequently cured. Moos, by means of an ordinary drill, opened up a closure caused by inflammatory hyperostosis of the meatus, and obtained a good result.

FORMATION OF BLOOD-CYSTS IN THE EXTERNAL MEATUS.

Extravasation of blood beneath the epidermis of the external meatus, *i.e.* an accumulation of dark fluid blood under the thin epidermic covering, is very rarely observed. Most frequently blood-cysts occur in acute inflammation of the middle ear and of the external meatus. The author observed a case in which such a blood-cyst had formed, accompanied by the symptoms of Menière's disease. It occupied the whole anterior wall of the meatus. Another case occurred in a patient, who suddenly became dull of hearing, but who had previously suffered from purulent inflammation of the middle ear. The cyst was situated at the inner end of the posterior wall of the meatus. In both of these cases the cysts disappeared after puncture.

CARIES AND NECROSIS OF THE OSSEOUS MEATUS.

The diseases of the osseous wall of the external meatus are caused either by otitis externa or by extension of inflammation from the cells of the mastoid process. Caries or necrosis causes loss of substance, and the pus is discharged through fistulous openings, at the margins of which granulations or polypi of varying size frequently form. The diagnosis of fistulous openings, when the formation of polypi is not too exuberant, can easily be made by means of the hook-shaped probe. After the polypi have been removed, they will persistently reappear so long as inspissated deposits lie deeply within the meatus. In such cases the growths can only be made to disappear by removing the deposits. For this purpose the author has found most suitable the 'metal tympanic tube' (Paukenröhre), which will be afterwards described (Chapter VIII.).

In the case of a female patient, the entire outer portion of whose meatus was filled with polypi, the author found that three *fistulæ* had formed in the neighbourhood of the ear, one above the mastoid process, one in the retro-maxillary fossa, and a third on the cheek. Being unable to remove the polypi by means of the snare, the tympanic tube was introduced behind them, and by syringing through it a large quantity of caseous pus was evacuated, and the polypi disappeared spontaneously. On examination, the whole posterior wall of the meatus was found destroyed, the external meatus, the tympanic cavity, and the mastoid forming one large cavity.

Treatment.—The treatment of carious processes in the external meatus should be confined simply to careful cleansing and disinfection, all irritation being avoided. In the case of narrow openings, or when the caries is superficial, it is of advantage to use the sharp spoon. We must not omit the treatment of constitutional affections or of mal-nutrition in such cases.

CHAPTER VII.

DISEASES OF THE MEMBRANA TYMPANI.

ANATOMICAL.

THE *membrana tympani* measures 9 mm. in extent from above downward, 8 wide, and 0·1 thick. Its function is to receive from the external air the waves of sound entering the auditory meatus, and to convey them through the ossicula to the labyrinth. It is conically depressed inward, and is inserted by its somewhat thickened border, the *annulus cartilagineus*, into a groove, the *sulcus tympanicus*, situated at the inner extremity of the meatus. In the anterior-superior part of this groove is the so-called *Rivinian notch*, and at this point the membrane is attached to the *margo tympanicus* of the squamous portion of the temporal bone. That part of the membrane which is situated directly above the short process of the malleus is called the *membrana flaccida Shrapnelli*. The membrane is inclined forward and downward in such a manner that it forms an angle of 140° with the superior as well as with the posterior wall of the meatus.

The membrana tympani consists of three layers :—(1) the *cuticular layer*, formed by epidermis and the connective tissue underlying it ; (2) the *membrana propria*, with its external radiating and its internal circular fibres ; (3) the *mucous layer*, furnished with peculiar vascular papillæ and pavement epithelium. The blood-supply of the membrane is chiefly by a branch of the *arteria auricularis profunda*, which, accompanied by two veins, extends along the posterior margin of the handle of the malleus to the *umbo*, and radiates thence along with the veins. The radiating twigs flow into the venous corona of vessels around the margin of the membrane. The blood-vessels of the mucous layer and of the cutis of the membrana tympani are connected with each other by a capillary network penetrating the membrana propria (Kessel). Moos has further ascertained by careful examination that the vessels communicate with each other along the whole periphery of the annulus, along the handle of the malleus, and through the membrana flaccida. Sensory nerve fibres are supplied by the *ramus meatus auditorii externi* of the *trigeminus*.

The *handle of the malleus* is situated upon the inner surface of the membrane, to which it is firmly united. It extends nearly from the anterior-superior border of the membrane to its centre, the *umbo*. Near the superior border *the short process* is visible upon the outer surface of the membrane as a distinctly projecting small white knob, and from it extend backward and forward to the margin of the membrana tympani two or three folds, the so-called 'folds of the membrane' (most marked when the membrane is pathologically indrawn). On the inner surface the angular spaces between the handle of the malleus and each fold of the membrana tympani are occupied with membranes situated parallel with the membrana tympani, and forming with it two pouches opening downward, the so-called 'Pockets of Von Tröltsch.'

Most diseased conditions of the external meatus and tympanic cavity are accompanied by similar conditions of the membrana tympani, on account of the continuity of the coverings of these two parts with the inner and outer layers of the tympanic membrane. As the diseases of this membrane occur simultaneously with those of the meatus and middle ear, they must be described together, so we will here confine our attention to the independent diseases of the membrane.

ACUTE INFLAMMATION OF THE MEMBRANA TYMPANI.

(SYNONYM : *Myringitis acuta*.)

Independent acute inflammation of the membrana tympani is a somewhat rare disease; along with acute catarrh of the middle ear, or with otitis externa, it occurs very frequently. It is mainly caused by cold arising from a draught, or by the entrance of cold water into the ear, especially while bathing.

The disease makes its appearance very suddenly, with great pain, accompanied by a feeling of tension, pulsation, and heat. To this is added annoying tinnitus; but, unlike the effect of acute inflammation of the middle ear, the hearing becomes only slightly impaired. Generally the disease only continues one or a few days at its height, after which the symptoms rapidly subside and recovery takes place. As a rule, it is only unilateral.

On examination the membrana tympani is found much reddened. At first the individual engorged vessels, especially along the handle of the malleus, can be observed. Diffuse reddening and swelling soon set in; the outline of the malleus becomes obliterated, the surface of the membrane being very lustrous and of a bluish-red colour. Sometimes extravasation of blood occurs beneath the epidermic layer, serous or purulent vesicles being more rarely observed. The adjoining portion of the external meatus is also hyperæmic. Either a cure takes place by simple subsidence of the hyperæmia and swelling, or desquamation of the superficial epidermis occurs, along with slight exudation sometimes containing an admixture of blood. When the membrana tympani becomes perforated the tympanic cavity may also be affected.

Treatment.—As with any other acutely inflamed organ, the first rule is to avoid all irritation. Syringing and the air-douche ought therefore not to be employed, and the treatment should be confined to warm instillations of oil or water, to which a few drops of tincture of opium may be added : a solution of cocaine (6—10 per cent.) should be tried. In addition, blood-letting in front of the ear may be resorted to, as also strong purgatives for the purpose of determining blood to the bowel. Bonnafont recommends scarification, and Schwartze, paracentesis.

In the case of a soldier who, suddenly, after bathing, was seized with violent pain in the ear, the author found on examination a bright-yellow lustrous vesicle almost as large as a pea protruding into the meatus from the posterior part of the membrana tympani. On puncture a drop of serous fluid was evacuated and the severe pain immediately abated. Two days afterwards the raised epidermis had completely re-applied itself to the surface, and the place of incision could be seen as a linear cicatrix.

CHRONIC INFLAMMATION OF THE MEMBRANA TYMPANI.
(Synonym: *Myringitis chronica*.)

Chronic inflammation of the membrana tympani occurs, especially in constitutionally weak persons, without any particular symptoms, sometimes with sensations of tension and itching in the ear, and more rarely with pain. It is mostly caused by foreign bodies, as ceruminal accumulations or exudation products, lying in contact with the membrana tympani. A slight exudation appears, either serous or purulent in character, with a very bad odour. This matter by drying becomes thicker, and forms a crust, below which any decomposed exudation acts as a continuous source of irritation upon the membrane, and so granulations form which prevent healing. The hearing, as a rule, is only slightly impaired.

After thorough cleansing, the membrana tympani appears lustreless, dull, and of a dirty-white colour; it is either denuded of epidermis and swollen at various spots, or over a large part, and even in its whole extent it may present a reddened granular surface.

Treatment.—In slight cases a cure may be effected by thorough cleansing, or by one or more applications of powdered alum or boracic acid. For granulations, the tincture of the perchloride of iron and nitrate of silver may be used with advantage. The former remedy produces no reaction and no pain, and should be employed first, a small drop being applied to the different granular spots by means of the probe. Caustic acts more powerfully, and a careless application may lead to inflammation and perforation of the membrane.

EXTRAVASATION OF BLOOD IN THE MEMBRANA TYMPANI.

In rare cases extravasation of blood takes place between the layers of the membrana tympani, especially when great hyperæmia occurs in the course of inflammation, as also in cases of severe concussion.

Urbantschitsch observed extravasations after the air-douche. Such are visible either only as points or as larger spots; in the most severe cases little blood-cysts form.

In one instance the author found very troublesome tinnitus, caused by an extravasation of blood, occupying the posterior part of the membrane. On its removal by careful scraping with a sharp spoon, the tinnitus permanently disappeared.

The absorption of extravasations occurs spontaneously. Von Tröltsch first observed the extension of extravasation from the centre of the membrana tympani to the periphery and to the adjoining wall of the meatus.

RUPTURE OF THE MEMBRANA TYMPANI.

Rupture of the membrane may be caused as follows :—

1. By sudden compression of the column of air in the external meatus, as in the case of a very loud sound or of explosions, and from the condensation of air in the meatus itself, as by blows on the ear.

2. Frequently the membrane is injured by solid bodies introduced into the meatus, either for the purpose of cleansing, or by accident, such as knitting-needles, straws, etc.

3. By condensation of air in the tympanic cavity in violent sneezing, coughing, or in applying the air-douche.

4. By concussions and fractures of the cranial bones.

Although it was doubted by the older writers whether rupture of the healthy membrane might occur in consequence of the violent action of loud sounds, this has now been unquestionably proved. A case came under the author's notice, in which, during gun-practice, a grenade exploded, causing rupture of the tympanic membranes of three artillerymen, who were sitting together, that side which happened to be turned towards the bursting grenade being the one affected. Ruptures in consequence of blows on the ear are mostly met with in the left ear, as they are generally inflicted by the right hand of the assailant standing in front.

Not unfrequently a rupture takes place on plunging or diving suddenly under water, as the air in the external meatus is thereby condensed. Pathological alterations of the membrane favour the occurrence of rupture; in such cases it may even be produced by the condensation of air in Politzerising or catheterising.

If the force of the air be slight, the injury may be limited only to rupture of blood-vessels in the membrane, causing extravasation under the cutis. As a rule rupture occurs in the inferior half of the membrane; most commonly only one perforation forms, but sometimes several.

Violent concussion of the cranial bones in the case of a blow or a fall, may alone cause a breach of the membrane, and it may also result from fracture of the temporal bone. In such cases fissures frequently form in the posterior wall of the meatus, proceeding outward from the region of Shrapnell's membrane, so that rupture generally occurs at that spot.

The occurrence of rupture produces the sensation of something bursting in the ear, and frequently a loud report is heard. Sometimes fainting occurs, but the pain is, as a rule, slight, and the hearing is affected according to the degree of injury and the simultaneous implication of the labyrinth. Subjective noises generally set in with great intensity. The tuning-fork placed upon the cranial bones is usually heard better on the affected side. But the reverse happens in the case of a simultaneous concussion of the labyrinth.

Lesions caused by foreign bodies may be accompanied by injury of the ossicula or the labyrinthine wall, as well as the membrana tympani.

In two cases which the author observed the injury was caused by a knitting-needle which had penetrated the posterior-superior quadrant of the membrane. Both patients fell down in an unconscious state, and although they quickly regained consciousness, they could not rise on account of great vertigo. Excessive vomiting also occurred at intervals, for one or two days, during which time the giddiness was so great that the patients were not able to sit upright in bed. It is remarkable that a moderate degree of giddiness remained for a long time after they had otherwise recovered. Usually in cases of perforation with a knitting-needle the consequent pain, tinnitus, dulness of hearing, and perhaps fainting, occur only at intervals. The author considered himself justified in diagnosing in these cases a dislocation of the stapes, with changes in the intralabyrinthine pressure.

The appearance of the membrana tympani in cases of traumatic rupture is generally characteristic when an examination is made shortly after the injury. As a rule, the breach is oval or round, due to the gaping of the edges of the wound, which are rarely cemented together by coagulated blood. Sometimes the rupture is like a fissure, its margins lying close to each other. The opening in the case of rupture is generally sharply defined, and, what is most important, its borders are lined with a narrow streak of coagulated blood of a lighter or darker colour. From traces of hæmorrhage, the traumatic nature of the lesion may be diagnosed with certainty during the first few days after its occurrence.

The several layers of the membrana tympani may be differently affected by the rupture, the edges of the wound in the cutis being wider apart than those in the deeper layers, which appear of a lighter colour than the rest of the membrane. The characteristic traces of bleeding are found at the margins of the wound in the cutis. In one case the author observed, the lesion was confined to the cutis.

The inner wall of the tympanic cavity is of a yellowish bone colour, and can be seen through the rent if sufficiently wide. With the auscultation-tube a blowing noise is heard when the Valsalvian experiment is made; perforations resulting from inflammation of the middle ear generally produce mucous râles.

The symptoms mostly disappear in a few days, followed by complete recovery. In rare cases rupture is followed by inflammation of the middle ear, with its symptoms. This may become chronic and give rise to discharge from the ear. In concussion of the labyrinth the prognosis is very unfavourable, as defective hearing generally remains; but even in such a case recovery may take place after a few days or weeks. As a rule the rupture heals in such a manner that the membrana tympani appears again quite normal, and the cicatrix can only be discovered with difficulty. Politzer has observed that a few days after the perforation a greyish-yellow membrane forms, which gives the observer the impression that it had spread over the rupture from the inside.

Treatment.—Therapeutic interference in order to promote or accelerate the healing of the rupture is unnecessary, as it takes place spontaneously when no inflammation occurs. All influences which might lead to inflammation must be avoided. The ear must be especially protected against cold, and should not be syringed. The insertion of antiseptic wool, either dry or soaked with carbolic solution, is all that is necessary.

Surgical wounds of the membrana tympani always heal like traumatic lesions. The attempts to keep them open permanently and safely have hitherto been unsuccessful. The author has repeatedly observed the restoration of the membrane, even after the malleus with a considerable portion of the membrana tympani had been removed.

Frank inserted a small gold tube, with a narrow rim on either end, into a perforation in the membrane, but failed to keep it open, and Politzer, who introduced an eyelet of vulcanite for the same purpose was also unsuccessful.

THE ARTIFICIAL MEMBRANA TYMPANI.

In cases of partial or complete destruction of the membrana tympani, the hearing may sometimes be materially improved by an artificial membrane. By this means pressure is exerted upon the remains of the membrana tympani and upon the ossicula, and the sound-conduction is increased. An artificial membrane should always be tried in cases where considerable destruction of the membrana tympani or of the ossicula has taken place, all exudation having ceased.

The oldest, simplest, and most suitable appliance employed for this purpose was suggested by Yearsley in 1848. It consists of a small pellet of wadding, which is placed in contact with the remains of the membrane by means of the forceps.

This pellet is impregnated with salicylic or boracic acid, or with thymol, is well pressed together, and then moistened in a mixture of glycerine and water (1 : 4). In 1853 Toynbee described his artificial membrane, which came rapidly into general use. This little instrument consists of a thin round india-rubber plate, to the centre of which a fine silver wire is fastened perpendicularly, which serves as a handle for its introduction and removal (Fig. 25).

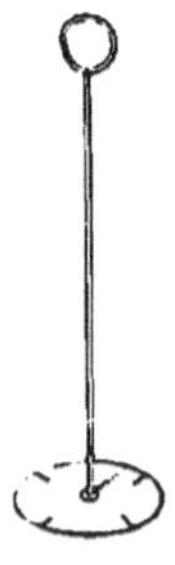

FIG. 25.

In introducing these artificial membranes the external meatus must be straightened by drawing the auricle backward and outward. They are then pushed downward to the bottom of the meatus with an inclination somewhat forward. Its proper introduction certainly requires some dexterity on the part of patients, but they succeed in most cases after instruction. These artificial membranes are removed in the same manner as they are introduced. The meatus is straightened, and the membranes are withdrawn by their handles. When Yearsley's cotton pellet is used, the forceps is introduced closed, then opened, and the cotton is caught and withdrawn. The small pellet remains better in position than other appliances; its application is very simple, and the cotton does not irritate but on the contrary acts as an aid to healing. In improving the hearing, wadding is not inferior to Toynbee's artificial membrane and its modifications; indeed, in some cases it is even more effectual, while sometimes certainly the reverse.

The improvement in hearing effected by artificial membranes is in many cases very considerable, while in others they produce no change at all. Their effect on the patient is most astonishing in a case where the hearing is so defective that he is unable to understand conversation, and when by means of the artificial membrane all at once he is enabled to take part in it. Even when the membrana tympani is completely destroyed, and the stapes is the only one of the ossicula remaining, a beneficial effect may be obtained by the artificial membrane.

While in many cases the artificial membrane may remain in the ear for several days without causing any bad symptoms, it often happens that its long-continued use produces tinnitus, a feeling of pressure and weight, or giddiness. Sometimes formerly existing exudation processes are renewed. At first, artificial membranes should therefore only be worn for a few hours, and this period should be gradually extended. Sometimes the ears of patients are so sensitive that their use has altogether to be dispensed with. Yearsley's cotton pellets are tolerated best. Knapp describes a case in which the pellet was worn for twenty-nine years, with considerable improvement in the hearing.

Instead of introducing the cotton pellet with the forceps, Hassenstein recommended a small holder, between the arms of which the little ball is held, and it remains with the wadding in the ear. Delstanche makes an artificial membrane in a very simple manner. He takes a small piece of soft wire, which he bends at one end. Around this wire the cotton-wool is wrapped in such a way that at the end a little ball is formed, while the rest of the wire is covered only by a thin layer of wadding. The author uses a small quantity of cotton-wool twisted into a small ball, and continued into a thin process, around which process a thread is wound, and the whole impregnated with a solution of wax (Fig. 26). Such little appliances are manufactured wholesale very cheaply. Kosegarten points out that in many cases pulverised substances, especially alum, insufflated into the ear, form into a solid disc, and thus act as an artificial membrane.

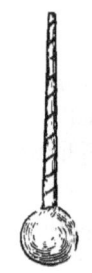

Fig. 26.

More recent authorities have altered Toynbee's artificial membrane in such a manner that the silver wire has been omitted, and simply a small india-rubber plate (Hinton), a round piece of linen (Gruber), or a small paper disc (Blake) is employed. These artificial membranes are also introduced with the forceps, and removed by them, or a thread is fastened to them, for the purpose of extraction. Lucae substituted for the silver wire of Toynbee's artificial membrane an india-rubber tube. The best way of introducing small plates of soft material, the most suitable of which is wax-cloth, is to fasten a thread to the centre, push the two ends of the thread through a thin straight tube, and hold them at the outer extremity. The little plate thus lies at the distal end at right angles to the tube, and can be introduced by means of it. When the ends of the thread are set free and the tube is withdrawn, the little plate with the thread remains in the meatus. In the same manner a cotton pellet fastened to a thread may also be introduced.

ANOMALIES OF TENSION OF THE MEMBRANA TYMPANI.

The tension of the membrana tympani may be diminished or increased.

Relaxation is caused by inflammation, especially when accompanied by a protracted inward curvature of the membrane. It may be so great that the membrana tympani lies upon the promontory, and that part of the ossicular chain formed by the long process of the incus and the stapes, so that they project through the membrane. Not unfrequently only a partial relaxation is found, especially in the posterior-superior quadrant.

Treatment.—Omitting useless instillations, the methods of treatment which have been recommended are multiple incisions (Politzer), galvano-caustic destruction of a portion of the relaxed membrane (Gruber), designed to form a firm cicatrix. McKeown recently proposed painting with collodion.

The folds of the membrana tympani are subject to abnormal tension. In many cases they project strongly, even without much indrawing of the other parts of the membrane. By incision of these folds (Politzer, Lucae) sometimes considerable improvement in sound-conduction is obtained. Particularly the subjective noises which accompany the abnormal tension are lessened or abolished.

For incising the membrane the so-called membrana tympani knife is used. The incisions are made between the umbo and the outer margin of the membrane, $1-2\frac{1}{2}$ mm. long, four or five times, at intervals of two to three days. The prominent folds are incised at right angles to their length.

Galvano-caustic destruction of a portion of the membrane is produced by bringing to a white heat a fine point inserted through a speculum well advanced into the meatus, the heated point by a slight rapid movement being pushed through the membrane. This instrument must be handled with precision, so that the proper part of the membrane be touched, and the inner wall of the tympanic cavity uninjured.

CHAPTER VIII.

DISEASES OF THE MIDDLE EAR.

ANATOMICAL.

THE tympanic cavity is lined with a very thin mucous membrane, and is of very small dimensions, its greatest height amounting to 15 mm., and its length from the *ostium tympanicum* to the entrance of the *antrum mastoideum* averaging 13 mm. Its width is greater at its upper part, being 4 mm., while between its inner wall and the membrana tympani there is only a distance of 1½ mm.; so that under pathological conditions the latter may easily come into apposition with the former.

In accordance with its shape the tympanic cavity has six walls (see Fig. 27). The inner wall consists chiefly of that somewhat projecting part of the labyrinthine wall, *the promontory*. In front of the promontory the inner wall is separated from the canal of the internal carotid only by a thin layer of bone. Above and in front of the promontory is the *processus cochlearis* for the tendon of the tensor tympani; behind and above, the *fenestra ovalis;* and behind and below, the *fenestra rotunda*. On inspecting the ear from the external meatus the two fenestræ are as a rule hidden behind the posterior border of the membrana tympani. Sometimes, however, when the membrane is absent, both fenestræ can be distinctly seen. Above and behind the fenestra ovalis, the outer wall of the canal of the facial nerve projects in the form of an arch. The outer wall of the tympanic cavity is formed chiefly by the membrana tympani, and above by bone, mainly consisting of air-cells. The superior wall consists of a thin plate of bone which forms the partition between the middle cranial fossa and the tympanum (*tegmen tympani*). The inferior wall has a rough surface; below it, and separated from it by an osseous layer of varying thickness, is the jugular fossa with the sinus of the internal jugular vein. The anterior and posterior walls form respectively by their upper parts the lower boundary of the orifice of the Eustachian tube and of the entrance to the antrum mastoideum.

The mucous membrane of the tympanic cavity is lined with ciliated pavement epithelium. Von Tröltsch was the first to trace isolated mucous glands near the ostium tympanicum tubæ.

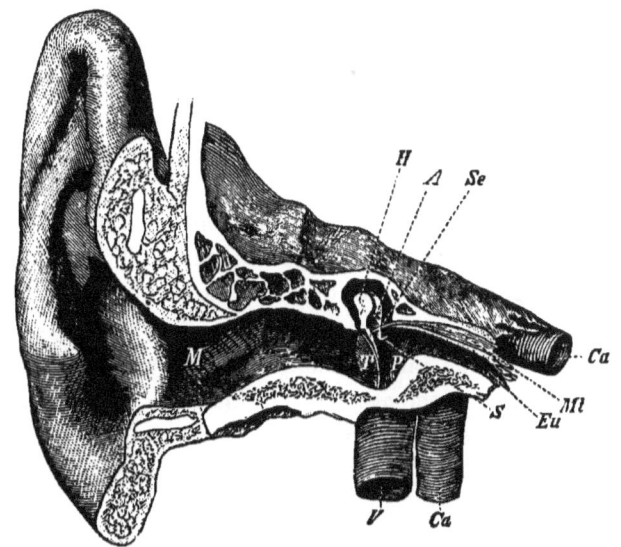

FIG. 27.

M. Meatus auditorius externus. *T.* Membrana tympani. *H.* Malleus. *A.* Incus. *S.* Stapes. *P.* Promontory. *Eu.* Eustachian tube. *Mt.* Tensor tympani. *Se.* Its tendon. *Ca.* Carotis interna. *V.* Vena jugularis.

Sound-conduction from the membrana tympani to the labyrinth is effected by the ossicula, the *malleus*, the *incus*, and the *stapes*, the latter fitting into the fenestra ovalis. As already seen, the malleus is united with the inner surface of the membrane by its handle, its neck bending at an angle, so that the head of the malleus extends freely into the highest part of the tympanic cavity. From the margin of the Rivinian segment ligamentous fibres (ligament of the axis of the malleus, Helmholtz) extend to the neck of the malleus, and fix it in its position anteriorly and posteriorly. The head of the malleus is attached to the upper wall of the tympanic cavity by the superior ligament. Above the short process of the malleus, between the head and the outer wall of the tympanum, are minute spaces formed by the membranous strands which connect these two parts. Shrapnell's membrane forms the outer boundary of the spaces adjoining the short process. That surface of the head of the malleus directed backward forms with the incus a peculiar check joint, by which the articulating surfaces are firmly pressed together by movements of the membrana tympani in an inward direction, while movements in the opposite direction can take place unchecked. Of the two processes with which the incus is furnished, the short one is directed straight backward to the entrance of the antrum mastoideum, while the long one extends, parallel with the handle of the malleus, backward and downward. The end of the long process is articulated by means of a convex surface (*processus lenticularis*) with the concave capitulum of the stapes. The two crura of the stapes occupy a horizontal plane, the foot-plate being fixed into the fenestra ovalis by means of a small circular membrane.

The surface of the membrana tympani is 15—20 times greater than that of the fenestra ovalis. The distance of the end of the handle of the malleus from the axis of rotation is once and a half as great as that distance from the end of the incus which presses upon the stapes. The pressure upon the stapes is therefore once and a half as great as the force exerted upon the end of the handle of the malleus.

The mechanical function of the tympanic apparatus is to convert a vibration of great amplitude and slight force exerted upon the membrana tympani into one of less amplitude and greater force, which is then communicated to the labyrinthine fluid (Helmholtz). The excursions of the foot-plate of the stapes, according to Helmholtz's measurement, do not in any case exceed $\frac{1}{10}$ mm.

The ossicula are furnished with two muscles, which influence their position and tension:—1. The *tensor tympani* arises in the canal running parallel with the Eustachian tube. It forms a thin tendon, leaving the canal at the processus cochlearis on the inner wall of the tympanic cavity in a direction almost at right angles to the rest of the muscle, extends transversely across the tympanum, and is inserted at the upper end of the handle of the malleus. 2. The *stapedius* is enclosed in the eminentia pyramidalis on the posterior wall of the tympanum. Its tendon passes through a small opening, and is inserted on the posterior margin of the capitulum of the stapes. Politzer proved by experiments that the tensor tympani is supplied by the motor portion of the trigeminus, and the stapedius by the facial nerve. Many persons are able to contract the tensor tympani simultaneously with the masseteric muscles, creating a peculiar crackling noise.

The tympanic cavity is supplied with *blood-vessels* as follows:— 1. The stylo-mastoid branch of the posterior auricular artery passes through the Fallopian canal, and gives twigs to the mucous membrane of the tympanic cavity and the air-cells of the mastoid process. 2. The tympanic artery from the ascending pharyngeal enters with the nerve of the same name through the floor of the tympanic cavity. 3. Small branches of the middle meningeal enter the tympanum through the petroso-squamosal suture. 4. The internal carotid supplies one or two minute vessels as it passes through the petrous bone. The veins empty their contents into the middle meningeal vein and into the venous plexus surrounding the maxillary joint. Anastomoses form with the vessels of the external meatus as well as with those of the labyrinth (Politzer).

The glosso-pharyngeal nerve chiefly supplies the middle ear with sensory fibres. Its small branch, the tympanic or nerve of Jacobson, enters through the floor of the tympanic cavity, extends in a groove, frequently partly bridged over, to the promontory, and then distributes itself upon the mucous membrane of the tympanum. This nerve is connected on the one hand with the otic ganglion of the trigeminus by the small superficial petrosal nerve, which extends below the canal of the tensor tympani muscle, and on the other hand with the sympathetic by small twigs from the internal carotid plexus. The system of nerves thus consisting of fibres of the glosso-pharyngeal, trigeminus, and sympathetic is called *the tympanic plexus.*

The facial nerve gives off the *chorda tympani* in its canal before it issues at the stylo-mastoid foramen. It enters the tympanum in a direction curving forward and downward upon the inner surface of the posterior pocket of the membrana tympani, passes above the

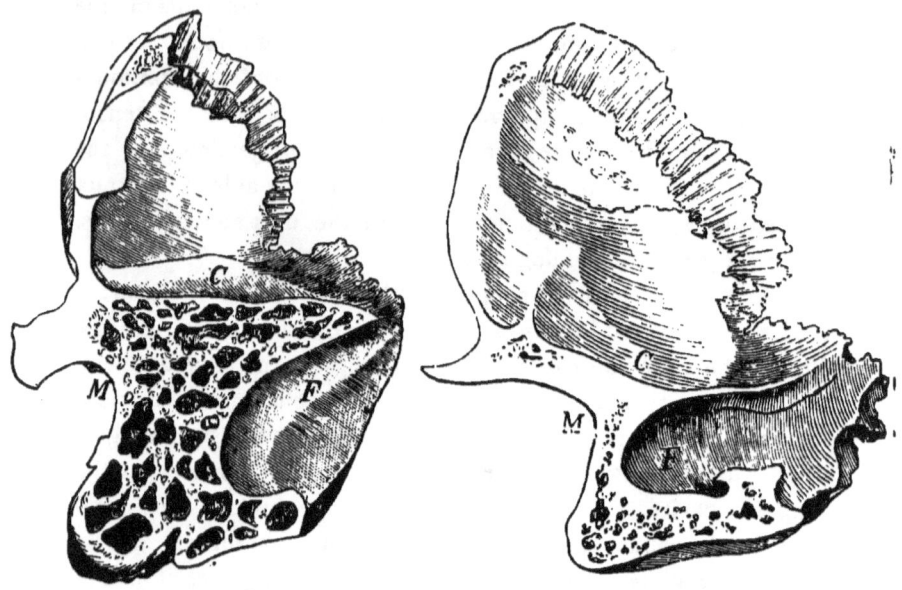

Fig. 28.   Fig. 29.

F. Fossa sigmoidea.   *M.* Meatus auditorius externus.   *C.* Cavum cranii.

tendon of the tensor tympani, and over the neck of the malleus, leaving the tympanum by descending through the fissure of Glaser, and then uniting with the lingual branch of the trigeminus. The chorda tympani contains gustatory fibres supplying the anterior part of the tongue, and also fibres influencing the secretion of the salivary glands. By experiments on animals, Gellè and Berthold have proved that the tympanic cavity is supplied with trophic fibres by the trigeminus. The latter in particular ascertained by numerous experiments that inflammatory symptoms are produced in the middle ear by section of the trigeminus, either in its course or at its origin. No changes are caused in the tympanum by removal of the glossopharyngeal or by extirpation of the superior cervical ganglion.

Posteriorly and externally the tympanic cavity is connected with the air-cells of the mastoid process, which, before they pass into the tympanum, form a common cavity, the *antrum mastoideum*. It lies at the posterior and upper part of the inner half of the osseous meatus, and is separated from it by an osseous layer 3—4 mm. thick. The air-cells extend over the whole mastoid process, and are also frequently met with between the superior wall of the meatus and the middle cranial fossa. Their total extent chiefly depends upon the conformation of the lateral sinus running into the sigmoid fossa, and also that of the middle fossa of the cranium. According to the author's measurements,[1] which agree with those of Bezold, the distance between the sigmoid fossa and the posterior wall of the meatus is frequently only a few millimetres. The

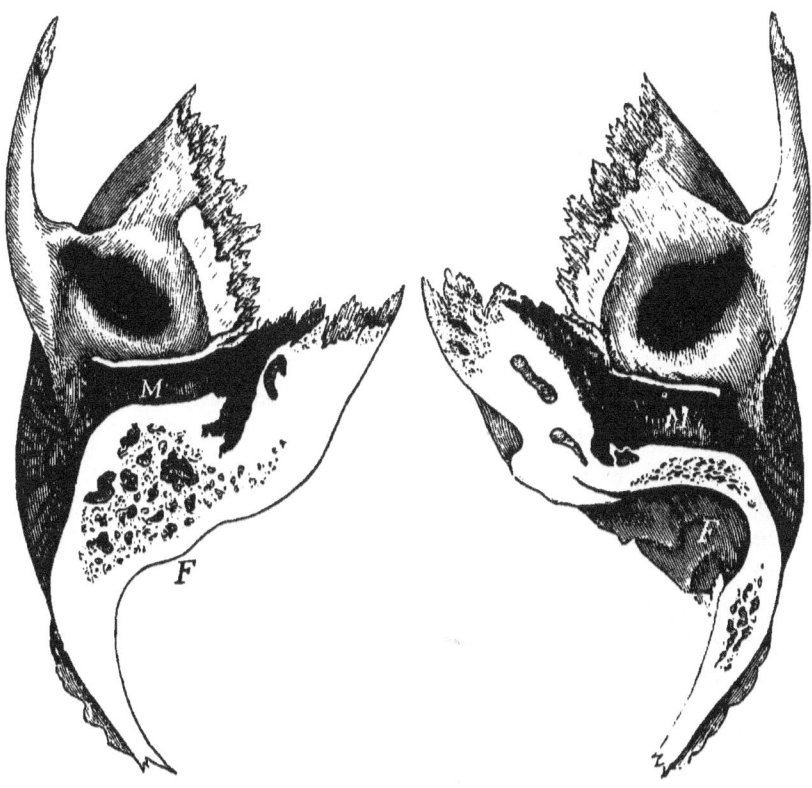

FIG. 30. FIG. 31.

M. Meatus auditorius externus. *F.* Fossa sigmoidea.

variations which are met with in this respect are very considerable, as is seen in Figs. 28 and 29, which represent sections made per-

[1] Von Langenbeck's *Archiv für Chirurgie*, vol. xxi.

pendicularly to the axis of the meatus, and in Figs. 30 and 31, which are sections made horizontally through the middle line of the meatus, the one showing a shallow and the other a deep excavation of the sinus. When this excavation is great, and the middle cranial fossa is only separated from the superior wall of the meatus by a thin layer of bone (a condition which the author has described as 'a low-lying middle cranial fossa,' Fig. 29), the space occupied by cell-cavities is greatly reduced. When the lateral sinus advances strongly forward, it at the same time assumes an outward direction (Fig. 31), so that, in extreme instances, like the two represented, the mastoid process is excavated in the direction of its outer surface, and the lateral sinus is to that extent deprived of its bony protection below and behind the auricle. There are also other deficiencies in the thickness of the mastoid process—so-called dehiscences of the bone, which may give rise to emphysema of the skin covering it.

The *Eustachian tube* extends from the tympanic cavity in a direction forward and inward, forming a canal 1 mm. high and 2 mm. broad. It lies above the canal of the internal carotid and below that of the tensor tympani muscle, and measures 12 mm. in length. The osseous portion of the Eustachian tube is continued by a cartilaginous and membranous tube measuring 24 mm. The latter portion consists mostly of cartilage, which, in the shape of a groove opening downward, forms the anterior, posterior, and superior wall of the canal. Forward and downward it is closed by soft tissues.

The chief function of the tuba Eustachii is to maintain a regular exchange of air between the tympanum and the surrounding atmosphere. In closed cavities of the body, absorption or decomposition of the air contained therein takes place, producing rarefaction, so, in order to preserve a state of equilibrium, frequent renewal of air must take place. As a permanently open tube would affect the vibrations of the membrana tympani, this change of air does not continually occur, for the tube is only made permeable by the action of certain muscles. In a state of rest, the walls of the membranous portions of the tube lie loosely in contact with the cartilaginous roof. As the author's investigations in the pneumatic cabinet [1] have shown, no air enters through the tube into the tympanic cavity under the influence of strong air-pressure, but, on the contrary, when the surrounding air is rarefied, a slight alteration in the air-pressure is sufficient to exhaust the tympanum of air through the tubes. By every contraction of the muscles patency of the tubes is produced.

While the *tensor veli muscle* or *dilator of the Eustachian tube* chiefly effects the withdrawal of the membranous wall from the cartilaginous roof, *the levator veli*, which extends along the floor of the tube, seems mainly to perform the function of making it permeable by contraction of its walls. Simultaneous with the action of these two muscles is the occurrence of tension and elevation of the soft palate. The different positions of the membranous wall of the tube as well as of the soft palate are indicated in the following diagram.

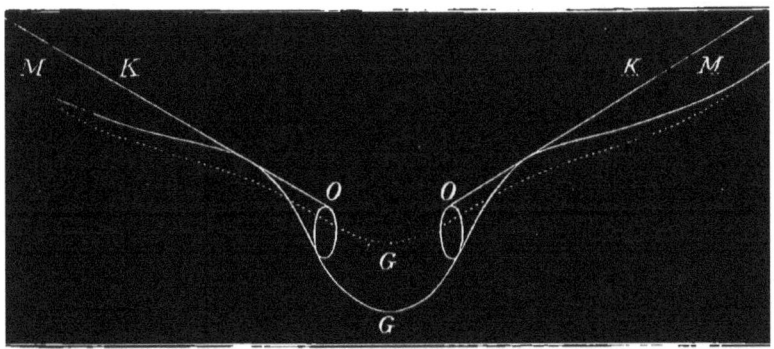

FIG. 32.

The pharyngeal orifices (ostia pharyngea) are marked *O, O*, the cartilaginous roof *K, K*, the membranous wall of the tubes *M, M*, and the soft palate *G*. The state of rest is indicated by white lines, the changed position during an act of swallowing by the dotted line.

1. When the muscles are at rest, the pharyngeal orifices are gaping wide, the soft palate lies low, and part of the membranous wall of the tube lies in contact with the cartilaginous roof. When

[1] The author entered the pneumatic cabinet with twenty-two adults, and the air-pressure was increased to such an extent (200 mm. mercury) that the pain in the membrana tympani could not be borne any longer. Air only enters the tympanum when an act of deglutition is performed.—*Experimentelle Studien über die Funktion der Eustachi'schen Röhre*, etc. Leipzig, 1879.

the air is compressed in the naso-pharynx (as in the pneumatic cabinet) no air enters the tympanum.

2. During the act of deglutition the pharyngeal orifices become greatly narrowed, apparently closed; the soft palate is markedly elevated; and the membranous wall is in its whole extent withdrawn from the cartilaginous roof. By manometrical experiments the author succeeded in proving that during the act of swallowing the tubes are opened, as air then enters into the tympanic cavities in the case of the slightest air-pressure in the naso-pharynx. If such pressure be insufficient to force the air into the tympanic cavity, it must be assumed that some defect has taken place in the normal ventilation of that cavity. The opening of the tubes takes place in such a manner that the superadded action of the muscles promotes their permeability.

ACUTE INFLAMMATION OF THE MIDDLE EAR.
(SYNONYM : *Otitis media acuta.*)

Most of the acute diseases of the ear occur simultaneously with acute catarrhs of the mucous membrane of the nose, and of the pharynx generally, in consequence of cold. These form chiefly the slighter forms of inflammation, such as are most frequently observed in children. The severe purulent form of inflammation, however, is mostly caused in children, as well as in adults, by the exanthemata, measles, scarlet and typhoid fever, and small-pox.

In the majority of cases only one side is affected, and, if both, they may be so to a different degree. When the inflammation is of a high degree, the effects on both sides are sometimes alike. Weak scrofulous persons, and all who are subject to affections of the mucous membrane, are particularly predisposed to acute diseases of the middle ear.

An attempt has been made to subdivide acute diseases by the circumstance whether the membrana tympani is perforated or not, calling the inflammation accordingly perforative and non-perforative; but as a perforation may take place even in the case of very slight inflammation, such a classification appears untenable. The distinctions depend rather upon the violence of the attack and the character of the exudation. We therefore distinguish between acute catarrh or acute simple catarrh, with muco-serous exudation, and acute inflammation or acute purulent inflammation with a discharge of pus. We must, however, not forget that the two forms are only different in their intensity and mode of attack.

In simple catarrh the vessels of the mucous membrane of the middle ear are injected, the mucous covering itself is moderately swollen, and, in the early stage, a serous, and afterwards a mucous, exudation appears. In the case of higher degrees of inflammation, very considerable swelling of the mucous membrane sets in, with great dilatation of the blood-vessels, and, instead of mucus, pus forms. According to Toynbee, if the mucous membrane of the tympanum be examined during an attack of acute inflammation, it will be found that the blood-vessels are so large and numerous that, on a cursory inspection, it seems as if the membrane were covered by a layer of dark-coloured blood. On closer examination, however, it will be noticed that this blood is contained in the vessels, and that they are greatly dilated.

ACUTE CATARRH OF THE MIDDLE EAR.

(SYNONYM : *Otitis media catarrhalis acuta.*)

As a rule this disease commences suddenly with a sharp pain. The patient has a feeling of obstruction and closure in the ear. This is followed by subjective noises, hissing or rushing, or sometimes a beating synchronous with the pulse. The hearing is impaired at first only in a slight degree, but considerably so when exudation has taken place. The impaired hearing is the chief mark of distinction between this disease and *myringitis acuta*. Not unfrequently the patient hears his own voice louder, or resounding in the affected ear. Especially in the case of children, there is fever and constitutional disturbance from the beginning. The pain generally becomes very violent, and is greatest at night, while during the day it may completely cease. It is felt not only in the ear, but over the whole corresponding half of the head. The movements of the maxillary joint produce pain, also pressure upon the mastoid process when its cells, as is so frequently the case in children, are implicated.

The symptoms set in rapidly, remain at their height one or several days, and disappear again as quickly, especially when perforation of the membrana tympani and a discharge from the ear take place. The pain generally continues for some time, as well as a sensation of fulness and pressure in the ear, along with dulness of hearing and tinnitus. In slighter cases the disease may limit itself to simple hyperæmia without exudation. Pain and subjective sounds occur. Especially in children, such acute hyperæmia is of a very marked character, and is called 'Earache.' It may entirely disappear again after a few hours. In other cases perforation of the membrana tympani takes place during the first night, a copious discharge of serum mixed with blood occurs, subsequently becoming mucous. After the occurrence of perforation, the inflammatory symptoms generally abate. The exudation may cease after a few hours, and the perforation rapidly close.

On examination, the membrana tympani is found to be more or less inflamed. When the hyperæmia is chiefly confined to the mucous membrane of the tympanum without much inflammation of the tympanic membrane, the latter assumes a diffuse bright-red colour, by reflection from the reddened mucous membrane of the promontory. But, as a rule, the tympanic membrane itself is attacked by the inflammation, and exhibits the same appearances as those which have been described under acute myringitis. At first, hyperæmia of the vessels sets in, then diffuse reddening and swelling. In consequence of the soddening and loosening of the epidermis, the surface becomes opaque, and appears as if it had a grey covering. Frequently the posterior-superior half of the membrana tympani is found to be most reddened, and strongly bulged out towards the meatus by the pressure of the exudation lying upon its inner surface. Sometimes cysts form in the membrana tympani, like those occurring in myringitis. The perforation of the membrane may take place in its superior or inferior half, generally in front and below. In the case of slighter degrees of inflammation, it is, as a rule, small, of the size of a pin-head or slightly larger, so that healing may rapidly take place.

After the symptoms have subsided, the membrane remains opaque for some time, and the vessels injected; but it soon assumes its normal appearance. In rarer cases, especially after recurrence of the inflammation, thickening, opacity, calcareous deposits, or atrophy are observed. Sometimes absorption of the exudation in the tympanic cavity does not take place, and thus a condition is created, which will be described under chronic catarrh of the middle ear. Only rarely does a perforation in the membrana tympani become permanent, and the acute inflammation chronic, with purulent degeneration of the exudation.

Even after a complete cure the ear remains a *locus minoris resistentiæ*, and the disease recurs readily.

ACUTE PURULENT INFLAMMATION OF THE MIDDLE EAR.

(SYNONYM: *Otitis media purulenta acuta.*)

Catarrhs of the nose and the pharynx are the most frequent causes of acute purulent inflammation of the middle ear. Thus, Knapp,[1] out of the large number of 8229 patients, found 564 cases of acute suppuration of the middle ear (6·85 per cent.). In 64 per cent. of the cases of suppuration the cause could be traced to catarrhs of the nose and pharynx. The severest forms of inflammation occur in the course of, or in consequence of, the exanthemata. Burckhardt-Merian gives the percentage of cases of inflammation of the middle ear during two scarlet fever epidemics; during the one, this complication occurred in 33·3 per cent. of the fever patients, and during the other in 22·2 per cent. Bezold[2] found among 1243 cases of typhoid fever, 48 (4 per cent.) with acute inflammation of the middle ear, and in 41 of these there was perforation of the membrana tympani. The inflammation may also be caused by direct irritation of the ear, injuries from foreign bodies, operative interference, and the entrance of cold water or irritating chemical substances, alcohol, etc. Such a result will arise also from fluid entering the tympanic cavities through the Eustachian tubes

---

[1] *Zeitschrift für Ohrenheilkunde*, vol. viii. p. 36.
[2] Ueber die Erkrankungen des Hörorgans bei Ileotyphus, *Archiv für Ohrenheilkunde*, vol. xxi. p. 8.

during the improper use of the nasal douche. The author has observed several cases of severe inflammation of the middle ear produced by plugging the posterior nares in cases of epistaxis. One-third of Knapp's cases occurred in children under ten years of age.

The symptoms described as occurring in acute catarrh appear with still greater severity in purulent inflammation. The pain is exceedingly violent and continuous, the subjective noises are unbearable, the pulsations of the arteries are like hammer strokes, and every sound increases the pain, which is not confined to the ear, but extends over the whole head, or only the affected side, and is particularly severe during the night, producing absolute sleeplessness. This pain is also aggravated by movement, shaking of the surroundings, excitement, and by stimulating diet. Frequently movements of the lower jaw are accompanied with such pain that opening of the mouth in speaking or masticating is rendered difficult, and the patient is compelled to take only fluid food; pressure upon the region of the maxillary joint also causes pain. The patient complains of a feeling of dulness, pressure, and heaviness in the head. Cerebral symptoms may also set in, such as vertigo and delirium. Such cases may be mistaken for meningitis, and errors in diagnosis, especially in children, are therefore of frequent occurrence. The fever is often very high, and generally accompanied by rigors. When the congestion extends to the labyrinth, and inflammation occurs there also, the dulness of hearing, resulting from the inflammatory changes in the tympanic cavity, is increased, and total deafness may follow. Neither words shouted into the ear, the watch, nor the tuning-fork placed upon the cranium are heard.

In the first stage of the inflammation the appearances in the membrana tympani are the same as in myringitis and simple catarrh. Generally the external meatus is also swollen and scarlet-red. But the surface soon changes its appearance, the loosened epidermis forming greyish-white flakes lying in the meatus. After a few days, on the average two or three, but sometimes on the first, or only after a lapse of fourteen days or more, the membrane is perforated. There may have been previously no exudation, or only a slight amount, due to the inflammation in the external meatus, but now a copious discharge takes place, at first of a serous character, afterwards muco-purulent, or purulent. The exudation is, as a rule, very copious, as it flows from the ear almost continually. The perforation may be recognised easily by the light-reflex (see page 15) at the innermost part of the meatus, when the exudation is only slight. It is not advisable to expose the perforation to view during the first stage of the inflammation by syringing or drying with cotton-wool, as by such manipulation the pain and inflammation may be aggravated.

In the way of destruction of the membrana tympani, either small perforations exist or very extensive losses of substance occur, resulting from the soddening effect of the discharge. A narrow border of the membrane and small remnants at the handle of the malleus are left, or it is destroyed in its whole extent. Frequently the inflammation has a destructive effect on the ossicula, causing their disarticulation and removal. As a rule, only the malleus and incus are affected in this way.

As soon as the membrane is perforated, the symptoms, which previously have been very severe, generally abate; the pain becomes less, the subjective noises decrease, as also the fever, and the cerebral symptoms which may have been present disappear rapidly. But the symptoms do not always abate when the membrane has ruptured; occasionally the pain and the other symptoms remain for some time in their former intensity.

When thickening of the membrana tympani has been caused by a former inflammatory attack, so that it offers increased resistance to the exudation in the tympanic cavity, perforation is delayed, and the symptoms remain at their height, until either a spontaneous perforation takes place or the membrane is incised.

The naso-pharyngeal catarrh accompanying or causing the inflammation is very severe in many cases, and is associated with obstructed breathing and copious secretion. Simultaneously with the naso-pharyngeal affection the mucous membrane of the Eustachian tube is also involved and becomes swollen, so that, in Politzerising, the air can only be made to pass with difficulty. Along with the inflammation of the middle ear, the external meatus may be very much inflamed and greatly swollen. Frequently the lymphatic glands in front and below the ear are also acutely inflamed and enlarged. Often diffuse swelling in front of the ear occurs. The inflammation sometimes spreads to the cells of the mastoid process, pressure upon which causes pain. Either œdematous swelling of the skin takes place, or periostitis, with formation of pus, which makes its way towards the surface. The complication of periostitis is generally developed when the free discharge of purulent matter is obstructed.

The results of acute purulent inflammation of the middle ear are the following :—

1. Complete cure, with no perceptible changes.
2. Cicatrices, perforations, or adhesions of the membrana tympani to the wall of the labyrinth.
3. Loss of the ossicula, or impairment of the vibratory power of the sound-conducting apparatus, due to processes of thickening and sclerosis of the mucous membrane covering the ossicula and their articulations.
4. A high degree of dulness of hearing through permanent defects in the labyrinth.
5. Continuance of the exudation, producing chronic inflammation with its consequences, which will be described afterwards.
6. Death may ensue if the inflammation spread to the meninges. Particularly in the case of children, in whom the petro-squamosal suture is not yet completely ossified, this may readily occur.

We are indebted to Burckhardt-Merian[1] for detailed communications regarding the occurrence of inflammation of the middle ear in scarlet fever. A distinction must be made between the slight cases which take a regular course, and the severe cases caused by extension of diphtheritic inflammation from the pharynx through the Eustachian tubes to the tympanic cavity. In the great majority of cases, the stage of desquamation is accompanied by earache, which at first occurs in paroxysms, but soon assumes an entirely neuralgic character, a previous rise in the temperature having taken place. Generally great dulness of hearing rapidly follows. Glandular swelling in the region of the ear is rarely absent. With the occurrence of perforation of the membrana tympani the fever dis-

[1] Volkmann's *Sammlung klin. Vorträge*, No. 182, 1880.

appears, as well as the pain, and the drowsy state of the patient which is sometimes observed. This disease is distinguished from ordinary inflammation of the middle ear by the rapidity with which great loss of substance of the membrana tympani takes place. Burckhardt-Merian observed the entire destruction of the membrane in 34·3 per cent. of his cases. 'The prognosis is the more unfavourable the longer the process is allowed to remain without treatment, while the sooner a rational treatment is commenced the more intact will be the organ of hearing after the scarlet fever.' On examining an ear affected with diphtheritic inflammation, it is found that in the first stage of the disease the meatus is filled with membranous masses, which make their way from the middle ear through the destroyed membrana tympani, and are adherent to the walls of the meatus. These masses are firmly attached by their surface, and can only be removed with great difficulty. At first the exudation is very slight, but increases considerably after detachment of the membranous masses.

While it is probable that inflammation of the middle ear connected with pharyngeal diphtheria is caused by extension of this disease through the Eustachian tubes, we must assume that inflammation of the middle ear, occurring simultaneously with other infectious diseases, arises in a different manner. In an article on disease of the ear in typhus fever, the author[1] has shown that the organ of hearing largely participates in the general hyperæmia which in this disease exists in various parts of the head. The ear affection sets in if hyperæmia remain in that organ, and extravasation of the corpuscular elements of the blood and transudation of fluid take place. Moreover, it is held that the specific germs of infectious diseases show a particular predilection for the ear, and that the exciting causes of inflammation reach the middle ear from the naso-pharynx.

Treatment.—Various authors give separate descriptions of the treatment of simple acute catarrh and of acute purulent inflammation; but, as they are only degrees of the same inflammatory process, and as both ears may be simultaneously but differently affected, the two diseases may be described separately, while their treatment

[1] *Zeitschrift für Ohrenheilkunde,* vol. viii. p. 212.

must be on the same principle. In order, therefore, to avoid repetition the author prefers to discuss the treatment of both together.

In the first place, the ear must be protected from everything likely to increase the inflammation. Patients must keep their room, in order to avoid changes of temperature, and, if the inflammation be of a purulent character, with fever, they must keep in bed. As in acute inflammation of the external meatus and of the membrana tympani, stimulating food, alcoholic liquors, mental excitement, and physical exertion, must be strictly forbidden. Irritating manipulations, syringing, and the air-douche must be dispensed with in the first stage of the disease.

The application of heat or cold is most important in the treatment of acute inflammation. Although, with regard to inflammations in general, it holds good that they are reduced by the application of cold and increased by warmth, this rule cannot altogether be applied to the ear, as cold acting directly upon the ear, in the form of instillations of cold water or ice-compresses, sometimes increases the pain; while, on the other hand, warm ear-baths and poultices generally afford relief. But, by the continued influence of heat, the ear is kept in such a state of congestion that the destructive process caused by the inflammation assumes greater activity, and the cure is retarded. While formerly the usual treatment of all acute inflammatory affections of the ear consisted in the application of warmth, especially of poultices, aural surgeons have recently gone to the other extreme, and advocated that all such cases should be treated with ice. In many cases the application of cold has the effect of rapidly lessening the inflammation and accelerating recovery, especially when the cold is not made to act directly upon the ear, but is applied to the surrounding parts. The best way is to place small longitudinal or kidney-shaped ice-bags below and behind the ear.

The author has found the combined application of warmth and cold to be of great service in many cases of acute inflammation of the middle as also of the external ear. The region below the auricle is covered with cold compresses or an ice-bag, and at the same time warm fluids are instilled into the external meatus, or warm sponges are placed upon its orifice. If the patient cannot bear the application of cold, or if it be not effective, as often happens in cases complicated with violent catarrhs of the nose and pharynx, the author confines the treatment to Priessnitz's compresses, or to covering the region of the ear with a layer of wadding, which suffices especially in simple catarrh.

For warm instillations, water, with or without the addition of a few drops of tincture of opium or warm oil, may be employed. The latter has the advantage that its action is more lasting. The introduction of steam through funnels, which is a remedy often popularly resorted to, proved useful to Knapp in cases in which the exudation was diminished after the membrana tympani had been perforated, but where the earache and headache returned.

When the inflammatory symptoms have become still more aggravated, and the pain is severe, the air-douche must not be employed, as the pain may thereby be increased. When pain and inflammation are slight, or when the latter is already past its height, the air-douche may be employed, even although no perforation of the membrane has taken place. But it must be employed in the most careful manner, with very slight pressure. When the patients bear this treatment well they experience at once a great improvement, the cure and restoration of the hearing being much accelerated.

Paracentesis of the membrana tympani, recommended by some authors for all cases of acute disease of the tympanic cavity, is unnecessary in the slighter affections—in simple catarrh and where there is only a moderate degree of pain. It is indicated, however, when the membrane is strongly bulging outwards, in consequence of the exudation upon its inner surface, and offers resistance to spontaneous perforation, while pain and feverishness continue. Moreover, paracentesis must be performed, when, after the inflammatory symptoms have subsided, a high degree of dulness of hearing still remains, caused by exudation in the middle ear.

Paracentesis is performed by means of the membrana tympani knife (Fig. 33). This instrument consists of a handle, furnished at one end with a holder at an obtuse angle, in which the knife can be fixed firmly in position. The same handle serves for holding (*a*) a small hook for the removal of foreign bodies, (*b*) a curette,

(c) a sickle-shaped knife, and (d) a blunt-pointed knife; also tenotomy knives, spatula-shaped instruments for the detachment of adhesions, and other appliances. Burckhardt-Merian recommends a small handle, which can be held between the thumb and forefinger. After anæsthetising the membrane with a 5—20 per cent. solution of cocaine, the incision is made at the point where the surface is most prominent. When it bulges uniformly, the artificial opening is made in the posterior-inferior part, as the distance between the membrana tympani and the inner wall of the tympanic cavity is greatest in that situation. After incision the air-douche is employed for the removal of the exudation. Sometimes such an opening closes so quickly that paracentesis must again be performed.

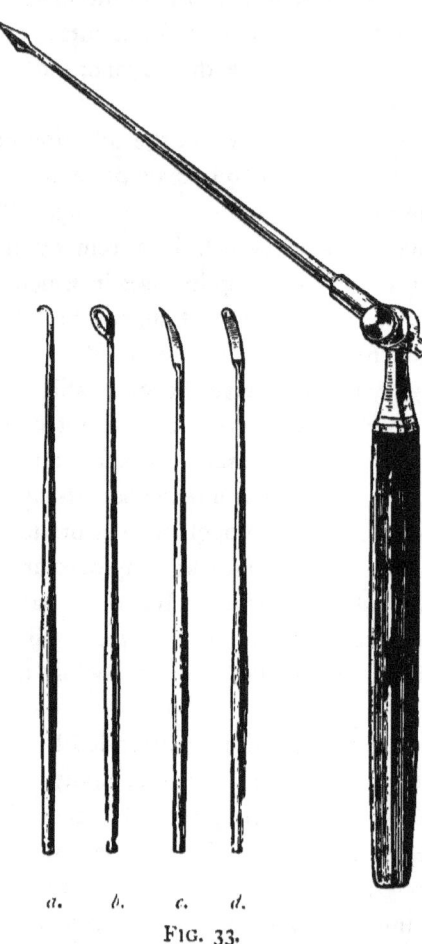

a. b. c. d.
FIG. 33.

The most varied remedies have been recommended for the pain which frequently continues after the membrane has become perforated, and especially for the nightly exacerbations. As a rule, narcotics, such as opium and morphia, are not very effective. Hydrate of chloral is more useful, and sometimes the pain is alleviated by a solution of iodide of potassium in doses of $\frac{1}{2}$—1 gm. Instillations of a $\frac{1}{2}$ per cent. solution of atropine, five drops being used several times daily, the author has often found of great service. For relieving pain, especially in children, Bendelack-Hewetson has recently recommended instillations of carbolised glycerine (1 : 5). In many cases, instillations of a 5—20 per cent. solution of cocaine relieve the pain at once, but sometimes this remedy is useless. In cases of neuralgic pains, with sleeplessness, the author obtained very good results from the application of the induced current upon the side and back of the cervical region. For cases where, in spite of treatment, the pain still continues after the membrane has been perforated and the suppuration is not checked, and for those in which the membrane presents a nipple-shaped elevation at the place of perforation, as also for cases of painful inflammation of the mastoid process, Politzer recommends injections of warm water through the catheter into the middle ear.

In order to reduce the hyperæmia, in slight cases purgatives are employed, and in the severer forms also blood-letting. In the former, compound infusion of senna (Ger. Ph.), castor-oil, or mineral waters may be ordered. Blood-letting is most effective when the disease is confined to the ear, while in the simultaneous affection of the mucous membrane of the nose and pharynx it is frequently of no use. It is performed in the manner described at page 68. When pressure upon the mastoid process elicits pain, or when the cutis covering it is hyperæmic, rapid relief will be obtained by blood-letting. When œdematous swelling exists at the same time, and when pus is suspected, or fluctuation can already be made out, an incision 2—3 cm. in length should be made over the mastoid process down to the periosteum,—the so-called 'Wilde's incision.' The head of the patient is first laid upon a firm cushion and is well fixed. Chloroform is only necessary in the case of particularly timid persons. The incision is made with a strong scalpel in a perpendicular direction, parallel with the line of attachment of the auricle, and 1—2 cm. behind it, by which the posterior auricular artery is avoided. The incision must be made at once through the whole thickness of the soft parts, which is sometimes very considerable when there is much swelling. If the soft parts be not completely cut through, the incision requires to be repeated. The bleeding, which is generally pretty profuse, may be stopped by inserting cotton-wool plugs into the wound, or the bleeding vessels must be caught by the artery-forceps and twisted or tied. After evacuating the pus a drainage-tube is inserted, and the wound is dressed antiseptically. Not unfrequently such incisions give immediate relief, pain, fever, and meningeal symptoms disappearing.

In the case of perforation of the membrana tympani the discharge soon diminishes by regular cleansing and employment of the air-douche. After it has ceased, the perforation begins to close. Whenever the most violent acute inflammatory symptoms have subsided, the insufflation of boracic acid may be commenced, which, without irritating, reduces the secretion and accelerates the cure. Strong astringents must not be used early. However, when pain is absent, and when the exudation has been thoroughly removed, they may be employed, being instilled in the form of a weak solution, as of sulphate of zinc (0·1 : 10—20). The entrance of instillations into the tympanic cavity is facilitated by pressure upon the tragus. In the same manner weak astringent solutions are effective when injected through the Eustachian tube by means of the catheter in cases where the membrana tympani has not been perforated.

When the symptoms indicate danger, namely, violent headache, stupor and high fever, due to the retention of pus in the mastoid cells or in the tympanic cavity, it may at once become necessary, after blood-letting and the air-douche have proved quite useless, to trephine the mastoid process, even although its outer surface is sound.

Acute naso-pharyngeal catarrh accompanying inflammation of the middle ear should be treated with gargles or inhalations by means of Siegle's well-known steam spray ; 1—2 per cent. solutions of the chloride or bicarbonate of soda or chlorate of potassium are used. At an advanced stage the application of borax as snuff is very efficacious. In the early stage of naso-pharyngeal catarrh, injections into the nose, or painting and cauterisation, should not be resorted to, as the inflammation may be increased thereby.

When the inflammatory symptoms in the ear have disappeared, but the exudation still continues, the remedies which will be detailed under chronic suppuration of the middle ear should be employed.

According to Burckhardt-Merian, the treatment of diphtheritic inflammation should consist in removing the tough fibrous coagula from the external meatus by the loop-snare or the curette, what remains being dissolved with a 10 per cent. solution of salicylic acid in spirit, or pure powdered salicylic acid may be insufflated. In addition, the meatus should be syringed several times daily with a 10 per cent. solution of salicylic acid and spirit in the proportion of 1—2 teaspoonfuls in 100 gms. of water. Under this 'unfortunately rather painful' treatment, the diphtheritic process is generally arrested in the course of a week, and the perforation closes with astonishing rapidity. Gottstein promotes the detachment and removal of the membranous coagula in a simpler and less painful manner by ear-baths of lime water. Moos and Wolf obtained good results from subcutaneous injections of pilocarpine (0·005—0·01 gm. at a time, once or twice daily). By this treatment a great quantity of watery discharge takes place, the process takes a favourable course, and the hearing is rapidly improved.

In cases of necrosis of the ossicles, the suppuration is sometimes kept up in consequence of their presence in the tympanum after becoming detached. The author has repeatedly succeeded in raising the ossicles with the probe from the situation into which they had sunk in the deep part of the tympanum, and then removing them by means of the syringe.

CONTRACTION AND CLOSURE OF THE EUSTACHIAN TUBE.

Acute as well as chronic inflammation of the middle ear is very frequently accompanied by catarrhal inflammation of the mucous membrane of the naso-pharynx. In both cases the catarrhal affection extends into the Eustachian tubes. It frequently occurs, however, especially in children, that the Eustachian tubes are affected without a simultaneous affection of the middle ear, only a mechanical interference with the function of the latter arising in consequence of a disturbance in the ventilation. According to Bezold, more than one half of the diseases of the Eustachian tubes occur in children.

Among the most important and most common diseases of the

ear are those which disturb or suspend the ventilation by the tubes, in consequence of contraction or closure. When the renewal of air between the tympanic cavity and the atmosphere through the tubes ceases, the quantity of air contained in the tympanum diminishes due to exchange of gases, and resulting in a preponderance of atmospheric pressure upon the outer surface of the membrana tympani, driving it inwards. Through the medium of the malleus the ossicula are also forced inwards, and the stapes is pressed into the fenestra ovalis. The dulness of hearing thus occasioned is generally very great. In addition, although not always, tinnitus and a feeling of stoppage and obstruction is complained of.

The causes which produce contraction or closure of the Eustachian tube are the following :—

1. Swelling of the mucous membrane in its whole extent or only in isolated parts. The pathological changes which cause swelling in the case of acute catarrh are hyperæmia and œdema, and, in chronic catarrh, infiltration of cells and new formation of connective tissue. The glandular structures situated in the mucous membrane of the tube, and consisting of adenoid tissue and acinose glands, play an important part in these changes. Especially in the middle part of the cartilaginous tube, these glands are present in such abundance that they occupy the whole thickness of the mucous membrane. According to Gerlach, this aggregation of glands should be called 'the tonsils of the tube,' corresponding with the tonsils of the pharynx. Swelling of the mucous membrane of the tube is almost without exception the consequence of naso-pharyngeal catarrh. Most frequently the tubes are implicated in syphilitic affections of the pharynx.

2. Closure of the tube, especially at its orifice, by products of secretion. The ventilation may be obstructed by viscid and inspissated secretion. Obstruction may also occur when its walls adhere together by means of secretion so that the lumen cannot be restored by the action of the muscles.

3. Not unfrequently contraction or closure is produced, without disease of the tube itself, by pressure of the surrounding structures upon its orifice. This may result from hypertrophy of the pharyngeal tonsils and of the glandular layer in Rosenmüller's fossa,

and from so-called 'adenoid growths' in the naso-pharynx. It is also caused by swelling of the posterior extremity of the inferior turbinated body, which may increase in bulk to such a degree that it covers the orifice of the tube. Growths encroaching upon the naso-pharynx from the nose, or developing there, affect the tubes in the same way. Swelling of the soft palate and of the tonsils is also concerned in constriction of the Eustachian tubes, but such a narrowing appears to be caused by a simultaneous affection of the tubes rather than by mechanical pressure; at least, it is frequently observed that there is no dulness of hearing even with the greatest hypertrophy of the tonsils.

4. Dieffenbach designates that condition of the tube observed in cases of atony of the muscles, and especially in cases of cleft palate, as 'collapse of the mouth of the tube.' As in these last cases the points of insertion for the muscles are wanting, the latter do not act upon the tube, and dilatation does not take place. But it must be noted that in most cases of cleft palate there is no dulness of hearing. Indeed, it is assumed by many that collapse of the walls of the tube happens also in other affections of the soft palate, especially in paretic conditions, but this diagnosis cannot always be made with certainty. The amount of resistance which the soft palate in its action offers to the influence of air-pressure can best be ascertained by the manometer. Von Tröltsch believes that defective action of the muscles may occur as a consequence of chronic pharyngeal catarrh.

5. After ulcerative processes, especially in syphilis, the mouth of the tube may be constricted, and even completely obliterated.

The diagnosis of affections of the Eustachian tube, without simultaneous disease of the tympanic cavity, is based upon the observation of the condition of the membrana tympani, and whether any marked improvement or complete recovery of hearing takes place after the air-douche.

On examination, the tympanic membrane is observed to be drawn inward in its whole extent, but retains its transparent character with smooth lustrous surface. (Fig. 34, normal membrana tympani; Fig. 35, the same, indrawn.) When the whole membrane is greatly indrawn, the handle of the malleus, being directed inward and backward, also assumes a more horizontal position, and appears shortened in perspective. The closer application of the membrane to the malleus causes the latter to project more strongly, its short process protruding like a white thorn. The folds are also well observed, extending from the short process forward and backward to the superior margin of the membrana tympani. The posterior fold is generally more prominent. Sometimes the membrane is closely applied to the articulation of the malleus and incus, which can be recognised as a white knob-like projection in the posterior-superior quadrant. When the central portion of the membrane lies upon the promontory it appears of a yellowish colour. As the extreme border of the membrane is of a somewhat firmer structure, it offers greater resistance to the atmospheric pressure. This causes a slight depression all round its periphery, to which Politzer first called attention, the extreme margin appearing less indrawn than the rest of the membrane. When an inward curvature exists for a long time, the continued stretching of the membrane produces thinning, especially in the posterior-superior quadrant. After the air-douche the thinned parts sometimes bulge out toward the meatus like vesicles, and may be mistaken for cicatrices. By the action of the air-douche, the membrana tympani, along with the handle of the malleus, regains the normal position, and the membrane at first protrudes even farther outward than the malleus, so that the latter is seen less distinctly. The surface of the membrane loses its smoothness and lustre, for, having been previously over-stretched, it now becomes shrivelled.

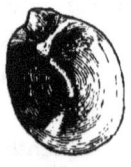 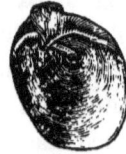

FIG. 34.   FIG. 35.

In the majority of cases, however, the effect of the narrowing of the Eustachian tube upon the middle ear is not purely mechanical. It becomes inflamed; hyperæmia, exudation, and processes of thickening set in, which will be discussed afterwards. Inward curvature of the membrane of long standing may cause contraction of the tensor tympani muscle, with secondary retraction of its tendon (Politzer).

The degree of narrowing or permeability of the tubes can be ascertained by measuring the pressure which is necessary to propel air into the tympanic cavity during an act of swallowing. While, as we have already seen, only slight pressure is required in the normal state, air will enter the tympanum only under a pressure of 100—200 mm. of mercury when the tubes are contracted, and it is quite impossible to force air into the tympanic cavity by Politzer's method, catheterism being necessary. When air passes through the catheter into the tympanum with slight pressure it may be concluded that the obstruction has its seat at the mouth of the tube. But when the current of air which is forced through the catheter, whose beak is inserted into the orifice of the tube, meets with considerable resistance, an obstruction may be assumed in the innermost portion of the tube.

The diagnosis of obstruction to the ventilation caused by defective action of the muscles of the tubes and the soft palate may be ascertained by observing the imperfect elevation of the soft palate during the acts of swallowing and speaking. But paresis of the muscles of the soft palate may also be ascertained by the manometer in the manner indicated by the author.[1] If during articulation, especially of the vowels, the air pass freely or with very slight pressure toward the inferior portion of the pharynx, it may be concluded that the action of the muscles is defective. If, on the other hand, the soft palate resist a pressure of 40—100 mm. of mercury its condition may be assumed as normal.

In order to ascertain thoroughly the state of the tubes they must be examined with the probe or with bougies, according to the method already described (p. 51). According to Urbantschitsch,[2] a constriction may exist, generally at the isthmus tubæ, while the permeability is apparently unimpaired.

The symptoms, especially dulness of hearing, caused by acute catarrh, usually appear very rapidly, so that, according to the statements of patients, the disease sets in quite suddenly. But the symptoms disappear just as quickly when the catarrh has subsided, as a powerful act of swallowing, blowing the nose, sneezing, or yawning is quite sufficient to make the tube again permeable. The entrance of air is generally accompanied by a crack or a report

---

[1] *Centralblatt für die med. Wissenchaften*, No. 15, 1880.
[2] *Wiener med. Presse*, Nos. 1, 2, and 3, 1883.

in the ear, and complete recovery may then take place. Sometimes this improvement is only of short duration, and the symptoms return after absorption of the air which had entered through the tubes. These symptoms continue until air again enters in sufficient quantity, and they then permanently disappear. In cases, however, in which a process of thickening of the mucous membrane has occurred, the vibratory power of the sound-conducting apparatus may be permanently impaired.

Complete closure of the Eustachian tube cannot be diagnosed, as was formerly done, from failure of the air-douche and bougies; the defective condition of its orifice should rather be ascertained by means of rhinoscopy.

Total closure is somewhat rare, and has been chiefly observed as a consequence of syphilis, with loss of a portion of the cartilage of the tube. Such cases have been described by Gruber, Lindenbaum, and Dennert (closure on both sides). The author also observed a case in which there was complete absence of the orifice of the tube, and of the inner extremity of its cartilaginous portion. The hearing distance for the watch was $\frac{20}{120}$ cm.; for loud speech, 3 m. In Dennert's case[1] the dulness of hearing was more marked, but he was successful in effecting a permanent improvement by incision of the membrana tympani and by the air-douche applied from the external meatus.

Treatment.—The first indication in treatment is to improve the hearing by forcing air into the tympanic cavity. In the slighter cases the obstruction to the passage of air is inconsiderable. The author, in the course of his air-pressure experiments, was astonished on observing that in Politzerising a pressure of 60—80 mm. of mercury is frequently sufficient to force air into the tympanic cavities, while in other cases, especially in opening the tubes for the first time, a much higher pressure is necessary. As pain is occasioned especially in the case of children, when the air-douche is applied under high pressure, and as great force is not required, and may prove injurious, the author considers it important that it should be applied with the least possible pressure. When the cause of obstruction to the ventilation consists only in accumulation

[1] *Deutsche Zeitschrift für praktische Medicin*, No. 44, 1878.

of mucus in the tubes, or agglutination of their walls, one or a few applications of the air-douche, either by Politzer's method, or, as is more rarely necessary, by the catheter, are sufficient to produce a complete cure.

It often happens that an apparent cure is produced by regular repetition of the air-douche, but when this treatment is discontinued, the dulness of hearing returns. This proves that the tubes have not yet been made permeable to the free passage of air, and that conditions still exist which require direct treatment.

When the swelling is of such recent occurrence, that it may be assumed no extensive infiltration has yet taken place, injections of astringent lotions may be employed, as a solution of sulphate of zinc (0·1 : 10—20 aq. destill.). When the inflammation is of longer duration, especially when the appearance of the mucous membrane of the pharynx indicates that the glandular structures of the mucous covering of the tubes are also implicated, stronger remedies must be used. In such cases the author uses either a solution of nitrate of silver (0·5 : 10—30 aq. destill.), or more frequently a solution of iodine and glycerine (potassii iodidi, 3 ; iodi puri, 0·3 ; glycer. pur. 10—30). The injection is made as follows :—A few drops of the solution are instilled into the catheter, and injected into the Eustachian tube by a weak pressure upon the air-bag, so as to prevent the fluid from entering into the tympanic cavity. Cauterisation is also performed by means of solid nitrate of silver, melted upon a thick silver wire and introduced through the catheter.

It is of great importance to treat simultaneous catarrhs of the mucous membrane of the nose and pharynx by means of the nasal douche, gargles, solutions applied with a brush, and cauterisation. These conditions also call for treatment which arise from pressure of the surrounding parts upon the orifices of the tubes, interfering with the ventilation, especially swellings and growths in the nasopharynx, hypertrophied pharyngeal tonsils, adenoid growths, and nasal polypi.

In the case of swollen conditions of the tube, as well as in exudative catarrh of the middle ear, the nose must always be most carefully examined ; for not unfrequently we find swellings at the posterior extremities of the lower turbinated body which cause ear disease, although the patients do not complain of any symptoms affecting the nose.

Most frequently the application of solutions with a brush, gargles, and inhalations are employed. For the first mentioned a solution of nitrate of silver (1 : 20—50), or solutions of iodine and glycerine, are used. Gargles act, on the one hand, upon the mucous membrane itself, and, on the other, they invigorate the muscles of the tubes and the soft palate, when the act of swallowing is simultaneously performed (Von Tröltsch). Solutions used for this purpose contain chlorate of potassium, alum, or tannin ($\frac{1}{2}$—2 per cent.). In order to act directly upon the muscles, the electric current, especially the induced current, is employed, by placing the one electrode externally upon the neck, while the other is placed in the mouth, upon the lower surface of the soft palate. Besides this, a wire, furnished at its end with a thin knob, may be passed through the tympanic tube (Paukenröhrchen), and made to act as an electrode. The tympanic tube thus armed is introduced through the catheter into the Eustachian tube, and in this way a direct action upon the latter is obtained. The swelling in the nose must be removed by the galvano-cautery, chromic acid, the cold snare, or in some other suitable manner.

Although the employment of bougies for dilating the tubes, to which the older aurists so frequently resorted, has almost been abandoned, they have recently been very highly recommended again by Urbantschitsch. He considers 'bougieing' of the Eustachian tubes to be indicated in all cases of chronic affections of the middle ear, in which, along with the symptoms of dulness of hearing and tinnitus, the lumen of the isthmus tubæ is less than $1\frac{1}{2}$—$1\frac{1}{3}$ mm. Not unfrequently 'bougieing' produces a better result than the air-douche. The success depends not only upon the fact that after 'bougieing' the air-douche is more effective, but because, as Urbantschitsch assumes in accordance with his experiments, the stimulation of the sensory twigs of the trigeminus in the tube, resulting from the 'bougieing,' has a reflex influence upon the sense of hearing.

The treatment of cicatricial formations is the most difficult. The older aural surgeons devised sharp instruments, which they introduced into the Eustachian tubes in order to incise the anterior wall. But good permanent results cannot be obtained thereby.

When the walls of the tube have become completely united, the condition may be alleviated by perforating the membrana tympani, and forcing air into the tympanic cavity by compressing the air in the external meatus. In this way, even although the artificial opening closes again, a permanent improvement may be effected. An attempt may be made to keep the perforation in the membrana tympani permanently open by extirpation of the malleus.

ABNORMAL PATENCY OF THE EUSTACHIAN TUBES.

(SYNONYMS: *Tympanophony*, *Autophony*.)

Generally, when the muscles of the tubes and the soft palate are at rest, and deglutition is avoided, even under very considerable pressure (100—200 mm. of mercury), no air passes through the tubes into the tympanic cavity; but, as the author has shown by experiments in the pneumatic cabinet, exceptional cases are found in which the passage of air takes place under slight pressure. In such cases, even by the Valsalvian experiment, the air passes through the tubes with very little pressure, and movements of the membrana tympani corresponding with inspiration and expiration can be observed, a free passage of air taking place between the tympanic cavity and the pharynx during respiration. Under such conditions it may happen that the tubes become temporarily more patent, and the symptoms called 'tympanophony' or 'autophony' arise, consisting of very much augmented loudness of the speaker's own voice, the sounds entering his ear with such intensity that pain is occasioned (Rüdinger). Jago reports that he suffers occasionally from undue patency of one of his Eustachian tubes, when he notices that the membrana tympani is forced outward with every expiration, and he hears his own voice much louder. Flemming can open his tubes by voluntary contraction of the muscles, and thus produce tympanophony, when every inspiration and expiration is accompanied by a loud rushing noise, and during phonation he hears a peculiar loud sound like the ringing of a bell. The author observed the symptoms of tympanophony in the case of an actress, who, when upon the stage and while playing her part, suddenly heard her own voice resounding unpleasantly loud in her ear, which greatly disturbed and annoyed her. After this had continued for a short time the normal condition returned.

In other cases autophony becomes permanent. The speaker's own voice enters the ear with a trumpet-like, pealing sound, and a loud rushing noise is perceived in the ear with every inspiration and expiration. Persons troubled in this way produce by their own speech such very disagreeable sensations that they carefully avoid speaking loudly. Brunner first drew attention to the fact that autophony is chiefly observed during phonation of the so-called 'resonants,' the consonants *m*, *n*, and *ng* (see p. 60). According to Brunner's observations, which the author has confirmed, autophony does not exist in a recumbent position or when the head is bent forward. As the valve-like closure of the tubes is effected by apposition of the anterior-inferior membranous wall of the tube to the cartilaginous roof, all processes which lead to lessening the bulk or elasticity of this wall may cause undue patency of the tubes and autophony. Such conditions may occur in acute and chronic inflammation of the naso-pharynx and the middle ear. The author has also observed it in cases where the general health was greatly reduced.[1]

A patient, whose constitution had been greatly reduced in consequence of extensive pneumonia, was troubled with autophony, which, however, disappeared when his strength returned. The author, therefore, concludes that in such cases the undue patency is occasioned by diminished bulk of the soft tissues situated below the cartilaginous portion of the tubes.

In order to convince himself whether tympanophony is caused by abnormal patency of the Eustachian tube, Poorten introduced into its orifice a catheter, perforated on the convex surface of the beak. When this perforation was closed the tympanophony ceased, but returned as soon as it was opened.

The prognosis is generally unfavourable, especially when atrophy

---

[1] Mitteilung in der otologischen Sektion der Naturforscherversammlung in Freiburg, 1883.

has been the cause, while in the cases of catarrh and a weakened state of the system the prospect of recovery is good.

Autophony is of rare occurrence; the author only observed it three times in more than 6000 patients.

Treatment.—When abnormal patency of the tubes arises from catarrhal conditions, treatment should be carried out in the manner already described, and the general health must be attended to. By various means which reduce swelling of the mucous membrane—the nasal douche, injections, or insufflations—autophony may be temporarily removed, but it returns when the swelling subsides. To render this symptom less troublesome to the patient, the author has found instillation of glycerine into the auditory meatus and firm plugging very useful. When the autophony is exceedingly troublesome, recourse may be had to closure of the Eustachian tube by inserting short catheter-like instruments.

NEUROSES OF THE MUSCLES.

Disturbances of the innervation and clonic spasms of the muscles of the ear belong to the class of affections which come under observation exceedingly seldom. The tensor tympani muscle, and the stapedius, as well as the muscles of the tubes, may be affected. Temporary spasms of the tensor tympani are sometimes observed after manipulations, especially after catheterism. They produce a series of crackling noises, which can also be perceived objectively. It has been already stated (p. 55) that Bremer[1] has related a case in which a person could produce the sound by voluntary contraction of the muscles 100—150 times per minute. As a rule, contractions of the tensor are accompanied by clonic spasms of the soft palate, or of the extrinsic muscles of the larynx. Schwartze observed in a patient a rapid succession of crackling noises synchronous with contractions of the soft palate. He simultaneously observed inward movements of the membrana tympani. In a case related by Böck, the noise and the elevation of the palate were synchronous with the pulse, without any movements of the membrana

[1] *Monatsschrift für Ohrenheilkunde*, No. 10, 1879.

tympani, which were also absent in a case described by Politzer, who succeeded in removing the noise by the faradic current.

Lucae first pointed out that, by a strong contraction of the facial muscles, especially of the orbicularis palpebrarum, the stapedius, which is partly supplied by the facial nerve, can also be made to contract. According to Hitzig, a low humming sound is thereby occasioned in the ear. During the spasm of the facial nerve sensations of sound were also observed at the same time, and we must assume that they were caused by the stapedius taking part in the spasm. In a female patient of Gottstein's,[1] attacks of blepharospasm were preceded by an intolerable rushing noise in both ears, which afterwards became continuous. As long as the finger was pressed upon a certain spot at the anterior-inferior part of the mastoid process, the tinnitus stopped, as also when the faradic current was applied, which permanently removed the noise. The author has observed mimicked facial spasm in the case of a female, who heard the rattling of a mill or the rustling of the wings of a large bird flying slowly. These different sensations afterwards changed into a deep humming noise. The induced as well as constant current had no effect in this case. According to Brunner,[2] a deep fluttering noise, like a bird with powerful wings rustling past our ears, occurs sometimes with glad surprises and in moments of deep emotion. The sensation of the rustling of wings corresponds with the duration of the different muscular contractions.

FOREIGN BODIES IN THE EUSTACHIAN TUBE.

The following cases of foreign bodies in the Eustachian tube have been observed. Fleischmann, at the autopsy on a man who had suffered for a long time from tinnitus, found a barleycorn in the tube. Heckscher discovered a raven's feather in it. Andry relates a case where an *ascaris lumbricoides* had travelled through the tube into the tympanic cavity, causing the most excessive pain. Reynolds recently described a case in which several *ascares lumbricoides* passed from the naso-pharynx out through the ear, the membrana tympani having been destroyed. After

---

[1] *Archiv für Ohrenheilkunde*, vol. xvi. p. 63.
[2] *Zeitschrift für Ohrenheilkunde*, vol. x. p. 176.

Schwartze had introduced laminaria bougies for the treatment of constriction of the tubes, it repeatedly happened that parts of them broke off and remained in the tubes (Mayer, Hinton). Meissner and Voltolini have described polypi, which had their roots in the tympanic cavity, and extended into the tubes. With these may be included plugs of inspissated cerumen, which sometimes close the tubes. Semeleder describes an interesting case of this kind observed by Dauscher. A yellowish-grey plug was discovered by means of the rhinoscope protruding 7 mm. from the orifice of the tube, and removed by syringing through the catheter. After its removal the patient was seized with pain and vertigo, preceded by a report as of a cannon, and the hearing was at once restored. While Schalle was applying the nasal douche by means of a vulcanite syringe, a small piece of vulcanite was broken off, 6 mm. long, and 1·5 mm. thick, and got into the tympanic cavity, where it set up acute inflammation, and was removed through the external meatus after perforation of the membrana tympani. Urbantschitsch describes an interesting case, in which the branch of a panicle of corn, 3 cm. long, travelled from the mouth to the pharynx, and through the Eustachian tube into the tympanic cavity, continuing its way into the external meatus after inflammation and perforation of the membrane, whence the patient removed it with a hair-pin. He relates another case communicated by Albers, in which a needle passed from the external meatus into the pharynx and was vomited.

CHRONIC CATARRH OF THE MIDDLE EAR WITHOUT PERFORATION OF THE MEMBRANA TYMPANI.

(SYNONYMS: *Otitis media catarrhalis chronica; Exudation in the middle ear.*)

The exudative form of chronic inflammation of the middle ear, without perforation of the membrana tympani, occurs either independently or in consequence of constitutional affections, more particularly the acute exanthemata. With trifling local symptoms, the lining membrane of the tympanic cavity assumes the condition of chronic inflammation, accompanied by hyperæmia, swelling, and increased secretion. This disease also appears very frequently along with catarrh of the mucous membrane of the naso-pharynx and affections of the

Eustachian tubes. In such cases the dulness of hearing is greater than in simple catarrh of the tube, and is only slightly improved by the air-douche. The exudation may also remain in consequence of acute catarrh or acute inflammation becoming chronic, because, after all the inflammatory symptoms have subsided, the exudation may neither become absorbed nor escape through the Eustachian tube.

The character of the accumulation cannot be inferred from the manner in which it originated. It may be either serous or mucous, whether the exudation has been caused by acute catarrh of the middle ear, with or without naso-pharyngeal catarrh, or whether it has occurred independently. Out of 97 cases of chronic accumulation of exudation, Schwartze,[1] after paracentesis, found it to be serous in 8, muco-serous in 14, purely mucous in 67, and muco-purulent in 8 cases. In cases of very long standing, the accumulation is most frequently of a mucous character. This mucus is as a rule viscid, consistent, and colourless.

Politzer in particular, to whose description we substantially adhere, has done much to define the appearances of the membrana tympani, and to explain their significance. When the tympanic cavity is entirely filled with exudation, the colour of the membrane appears darker and more deeply impregnated in the tissues, and frequently a faint bottle-green tint is added to its grey colour. From muco-purulent exudation this darker colouring receives a yellowish tinge, which is most marked behind the umbo in the region of the promontory. This yellowish colour, which is caused by the exudation shining through the membrane, may be mistaken for the appearance which the membrane presents when it lies upon the promontory in cases where it is greatly indrawn. If there be any doubt, the diagnosis can be established by carefully touching the membrane with the probe. When only a slight quantity of secretion is present in the tympanic cavity, the membrana tympani, if not opaque, exhibits a sharply defined line, representing the level of the fluid, as was first recognised by Politzer, but which comes very rarely under observation. By bending the head backward or forward, this line alters its position

[1] *Archiv für Ohrenheilkunde*, vol. vi. p. 182.

according to the change in the level of the exudation. The portion of the membrane lying below the line is of a dark colour, while above it the colouring is light, due to the air-space behind. After the air-douche, bubbles can be observed. When the membrane is opaque, no information regarding the presence of exudation can be obtained.

The membrana tympani varies very much in appearance. It is strongly indrawn in the case of constriction of the tubes or obstruction by a slight quantity of viscid secretion, and uniformly flat, especially when the latter is copious and muco-purulent. The most flaccid portion of the membrane, the posterior-superior quadrant, in the presence of a very large amount of exudation, projects strongly, sometimes resembling a semi-globular cyst. In this way the membrane assumes the appearance which was described as occurring after the action of the air-douche, in the case of atrophy of the membrana tympani, resulting from obstructed ventilation.

Auscultation is not always a certain test with regard to the presence of exudation in the tympanic cavity. The râles which are heard may be caused by mucus driven from the tubes into the tympanum. When the accumulation of mucus in the tympanum is of a viscid character, no râles will be heard. On the other hand, from the very distinct sound caused by the air striking against the walls of the tympanum, a conclusion may be drawn that no exudation is present. The most reliable test, however, is an exploratory incision in the tympanic membrane, which may be made without fear of injurious effects.

An accumulation of exudation in the tympanic cavity, especially when complicated with swelling of the Eustachian tube and abnormal tension of the sound-conducting parts, produces a very marked degree of dulness of hearing. The labyrinth may remain unaffected, while the bone-conduction may be quite perfect. Not unfrequently peculiar noises are heard in the ear, such as crackling, rattling, or snapping. When the head is moved, the sensation is sometimes felt as if something were moving backward and forward in the ear. In many cases the hearing is considerably improved while lying, and becomes worse again on assuming the upright position, such symptoms being caused by the movements of the exudation in the tympanic cavity. The other subjective sensations of hearing vary; sometimes, however, tinnitus and vertigo are present in a high degree.

Purulent exudation may lead to caries of the walls of the tympanum, without perforation of the membrane, and may prove fatal by extension to the cranial cavity. Most frequently such purulent accumulations are found in cases of pulmonary phthisis and after typhoid fever. Muco-purulent exudations occur with astonishing frequency in the tympanic cavities of newly-born children.

Treatment.—The treatment has for its objects, (1) removal of the exudation, (2) of its causes, and (3) improvement of the condition of the mucous membrane.

In many cases a thorough removal of the exudation is sufficient to bring about a permanent cure. But if the causes which originated the accumulation remain unchecked, the exudation will continue. This is especially the case in affections arising from naso-pharyngeal catarrh, with swelling of the Eustachian tube. The exudation may be removed in various ways. While air is injected through the tube into the tympanic cavity, the head of the patient being inclined forward and toward the opposite side (Politzer), the exudation is thereby displaced, and passes into the naso-pharynx. This method is more successful when the exudation consists of thin fluid, in which case the air-douche being repeated several times will effect its complete removal. The difficulty is increased by simultaneous swelling of the tube; and, when the exudation is thick and viscid, its removal by the above method is impossible, so that paracentesis [1] of the membrana tympani is necessitated. After making an ample opening, the exudation should be driven into the external meatus by means of the air-douche, which in many cases, however, is not sufficient, and the removal can only be effected by injecting tepid salt water (1 per cent.) through the

---

[1] Frank, in his text-book (*Erlangen*, 1845), laid down the rule of practice always to perforate the membrana tympani when the symptoms pointed to a mucous accumulation in the middle ear. In addition, he recommended paracentesis in cases of impermeability of the Eustachian tube, of hæmorrhage into the tympanic cavity, and of thickening of the tympanic membrane. Thus the indications for this operation were the same then as now. Fabricius considered the operation also necessary for diagnostic purposes.

catheter (Schwartze), but inflammation is frequently occasioned thereby.

Some have proposed to remove the exudation by suction, either from the meatus through an artificial perforation in the membrana tympani (Hinton, Schalle), or from the Eustachian tube. For the former purpose Pravaz's syringe, with a thin tube for a nozzle, or some other instrument, such as Schalle's exudation-aspirator, is employed. For the latter purpose, the so-called 'tympanic tube' (Paukenröhrchen) may be passed through the catheter into the tympanic cavity (Weber-Liel). Both methods are seldom employed, because, when the exudation is thin, they are not necessary, and when it is of thick consistence, it is too viscid to be removed through a very narrow tube even by applying strong suction. In order to effect the thorough removal of the deposits of secretion the metal tympanic tube should be used, of which a detailed description will be given under the head of chronic purulent inflammation of the middle ear.

The membrana tympani knife used for performing paracentesis (see page 138) is employed after anæsthetising the membrane. To facilitate the escape of the exudation, the perforation is made in the inferior half of the membrane, generally in its posterior part. By the subsequent employment of the air-douche or syringing, sometimes large masses of thickened secretion are discharged from the tympanic cavity and the mastoid process. As a rule, the perforation closes after a few days, and only remains for a longer period when reactive inflammation sets in. During the first few days after paracentesis and removal of exudation, the air-douche is employed in order to expel any remaining fluid, and to re-establish the membrane in its normal position. Inflammatory reaction only occurs in rare cases, generally on the second or third day, and as a rule quickly disappears.

The simultaneous swelling of the Eustachian tube, which sometimes causes obstruction of the ventilation, must be treated in the manner already described. Diseases of the nose and of the nasopharynx must be specially attended to.

In order to promote the absorption of any remaining exudation, we inject through the Eustachian tube alkaline solutions, consisting of bicarbonate of soda (1 : 100 aq. destill.), or preferably liquor potassæ (gtt. 3 : 30 aq. destill.). For hyperæmic swelling, astringents are used, such as sulphate of zinc (0·1—0·2 : 20 aq. destill.).

CHRONIC PURULENT INFLAMMATION OF THE MIDDLE EAR.

(SYNONYM : *Otitis media purulenta chronica.*)

When the discharge from the ear is of a purulent character, we infer, in the majority of cases, that we have to deal with disease of the tympanic cavity, along with more or less destruction of the membrana tympani. Only in a very small number of cases does the exudation originate in the external meatus from independent inflammation.

The most frequent cause of chronic suppuration is acute inflammation of the middle ear, which, in consequence of insufficient treatment and the long-continued action of injurious influences, along with unfavourable constitutional conditions, degenerates into the chronic form. The cure of acute inflammation is rendered particularly difficult when the membrana tympani has been destroyed to any considerable extent, as is often the case, in the exanthemata. In the majority of cases, therefore, scarlet and typhoid fever, and measles, are given in the history of cases as the cause of the disease.

The character of the discharge varies, being sero-purulent, muco-purulent, and purulent. On examination it is frequently found that the whole external meatus is filled with the exudation, which is either of uniform consistence or mixed with inspissated masses, or detached epithelium. In many cases the discharge is exceedingly profuse, so that the plugs of cotton-wool which are inserted are very often saturated with it and have to be changed frequently. In other cases it is very slight, so that on examination only a small quantity of pus is found at the bottom of the meatus or in the tympanic cavity. When the discharge is obstructed, as by small perforations, swelling, or polypi, it becomes inspissated, in course of time forming crumbling, shreddy masses, mixed with thin purulent fluid. These masses are to be found especially in the superior and posterior parts of the tympanic cavity, as well as in the antrum mastoideum.

The exudation from the middle ear, when exposed to the atmosphere and still under the influence of the temperature of the body, presents a very favourable soil for putrefactive processes, organisms being developed which are always present in enormous amount in fœtid exudation products.

The odour of the exudation is of a sweetish putrid character, and, in the case of old-standing otorrhœa, is exceedingly disagreeable. When putrefaction sets in, the smell becomes very pungent, like rotten cheese. In such cases it often happens that the silver probe assumes a brown colour, due to the action of sulphuretted hydrogen. On account of the disgusting odour of the discharge, a patient suffering from otorrhœa is frequently avoided. In many cases such patients complain both of a disagreeable smell and taste, on account of the matter flowing through the Eustachian tube into the pharynx. In this way the digestion may be affected.

Perforations of the membrana tympani vary greatly in extent, being scarcely the size of a pin-head in some cases, while in others the whole membrane is destroyed. Generally, there is only one perforation, rarely two or more. In the case of large perforations, the border of the membrane is generally preserved, remnants of it being left at both sides of the handle of the malleus, which is frequently drawn inward to such an extent that it assumes a horizontal position, and on examination only the strongly projecting short process can be seen. Sometimes, however, the malleus retains its normal position, and projects freely downwards. The remains of the membrane are usually thickened, and frequently contain calcareous deposits. Variations likewise occur in the appearance of its surface, the whole membrane, or only portions of it, being drawn inward, and it is frequently adherent to the inner wall of the tympanic cavity.

After removing the exudation, the small perforations appear black and sharply defined when examined with ordinary light; but when they are large the mucous membrane of the tympanum is visible in the background. Chronic inflammation produces in the mucous membrane hyperæmic swelling, cell infiltration, and new growth of connective tissue, either a uniform swelling occurring with a smooth surface, or circumscribed hypertrophy in various parts, producing a granular appearance of the surface. In many cases the mucous membrane is atrophied. In order to ascertain the condition of the mucous membrane, the probe may be employed.

Perforations of Shrapnell's membrane[1] require special attention. In the anatomical review of the middle ear, we have drawn attention to the cellular spaces (Politzer) between the upper part of the head of the malleus, on the one hand, and Shrapnell's membrane and the outer wall of the vault of the tympanum, on the other. In these spaces, suppuration, caseous deposits, granulations, and caries may exist. In most cases disease of this part of the tympanum remains after the other parts have been cured, and may produce headache, vertigo, giddiness, and even symptoms of paralysis. Granulations and carious spots can be discovered by means of the probe. In the great majority of cases no free communication with the tympanic cavity is possible, so that the air-douche is ineffective in forcing air or exudation into the external meatus. When the perforation in Shrapnell's membrane is accompanied by purulent inflammation of the tympanum and of the cells of the mastoid process, complications, to be afterwards discussed, may arise in consequence of obstruction to the escape of the discharge. In a case observed by the author an enormous abscess formed over the mastoid process. An opening having been made, a sequestrum was found in the antrum mastoideum, the cavity itself as well as the tympanum being filled with a caseous substance. Death ensued with meningitic symptoms.

In the normal state the mucous membrane of the tympanic cavity is protected by the membrana tympani against external influences; but when this structure is absent, it is exposed. Not unfrequently, therefore, in the course of chronic suppuration of the middle ear, acute exacerbations occur. While these attacks

---

[1] See Burnett, *American Journal of Otology*, vol. iii. ; Morpurgo and Hessler, *Archiv für Ohrenheilkunde*, vol. xix. and xx.

continue, the exudation is temporarily diminished; but on the second or third day it becomes more copious than ever. The tympanic cavity and the membrane are inflamed afresh; intense pain sets in at the same time, accompanied by tinnitus, pulsation, and increased dulness of hearing. Such reactive inflammation is often the consequence of treatment, and occurs after operations or irritating applications. Even when the inflammation of the mucous membrane has entirely subsided, a disposition to renewed attacks of the disease remains in the case of loss of substance of the membrana tympani. Most frequently such an attack is caused by the entrance of cold water into the meatus while bathing or washing.

In purulent inflammation of the middle ear, the dulness of hearing depends partly only upon the size of the perforation of the membrana tympani. It depends chiefly upon the remaining degree of vibratory power of the labyrinthine fenestræ, so that very great dulness of hearing may exist with a small perforation, while, on the other hand, when the entire membrane, as well as the malleus and incus are wanting, the hearing may be good. As a rule, the bone-conduction is preserved, and even increased. When it is markedly diminished, it must be concluded that the labyrinth is implicated. The hearing is generally remarkably good in cases of perforation in Shrapnell's membrane.

Subjective noises and pain in the ear are sometimes complained of, but these symptoms are generally absent. They may occur in consequence of extension of the inflammation or destruction, and also, as the author feels justified in inferring from the postmortem examinations he has made, in consequence of processes of condensation in the bone, and sclerosis of the mastoid process. Neuralgia of the trigeminus may also arise in the course of purulent affections of the middle ear, to which Moos first drew attention. It is generally confined to a single branch of the trigeminus—most frequently the first, more rarely the second or third, and always only on the side of the affected ear. According to Moos, neuralgia of the trigeminus occurs with the following ear diseases: acute purulent inflammation of the tympanic cavity, chronic inflammation of the mastoid process without phlebitis of the lateral sinus, and cholesteatoma in the tympanum. In the Otological section of the meeting of the Natural History Congress, in Freiburg, Moos related a case in which neuralgia arose from an exostosis in the external meatus.

Mosler[1] observed a case of very troublesome sneezing, arising from purulent inflammation of the middle ear, about 30 successive paroxysms occurring, with intervals of only a half to one minute. While these attacks lasted the woman was in a most pitiable condition. By pressure upon the inflamed ear, the fits were aggravated; as the ear affection got worse they increased, but occurred seldomer as improvement set in.

Very frequently (in 46 out of 50 cases) Urbantschitsch found anomalies of taste upon the surface of the tongue on the side of the diseased ear, in cases of purulent inflammation of the tympanum, caused by implication of the chorda tympani; even entire loss of taste upon that half of the tongue has been observed. In one case in which the author scraped the stump of a polypus from the posterior margin of the membrana tympani, loss of taste occurred upon the anterior two-thirds of the surface of the tongue on the same side, due to injury of the chorda tympani, which supplies this part of the tongue with gustatory fibres.[2]

From direct irritation of the chorda tympani, as in syringing, insufflation of powders, touching with the probe, and removing polypi, sensations of taste are frequently felt upon the corresponding half of the tongue.

By extension of the inflammation to the canal of the facial nerve, temporary or permanent facial paralysis may be produced. Either infiltration occurs or pressure is exerted upon the nerve from the walls of the canal. In both cases improvement or recovery may take place on abatement of the inflammation, absorption of deposits, or removal of pressure. In severe cases, softening and destruction of the nerve results from the suppuration. When the

---

[1] Virchow's *Archiv*, vol. xiv. p. 557.
[2] 'Die Beziehungen der Chorda Tympani zur Geschmacksperception auf den vorderen zwei Dritteln der Zunge,' von Ed. Schulte, *Zeitschrift für Ohrenheilkunde*, vol. xv. p. 67.

wall of the canal has been destroyed by caries, the prognosis is very unfavourable; but a cure generally takes place after removal of a sequestrum from the mastoid process. The prognosis is more favourable in the case of children than in adults.

Course and results.—The duration of this disease varies; a spontaneous recovery may take place after months or years, or a purulent discharge, varying in quantity, may continue during a whole lifetime. After healing sets in, the swelling of the mucous membrane subsides, the surface is covered with a coarse epithelium, and appears dry and of a light red or yellowish colour. The perforation of the membrana tympani either becomes permanent or closes. Frequently adhesions form with the inner wall of the tympanic cavity. When much destruction of the membrana tympani has occurred, along with loss of the ossicula, the formation of new tissue does not take place, but when the malleus remains as well as the margin of the membrane, even extensive losses of tissue may be replaced by cicatrisation. After healing, the remains of the membrane are generally much thickened, and often contain calcareous deposits. The mobility of the ossicula is markedly diminished or quite abolished, their covering of mucous membrane becoming sclerosed, and anchylosis taking place at the fenestra ovalis. The mucous membrane, likewise, covering the fenestra rotunda may lose its elasticity. In both cases the dulness of hearing is very great.

The prognosis of suppuration in the middle ear depends upon its extent, character, and complications, which latter should be kept in view in every case, and we should remember Wilde's words—'that so long as otorrhœa is present, we can never tell how, when, or where it will end, or what it may lead to.'

A person suffering from purulent inflammation of the middle ear is not eligible for life assurance or military service. A cure having taken place, with closure of the perforation in the tympanic membrane, the disqualification in the way of life assurance or military service does not hold. When a perforation in the membrana tympani becomes permanent, the mucous membrane being dry and of a dermoid character, the tendency to dangerous relapses is very slight, so that such a condition may be considered satisfactory for life assurance at an increased rate and for military service.

The continuance of the discharge from the ear may be caused by irritation of the mucous membrane, from the presence of deposits of matter, mostly in a state of decomposition. Frequently it is kept up by the growth of polypi or disease of the osseous walls (caries or necrosis). In not a few cases purulent inflammation of the middle ear proves fatal by extension to the neighbouring blood-vessels (phlebitis and thrombosis), or to the interior of the cranial cavity (meningitis and abscess of the brain). The occurrence of these complications arises from deposits and stagnation of the products of exudation in the tympanic cavity and its recesses, but especially in the mastoid process.

The following diseases of the ear render a man only conditionally fit for service (for the reserve) according to the regulations of the German Empire as applying to recruits :—' (*d*) Deafness in one ear after exhausted pathological processes ; (*e*) a moderate degree of dulness of hearing in both ears, the hearing distance for whispered speech (see page 24) being about 4 m. to 1 m.

Permanent unfitness is constituted by :—(28) the loss of an auricle ; (29) deafness or incurable dulness of hearing in both ears, the hearing distance being about 1 m. or less ; (30) pathological conditions of the ear which are serious or difficult to cure ; (37) dumbness and deaf-mutism.

Liability for field service of trained soldiers ceases when they become affected with the diseases enumerated above under (*d*) and (*e*). Field and garrison duty also ceases with those quoted under (28), (29), and (30).

Paragraph (30) formerly ran as follows :—' Permanent perforation of the membrana tympani, as well as other pathological conditions of the ear which are serious and difficult to cure.' According to the Annual Report for 1878—79, 462 soldiers in the service had to be dismissed from the Prussian army as unfit, owing to perforation of the membrane. In consequence of the alteration in this paragraph, it is now left to the chief military surgeons to decide whether a disease is dangerous, or only slight and uncomplicated, so that it constitutes no reason for declaring a man unfit who is otherwise healthy and strong. Chief military surgeons are therefore supposed to have acquired an exact knowledge of the pathology of the ear.

Treatment.—See page 181.

DEPOSITS OF EXUDATION PRODUCTS AND FORMATION OF CHOLESTEATOMATA.

Retention and deposits of the products of purulent discharge chiefly take place when its free exit is obstructed, as in cases of small, unfavourably situated perforations in the tympanic membrane, adhesion of the membrane with the inner wall of the tympanic cavity, polypi, and swelling in the tympanum or external meatus. Such obstruction to the discharge from the ear acts like a filter, the more solid constituents remaining behind and the fluid escaping. The pus subsequently becomes inspissated, and forms caseous, crumbling masses.

While the discharge continues, or after it has ceased, *Pearl-tumours* (Perlgeschwülste) and *Cholesteatomata* may form. The pearl-tumours consist of desquamated epithelium, either forming membranous masses, or they are globular in shape, being composed of concentric layers, and vary in size from a pea to a hazel-nut. These tumours contain large nucleated and flat epithelial cells, among which numerous cholesterine crystals may be found. The epithelial masses may be regarded as the product of the desquamative inflammation of the surface of the mucous membrane. Most frequently this desquamation occurs in the antrum mastoideum, more rarely in the tympanum. The deposits of exudation products forming cholesteatomata can generally be observed lying behind the place of constriction, especially in the deepest part of the tympanic cavity, and forming inspissated or membranous masses, which may be loosened with the probe and removed. Sometimes the tympanic cavity and the mastoid antrum are quite filled with these caseous or cholesteatomatous masses. Under these conditions the discharge from the ear is very slight or is absent altogether.

These deposits may produce sclerosis, atrophy from pressure, and caries and necrosis of the osseous walls. They may make their way to the surface of the mastoid process, the meatus, or to the neighbouring blood-vessels and the cranial cavity.

The symptoms arising from the presence of the deposits are a feeling of pressure and heaviness in the head, headache, giddiness, and fever. Frequently acute exacerbations occur with violent pain. After the accumulated masses have been removed, the symptoms disappear, if no further complications set in.

When the escape of the discharge from the ear is completely obstructed, the symptoms become greatly aggravated, namely, excessive pain in the ear and head, symptoms of meningeal irritation, giddiness, and vomiting.

Treatment.—See page 185.

POLYPI.

Aural polypi form chiefly in cases of neglected otorrhœa of long standing. They appear as small nodules upon the walls of the tympanic cavity, or they may fill the whole external meatus. The great majority of polypi originate on the outer wall of the labyrinth. Out of 100 cases, Moos and Steinbrügge[1] observed 75 polypi in that situation and 25 in the external meatus. They rarely arise from the margin of the membrana tympani. Sometimes the ossicula, especially the malleus, are imbedded in the polypous mass. They are attached either by a small, thin pedicle, or they grow from a broad base. In many cases a polypus growing from the tympanic cavity with a narrow pedicle makes its way through a small perforation in the membrane, and appears as if originating in the external meatus. Several cases have been observed of the growth of polypi in the tympanic cavity without perforation of the membrane. In 10 cases out of 100 Moos and Steinbrügge noted the formation of polypi associated with caries.

According to their structure, polypi may be divided into three kinds, namely, *granulations*, *fibromata*, and *myxomata*. The *granu-*

---

[1] *Zeitschrift für Ohrenheilkunde*, vol. xii. p. 43.

lations are most frequently observed, forming, according to Moos and Steinbrügge, 55 per cent. They consist of areolar connective tissue, in which are observed exudation corpuscles and connective-tissue cells, in more or less abundance, and contain numerous blood-vessels and mucous fluid. They are of a papillary structure, and when the papillæ develop strongly their extremities join together and form adenoid spaces or closed mucous cysts. The cellular elements develop into spindle-cells and connective-tissue fibres. The growth then assumes a firmer and denser character, some of the blood-vessels becoming obliterated. The granulation growth thus develops into a *fibroma*. The covering of such polypi when deeply situated consists of cylindrical epithelium, sometimes ciliated. The more the polypus grows outward, the flatter becomes the epithelium, and finally assumes an epidermoid character. The surface of the granulation-growth is generally uneven, resembling a raspberry; that of the fibroma is smooth. The colour varies according to the blood-supply and the epithelial covering. The rarest of aural polypi (5 per cent.) are the *myxomata*, which are of a gelatinous character.

Otorrhœa is aggravated by the presence of polypi, and can only be stopped by their removal. During manipulations in the external meatus, as in cleansing or syringing, the surface of the polypi is easily made to bleed. The discharge is also frequently mixed with blood, even without any interference, which is a notable point in the diagnosis.

Polypi may exist for years without any other symptoms than dulness of hearing and otorrhœa. They become dangerous when they obstruct the discharge of the purulent exudation.

Treatment.—See page 192.

DISEASE OF THE OSSEOUS WALLS.

(a) *Sclerosis.*—In a great many cases sclerosis of the osseous walls of the middle ear takes place, in consequence of chronic purulent inflammation through reactive processes. Especially is this the case in the mastoid cells, where an entire change of structure is effected by a uniform osseous substance as solid as ivory taking the place of the spaces surrounding the antrum mastoideum. In the dead subject the author has found the whole mastoid process composed of such a substance, while in other cases it only formed a concentric ring round the antrum.[1]

Wendt frequently observed on post-mortem examination that the cavities and cells of the mastoid process had been entirely occluded by swelling of their mucous membrane. In the most aggravated cases this gives rise to great pressure, causing violent pain. Buck also found the cells occupied by a reddish pulpy mass.

There can be no doubt that sclerosis arises from these pathological processes, accompanied by hyperplasia of the osseous tissue, termed *ostitis interna osteoplastica*. The osseous formation finally occupies the whole of the interior of the cells previously containing air. Both in the early acute stage of the process of inflammatory swelling, as well as in the later stage of sclerosis, the pain is generally very great, and is removed by trephining the sclerosed bone, or by chiselling into it, even without opening the antrum mastoideum. In two cases, in which there had been great pain confined to the region of the mastoid process long after the otorrhœa had ceased, the author found at the necropsy, sclerosis of the mastoid process, without inflammation of the mucous membrane, and formed the opinion that the pain was produced by pressure exerted by the newly formed bone upon the branch of the trigeminus distributed to the mastoid cells.[2]

Sclerosis of the mastoid process occurs both as independent periostitis and ostitis interna. The ostitis either develops after inflammation of the tympanic cavity has subsided, or co-exists

---

[1] 'Ueber Sklerose des Warzenfortsatzes,' *Zeitschrift für Ohrenheilkunde*, vol. viii.

[2] Hessler dissents (*Archiv für Ohrenheilkunde*, vol. xxi. p. 143) from this opinion, and erroneously assumes that the disease was acute in one of the above cases, and that the patient was convalescent from typhoid fever, while the report states that, owing to that fever, the woman had acquired purulent otitis, which had been exhausted two years before death. He then informs us at length that in these cases (acute) it must be assumed that the success of the operation results from direct blood-letting from the swollen mucous membrane of the cells of the mastoid process.

with the latter, being either stationary or progressive during its course.

While it was formerly assumed that in sclerosis a general enlargement of the mastoid process took place, the author has shown by preparations from the dead subject that this is not usually the case, but that the sclerosis is rather confined to the interior of the mastoid process. In the case of sclerosis combined with atrophy from pressure, an increase of the bulk of the mastoid process sometimes takes place.

(b) *Atrophy.*—By the pressure arising from their presence, deposits in the antrum mastoideum, especially cholesteatomata, may produce atrophy of the bone, and may eventually eat their way through the osseous wall. In a preparation in the author's collection, cholesteatomatous masses were found in the enlarged mastoid antrum, which were only separated from the external meatus by an osseous layer as thin as paper of the otherwise sclerosed bone. When such a thin layer is destroyed, a spontaneous discharge of cholesteatomatous material takes place into the external meatus. Such a discharge has repeatedly occurred in the direction of the surface of the mastoid process, more rarely towards the cranial cavity.

(c) *Caries and Necrosis of the Petrous Bone.*—These destructive processes in the osseous tissue occur mostly in persons of weak constitution, and scrofulous or phthisical subjects, who generally suffer from other affections. Caries or necrosis of the petrous bone may take place either in acute or chronic inflammation of the middle ear; its lining mucous membrane being destroyed, the bone is laid bare, and thereby ulcerative ostitis or caries superficialis results. The occurrence of caries is promoted by accumulated exudation products in a state of decomposition. When a portion of the bone is deprived of its blood-supply, necrosis follows, and thus a large part of the petrous bone may be destroyed and separated.

Destructive processes attack the walls of the tympanic cavity as well as the mastoid process, but especially the latter, whose spaces, owing to their construction and position, afford a favourable situation for the deposit of exudation. Most frequently the suppuration takes an outward course, carious canals forming toward the outer surface of the mastoid process. The most dangerous direction for pus to take is toward the cranial cavity, by destruction of the roof of the tympanum and the mastoid antrum, and opening into the middle cranial fossa, or by the formation of carious canals through the bone to the posterior cranial fossa. More rarely are the jugular veins or the internal carotid affected by destruction of the inferior or anterior wall of the tympanic cavity. Not only may hæmorrhage take place from these vessels, but from the cranial sinuses, and the middle meningeal and stylo-mastoid arteries. In the case of venous hæmorrhage, the stream of blood is dark red and uniform; in arterial, it is light red and intermittent. Hæmorrhage from the carotid may be so great that the blood flows from the external meatus in a thick stream. Such hæmorrhage may prove fatal in a few minutes.

The canal of the facial nerve may be opened, and facial paralysis may result. The labyrinth is protected by its dense osseous wall, which renders it capable of resisting destructive processes, if its membranous fenestræ have not been destroyed. But if such destruction has occurred, the suppuration extends, and may spread to its interior, and proceed through the meatus auditorius internus to the cranial cavity. Sometimes carious canals form all round the osseous capsule of the labyrinth, either backward and downward, as far as the posterior cranial fossa, or, in other cases, between the upper wall of the labyrinth and the middle cranial fossa.

When carious destruction thus occurs at different places, the labyrinth may be separated completely from the other portion of the petrous bone, and then expelled, which has very frequently occurred in the case of the cochlea. The whole labyrinth has been extracted by Crampton. In very rare cases the carious process extends below the superior semicircular canal through the *hiatus subarcuatus*, which in the adult presents an indication of the remains of the *fossa subarcuata* of infancy (Von Tröltsch), and from which blood-vessels run to the tympanum. Such cases have been reported by Voltolini, Odenius, and Von Tröltsch, and the author's collection contains a preparation of a fourth case.

When the suppuration makes its way to the surface of the mastoid process, great swelling and redness appear behind the auricle, which is itself raised from its attachments, and driven outward and forward. Sometimes very great infiltration of the soft parts takes place, so that on opening the abscess the bone is found lying as much as two cm. and more below the surface. Especially in the case of such abscesses occurring in children, it should be borne in mind that their chief cause is obstruction to the discharge of pus from the external meatus either by an insufficiently large perforation, by polypi, by inspissated masses of secretion, or a sequestrum, and that under such circumstances the pus seeks a way of escape through the mastoid process. Hence the treatment must not be confined merely to evacuating the abscess in the mastoid process, or, if necessary, to opening the bone with a chisel, but a free discharge from the tympanic cavity into the external meatus must also be provided for.

In acute as well as chronic purulent inflammation of the middle ear, abscesses may form on the surface of the mastoid process, having no communication with the mastoid cells. After incision, with antiseptic precautions, a cure may be effected in such cases *per primam intentionem.*

Abscesses upon the outer surface of the mastoid process without disease of the middle ear have generally been described as acute periostitis. If not incised, they may make their way into the external meatus.

Bezold has recently drawn attention to a peculiar form of extension of the inflammation upon the surface of the mastoid process to the inner aspect of its apex.[1] At this point the air-cells are frequently protected by an osseous layer as thin as paper, through which the discharge of pus may take place. After breaking through the surface of the mastoid process at its inner side, the pus extends along the muscles inserted upon it. According to Bezold, this first gives the impression that inflammatory infiltration of the attachments of the muscles has occurred, as they appear raised up. A swelling forms at both sides of the sterno-cleido-mastoid muscle as hard as

[1] 'Ein neuer Weg für Ausbreitung eiteriger Entzündung,' etc., *Deutsche med. Wochenschrift,* No. 28, 1881.

a board. The accumulation of pus forming at a considerable depth may break through either toward the neck or the meatus. The extension of the purulent accumulation internally may prove fatal by œdema of the glottis, by gravitating into the thoracic cavity, or by exhaustion.

In the case of children, a sequestrum often forms in the mastoid process. As a rule, the part of the bone between the antrum and the external meatus is attacked by necrosis.

In the temporal bone of the child a large cavity exists, the *antrum petrosum* (*A A*, in Figs. 36 and 37, representing sections

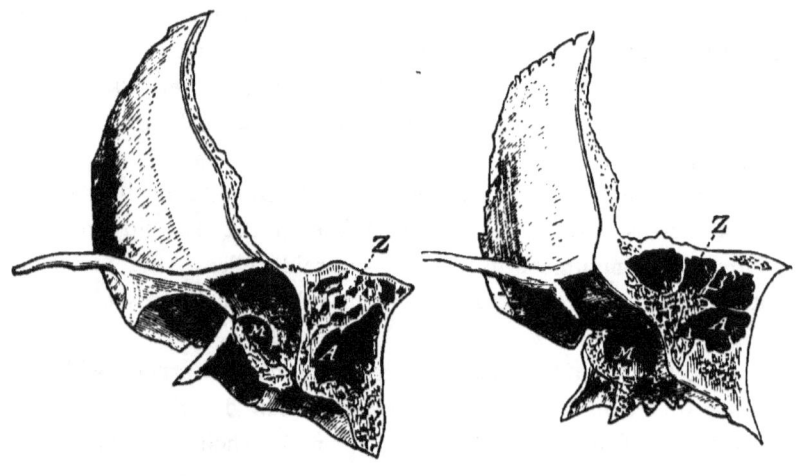

Fig. 36.   Fig. 37.

M. Meatus auditorius externus.   *A.* Antrum petrosum.   *Z.* Cell-spaces.

through the temporal bones of children of three years of age). Its walls are formed by the posterior wall of the external meatus (belonging to the squamous part of the temporal bone), the externa surface of the mastoid process, the wall of the lateral sinus, and that part of the petrous bone which encloses the labyrinth. This cavity diminishes in size by the growth of bony trabeculæ proceeding from the walls, and chiefly from the squamous part, so that finally only a relatively small space is left to form the *antrum mastoideum*. Necrosis leading to the formation of sequestra most frequently affects the part composed of cell-cavities (*Z Z*, Figs. 36 and 37).

The sequestrum is frequently 1—1½ cm. in diameter. A great number of cases of the formation of large sequestra have been recorded. In one of the author's cases [1] large sequestra were removed from both sides during life, consisting of the roof of the tympanic and mastoid cavities, the petro-squamosal suture being visible on the superior surface of each sequestrum.

The diagnosis of the presence of sequestra can only be made with certainty by feeling with the probe a piece of bone which is movable and denuded of its periosteum, but the existence of a sequestrum can also be assumed, although not with so much certainty, from the following series of symptoms :—

1. A long-continued purulent otorrhœa, having an offensive odour, and not amenable to ordinary treatment.

2. The presence of granulations growing from the tympanic cavity which after removal quickly re-appear.

3. Stenosis of the interior portion of the osseous meatus from bulging of the posterior wall.

4. The previous removal of small sequestra from the external meatus without lessening the discharge.

5. The present or past existence of fistulous openings behind the ear, the discharge being copious and of a bad odour.

6. When, under these circumstances, the region of the external ear is swollen, and accompanied by diffuse infiltration and abscess or swelling of the lymphatic glands.

From such symptoms we may form a diagnosis in regard to the presence of sequestra with almost absolute certainty, even without being able to obtain positive proof by means of the probe. In many cases the symptoms enumerated from 1—4 are quite sufficient for such a diagnosis.

The prognosis in cases of such destructive processes in the osseous structures must always be doubtful, as extension to the neighbouring organs is to be feared. When a breach of the outer covering of the bone has taken place, the prognosis is more favourable, as the discharge can then escape through it. In many cases a cure cannot be effected on account of unfavourable constitutional

---

[1] 'Ueber Sequesterbildung in Warzenteil des Kindes,' *Archiv für Augen- und Ohrenheilkunde*, vol. vii.

conditions, even when the most careful local treatment is carried out, which, under more favourable circumstances, readily brings about recovery. Sequestra of necrosed bone, when small, are frequently discharged spontaneously from the external meatus, this being particularly the case in children. But the sequestrum may remain for months or years *in situ*. Under these circumstances, the discharge is very copious and of a very bad smell. Swelling of the lymphatic glands is also found, along with abscesses, in the region of the external ear. General marasmus may even be present, due to the long-continued suppuration.

When the bone has become carious or necrosed as far as the cranial cavity, pus collects between it and the dura mater, on which granulation-tissue forms, and affords protection against the spread of the disease. After separation and removal of the sequestrum, the dura mater may be laid bare, or the lateral sinus also, if the sigmoid fossa be implicated. Whenever destruction of the dura mater and the wall of the sinus has taken place, a fatal termination results. Sometimes such a purulent accumulation spreads beneath the dura mater, especially toward the cranial nerves, which in such cases are found bathed in pus, their functions being nevertheless well maintained.

Treatment.—See page 195.

CEREBRAL ABSCESS.

Cerebral abscesses are not an uncommon complication of purulent inflammation of the middle ear. Out of eighty cases of cerebral abscess which Lebert compiled, twenty originated from the ear. R. Meyer (*Dissert*. Zürich, 1867) found 9 such cases out of 19. They are not only caused by direct extension of the suppuration to the brain, but by transmission through vessels and strands of connective tissue, so that healthy tissue is found between the original purulent collection and the secondary abscess. Caries is present in the great majority of cases. According to some observers, cerebral abscesses have developed in consequence of otitis externa.

Most commonly the extension of the suppuration takes place

through the tegmen tympani, and the abscess forms in the temporal lobe of the corresponding side. On post-mortem examination, the surface of the brain in the region of the tympanic cavity is found either united with the dura mater, or is quite intact. In other cases the abscess is accompanied by circumscribed or diffused meningitis. At the place corresponding with the tympanic cavity a dirty discoloration of the surface is as a rule observed. If an incision be made into this part, the abscess cavity will be reached, enclosed by a somewhat firm capsule, several millimetres thick. The author has frequently found these abscesses very extensive, sometimes being as large as a hen's egg, so that almost the whole temporal lobe has been destroyed. Their contents are of a greenish-yellow colour, of synovia-like, greasy consistence, generally of an acid reaction, and in the majority of cases inodorous. When destruction of bone has extended in the direction of the posterior cranial fossa, abscess forms in the cerebellum. Abscesses may also develop in situations at a distance from the original purulent deposit, and even in various parts of the brain. In two cases the author found them at the convexity. Abercrombie and Von Tröltsch have observed them in that side of the brain opposite to the diseased ear. It may be assumed that the micro-organisms which act as the exciting causes of the inflammation get into the vessels and produce metastatic abscesses. Fistulæ are sometimes observed between the abscess and the carious bone. Cases have been repeatedly observed in which the abscess communicated with the middle ear by means of fistulous channels which afforded a free passage for the pus. The old aural surgeons, therefore, distinguished a particular disease as *otorrhœa cerebralis*, and Itard, who assumed that in the case of a healthy middle ear a cerebral abscess could discharge its contents through it in an outward direction, even made a distinction between *otorrhœa cerebralis primaria* and *secundaria*. An abscess on the surface of the brain may burst into its interior, and occupy the ventricles. One case has been observed in which the abscess discharged into the nasal cavity (Rokitansky). Abscess may be associated with phlebitis of a sinus, with consequent thrombosis.

Cerebral abscesses may develop without any characteristic

symptoms. They may remain latent for a long time, without preventing the patient from following his daily occupation. In other cases, the formation of these abscesses starts with violent acute symptoms, being ushered in with rigors and a rapid increase in the temperature to 39°—40° C. (102°—104° Fah.). The fever remains at its height with slight variations; in this way it may be distinguished from pyæmia. In meningitis, on the other hand, the increase in temperature is generally slight, with irregular remissions. In the case of cerebral abscess, the high temperature is generally accompanied by very severe headache, localised as a rule in the situation where the abscess is forming, and is increased by pressure upon the surface of the cranium. The other symptoms consist of heat of the head, giddiness, vomiting, hallucinations, convulsions, and unconsciousness. Mental disturbances are not always present, but anæsthesia and paralysis are sometimes observed, limited to certain parts. As a rule, however, symptoms of localised disease of the brain are absent, owing to the situation of the abscess generally in the temporal lobe, through which run neither motor nor sensory nerve-tracts.

The different symptoms occur in variable order and intensity. The course of the disease is also somewhat irregular, apparent improvement alternating with the gravest symptoms. Not unfrequently does it happen that the symptoms are only trifling, and disappear in a short time, the abscess assuming a latent stage. Such an occurrence may take place several times until the symptoms become graver and the disease ends fatally. When an abscess which has been previously latent assumes the acute form on account of the action of some irritation, as injury or cold, we have the same set of symptoms presented as in the acute stage of abscess formation.

A most important point in the diagnosis is the continuous exceedingly severe headache, frequently confined to certain situations, which may continue even in the latent stage, along with the symptoms of cerebral pressure. The pulse is sometimes very sluggish, Toynbee having observed it numbering in one case 16—20 beats in the minute, and Wreden as few as 10.

The above symptoms either end fatally after a state of coma, or the abscess-formation assumes the latent stage, a firm capsule developing around it, which may be completed in three weeks or longer. Sometimes death occurs with apoplectic symptoms, especially when rupture takes place in the direction of the meninges or the ventricles of the brain. In a case which the author examined post-mortem, sudden death had been caused by hæmorrhage into the cavity of the abscess. When an abscess bursts through toward the tympanic cavity, the symptoms are temporarily alleviated, but they set in again with their former intensity whenever the orifice for the exit of the discharge closes. Leblanc has reported the cure of a case of such cerebral suppuration.

Treatment.—See page 197.

MENINGITIS PURULENTA.

Purulent meningitis arising from suppuration of the middle ear mostly affects the meninges of the base of the brain, and more rarely those of the convexity. It either occurs independently or simultaneously with the formation of an abscess in the brain, or an affection of parts closely related to the brain. The extension of the inflammatory process to the meninges takes place by means of carious processes, such as we have already described. In most cases the dura mater is perforated; but, as in the case of cerebral abscesses, meningitis is sometimes observed arising from purulent inflammation of the middle ear without caries or any direct communication with the cranial cavity.

The autopsy discloses a more or less extensive purulent infiltration of the pia mater, especially along the course of the vessels, and extending frequently far down into the vertebral canal, the substance of the cortex of the brain being also infiltrated with pus in a less degree.

Meningitis generally arises from special causes, such as injury, the influence of cold, and all conditions producing cerebral congestion, as excessive indulgence in alcoholic liquors and severe bodily exertion. It is particularly promoted by obstruction to the free discharge of exudation from the tympanic cavity. The writer observed a case of meningitis with a fatal termination in a patient who determined to stop the annoying purulent discharge from his ear by inserting a paper plug deeply into the meatus.

The fever accompanying purulent meningitis varies greatly. In cases running a slow course it is slight, with irregular remissions. The form assuming a more rapid course sets in with rigors, succeeded by a variable febrile temperature, very severe headache, giddiness, vomiting, constipation, along with mental irritability, delirium, and sometimes stiff-neck, paralytic, and pressure symptoms, such as slow pulse and impaired sensitiveness of the pupils to light. Drowsiness sets in early, and soon changes into a deep stupor, the patient being roused to temporary consciousness with great difficulty.

Meningitis sometimes develops very rapidly, causing death in a few days with cerebral symptoms, immediately preceded by convulsions. In other cases the disease lasts from 8 days to 3 weeks, with cerebral symptoms of moderate intensity, the sensorium remaining intact for a remarkably long time.

Treatment.—See page 197.

PHLEBITIS, THROMBOSIS, PYÆMIA.

Although the walls of the sinuses of the brain offer so great resistance to the pus surrounding them that an accumulation may exist for a long time between them and the carious or necrosed bone without affecting them, yet sometimes they are affected by inflammation or destruction, either partial, or so extensive that great hæmorrhage will arise, which may cause death. In the case of a slight degree of destruction, hardly discernible at the necropsy, phlebitis and thrombosis occur, along with the entrance of purulent matter into the blood. The diploetic veins in the petrous bone seem to play an important part in this process. On account of the thrombosis, engorgement occurs in the neighbouring veins. The thrombosis itself spreads in both directions, with simultaneous inflammation of the walls of the veins. By the reception of recently-formed or broken-down thrombotic material into the blood, pyæmic symptoms are produced, with the formation of emboli, producing mal-nutrition and inflammation in various organs of the body.

When the process extends to the surrounding veins, the thrombi break down and give rise to purulent meningitis.

Most frequently the lateral sinus is primarily affected, or the inflammatory thrombosis spreads from the superior petrosal sinus, extending along the superior border of the petrous bone to the lateral sinus. As distinguished from the formation of cerebral abscess, the most important and earliest symptom is severe rigors.

The pain is very great, limited to the region of the inflamed sinus wall, and increased on pressure. Great restlessness sets in early, with delirium, convulsions, and extreme prostration. Sometimes a temporary remission of the symptoms occurs, but the patient sinks, and coma and death ensue. In rare cases the symptoms abate in severity, and recovery follows.

According to the different veins attacked by thrombosis, various symptoms appear, by which the diagnosis of the seat of the disease may be established. The extension of inflammatory thrombosis from the lateral sinus to the internal jugular vein can be recognised by an œdematous swelling along its course in the neck, the vein feeling like a hard cord on digital examination, and the pain on pressure being generally very considerable. By inflammatory œdema in the region of the vein, especially of the sinus of the internal jugular, the neighbouring nerve-trunks, the vagus, the glosso-pharyngeal, and the spinal accessory may be affected, and consequent irritation or paralysis may result. In the case of obstruction of the mastoid vein, which inosculates with the lateral sinus, the œdema is limited to the region of the mastoid process, to which Griesinger first directed attention, and which Moos first demonstrated on the dead body. Implication of the facial veins produces an erysipelatous swelling of the cheeks and eyelids, which may be accompanied by the formation of vesicles. In the event of thrombosis extending to the cavernous sinus, œdema of one or both orbits sets in, along with exophthalmos and blindness, the neighbouring parts also being generally swollen. Of the nerves found in this situation in addition to the optic, the abducens, oculomotor, and trigeminus may be affected.

The extension of thrombosis to the longitudinal sinus causes vascular engorgement in the cortical substance of the cerebrum, producing unconsciousness, convulsions, and epileptic seizures. Sometimes epistaxis results from engorgement of the vein passing through the *foramen cæcum*, connecting the cells of the ethmoid bone and the mucous membrane of the pharynx. By the union of the two lateral sinuses at the internal occipital protuberance, the thrombosis may extend from one sinus to the other, and thereby produce at the opposite side the same conditions as existed at the place of origin.

Thrombotic material is carried away into the circulation, and gives rise to embolic phenomena in various parts of the body. The reception into the blood of the micro-organisms of the septic process of suppuration gives rise to pyæmia and its symptoms.

Treatment.—See page 197.

TUBERCULOSIS.

Von Tröltsch first pointed out that tuberculosis frequently occurs in the course of chronic otorrhœa, a fact which has been confirmed by various authorities. He assumes, however, that, according to Buhl's view, tuberculosis is produced by absorption from old purulent and caseous deposits. But after Koch's discovery of the tubercle-bacillus, we must explain general tuberculosis originating in the ear by the entrance of tubercle-bacilli from the outside into the deposits of pus, which find there a favourable soil, spread thence over the body, and thus produce general infection. In cases where the affection has existed longer than that of the ear, purulent otitis may be regarded as a localisation of the general infection originating in pulmonary tuberculosis. Direct transmission of tuberculosis from the sputum to the mucous membrane of the tympanic cavity may also take place through the Eustachian tube.

Tubercle-bacilli were first detected in the discharge from the ear by Eschle.[1] Nathan[2] found bacilli in 12 out of 40 cases of chronic otorrhœa, which Bezold had sent to him for examination. In 8 of these cases could a simultaneous tuberculosis of the

---

[1] *Deutsche med. Wochenschrift*, No. 30, 1883.
[2] *Inaug. Dissert.* München, 1884.

lungs be diagnosed. Schwartze and others have observed miliary tubercles in the mucous membrane of the tympanic cavity, and in the membrana tympani. Habermann has also detected the presence of tubercle-bacilli in such purulent collections.

Ear diseases associated with tubercular infection arise without definite symptoms. Mostly without inflammatory appearances, dulness of hearing and otorrhœa set in, with more or less extensive destruction of the membrana tympani, the mucous membrane of the middle ear, and its osseous walls.

Treatment of Chronic Purulent Inflammation of Middle Ear.

Having seen that every otorrhœa may prove fatal on account of the complications which may arise, it is our duty to point out to patients the danger likely to result from neglect. We must endeavour to stop the suppuration as early as possible.

The prime necessity in the rational treatment of chronic purulent inflammation of the ear is the careful removal of the exudation products, because applications can only come in contact with the mucous membrane after thorough cleansing. These products are removed by syringing, in the manner described at page 19, with a 1 per cent. solution of common salt, or Glauber's salts (sulphate of soda), or with antiseptic solutions, as carbolic acid, $\frac{1}{2}$—1 per cent.; salicylic acid, $\frac{1}{2}$—1 per cent.; boracic acid, 2—4 per cent. Exudation in the tympanic cavity lying below the level of the perforation in the membrane, as is especially the case with small perforations, cannot be removed by syringing. Such collections must first be driven into the external meatus by Politzer's method, and then removed. Or, after cleansing of the meatus, the exudation may be driven through the Eustachian tube into the naso-pharynx, by Lucae's meatus air-douche, consisting of an india-rubber bag furnished with an olive-shaped nozzle, which is inserted into the orifice of the meatus. In the case of children especially, this manner of removing the secretion is very effective, but sometimes it produces giddiness.

Cleansing may also be effectually performed by the dry method of removing the discharge with tampons of cotton-wool, either introduced by means of the forceps or on a holder. The introduction of the tampons must be repeated until they show no trace of exudation. This dry cleansing was formerly recommended by Yearsley, and recently by Becker. But it must be noted that inspissated matter cannot be removed in this manner, especially from the deeper parts of the tympanic cavity, and this mode of cleansing is therefore only of very limited application.

As the continuance of otorrhœa is sometimes caused by accumulation and stagnation of secretion in the tympanic cavity, besides regular cleansing with the syringe or with cotton-wool, the air-douche must be employed in order to effect a cure.

Considering the triumphs achieved in surgery by the antiseptic treatment, it cannot fail also to be effectual in purulent otorrhœa, for it is assumed that in such cases the development of low organisms plays an important part in promoting the exudation and the continuance of the inflammatory process. Therefore, in addition to the permanganate of potash formerly in use, the various antiseptics, carbolic acid, salicylic acid, thymol, and iodoform have been recommended. Boracic acid has proved to be the most effective, for the introduction of which into the therapeutics of aural surgery Bezold[1] deserves special credit. Its advantages lie in its easy, painless application, on the one hand, and its certain action on the other.

Before applying the boracic acid in the form of powder, the ear is cleansed with a saturated solution of it, other solutions, however, being also employed. After drying the meatus carefully, and using the air-douche, the powder is insufflated by means of the powder-blower. As much is used as fills about the inner third of the meatus, and the orifice is closed with antiseptic cotton-wool. The application of boracic acid should be repeated so long as the cotton is moistened with the discharge. Bezold's average time of treatment until the suppuration ceased was 19 days. In the case of a small perforation of the membrane, the effect of the acid is sometimes so limited that the opening requires to be enlarged by means of the membrana-tympani knife, or by the galvano-cautery.

Bezold achieved no success with patients suffering from advanced phthisis pulmonalis, in which cases we assume the presence of tuber-

[1] *Archiv für Ohrenheilkunde*, vol. xv. p. 1.

cular disease; but even in phthisical patients the writer has succeeded in stopping the suppuration. The cure may be hindered by perforation in Shrapnell's membrane, with formation of polypi behind it. Granular swelling of the mucous membrane must first be treated by cauterisation. Other complications, such as accumulation of exudation, polypi, and destructive processes in the bone, require the necessary attention before a cure can be effected.

In the complication of perforation in Shrapnell's membrane a cure can in most cases be brought about rapidly, by removing, in the manner to be described afterwards, the polypi which may be present, and the exudation products confined in the cellular spaces at the neck of the malleus. With regard to such cases the author's experience does not agree with the statement of Morpurgo and Hessler, who describe the cure as being exceedingly difficult and tedious. Their unfavourable results are due to the circumstance that they did not employ the metal tympanic tube, by which alone, in uncomplicated cases, a certain and complete removal of exudation deposits can be effected. The presence of carious processes will hinder the cure, and in such cases the malleus must be removed according to Schwartze's proposal. After cutting through the membrane at both sides of the handle, along with the axis ligaments, the malleus is caught in the loop of the snare, as high up as possible, and then extracted. In a case operated upon by the author in this manner, the watch was heard at a distance of 75 cm., and whispered speech at 5 metres, after healing had taken place.

When success does not attend the treatment by boracic acid, according to Schwartze, a concentrated caustic solution (0·5—1, argent. nitr.; 10, aq. destill.), or, according to Weber-Liel and Löwenberg, spirit may be used with good effect. The caustic solution is instilled into the ear, in the manner indicated at page 67, either daily or every second day (10—20 drops). It is allowed to remain in the ear 1—2 minutes, when it is syringed out. Schwartze recommends neutralising with a solution of common salt. Spirit (*Spiritus vini rectificatus*) may be instilled more frequently (2—3 times daily). If the instillation of spirit occasion much pain, it may be diluted with the same quantity of water. A cure may soon be effected by repeated employment of one or the other of these two remedies, but in some cases the treatment requires to be continued for several weeks. Both of these remedies, compared with boracic acid, have the disadvantage, that their application causes more or less sharp pain, sometimes producing reactive inflammation of the tympanic cavity or otitis externa.

Hagen and Menière have recommended carbolic acid (1 : 10 glycerine or olive oil). Iodoform has proved bad. Corrosive sublimate, in the proportion of 1 : 10,000, was recently recommended by Wagenhäuser, and powdered calomel by Gottstein.

For swelling of the mucous membrane, especially if granular, solid nitrate of silver (melted upon the probe) should be used, or liquor ferri perchloridi, of which a drop is applied by means of the probe. If these remedies do not suffice, the swelling may be treated with chromic acid. The galvano-cautery has also been recommended, but even its cautious application may produce mischief as the subjacent bone and the labyrinth may be injured.

When the otorrhœa is not of very long standing, and the swelling of the mucous membrane is not great, it is sometimes possible to stop the discharge by means of astringents. Those most frequently employed are solutions of sulphate of zinc (0·1—0·4 : 20 aq. destill.), sulphate of copper, acetate of lead, acetate of alumina, tannic acid—which latter, however, have no advantage over zinc.

One remedy has still to be mentioned, which may prove useful, especially in cases of extensive destruction of the membrane, namely insufflation of powdered alum, as first recommended by Erhard, and subsequently by Politzer; it may be used alone or along with a caustic solution. Unfortunately the treatment with alum has the drawback, that it causes the formation of a solid coagulum with the exudation, which it is difficult to remove. Frequently the masses thus formed require to be first loosened with the probe, and then removed by repeated syringing. The action of the alum is quite as reliable as that of boracic acid, and is in many cases effective where boracic acid has failed.

After cure of the inflammatory process, the defective hearing due to loss of substance of the membrane can in many cases be improved by the employment of artificial membranes, which we have previously described, page 116.

TREATMENT OF EXUDATION DEPOSITS.   185

In cases of union by means of connective tissue between the membrana tympani, the ossicula, and the walls of the tympanum, as well as in cases of permanently cicatrised perforations, Politzer noticed an improvement in the hearing resulting from instillations of rectified spirit twice daily into the meatus, allowing it to remain in the ear from ½—1 hour.

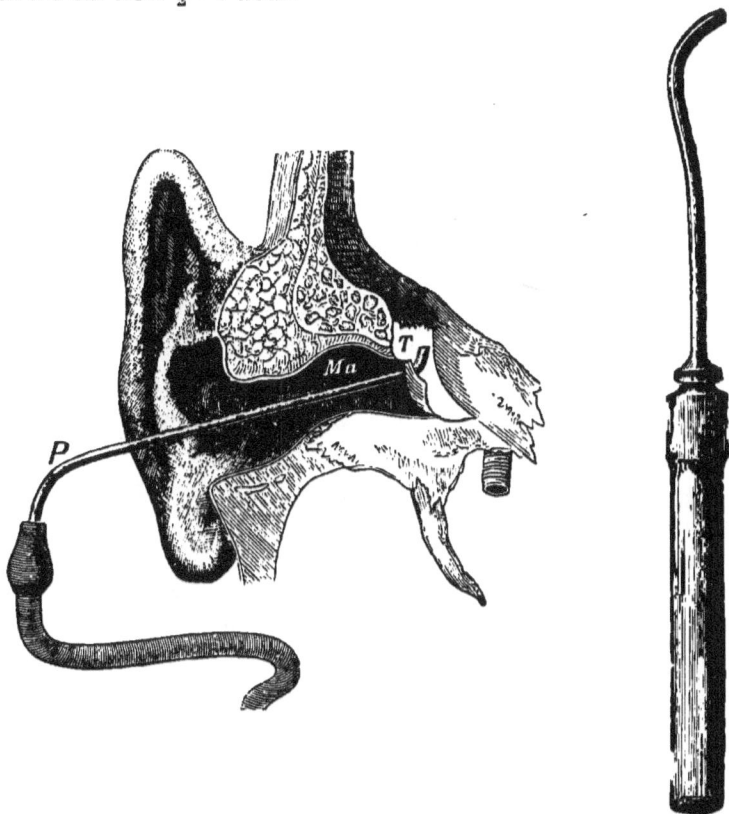

FIG. 38.   FIG. 39.

Ma. Meatus auditorius externus.   *P.* Tympanic tube (Paukenröhre).
T. Tympanum.

Treatment of Exudation Deposits and Cholesteatomata.

In the first place we must endeavour to give free exit to any discharge, by removing every obstruction : polypi must be removed, perforations of the membrane which are too small enlarged, and constrictions of the external meatus treated according to their character; any accumulation of matter must also be cleared away.

We cannot reach exudation deposits located in the posterior-superior part of the tympanic cavity, or in the mastoid process, by the ordinary manner of syringing from the meatus, or by a stream passed through the Eustachian tube into the tympanum by means of the catheter. We therefore make use of a metal tube, suitably bent, for the purpose of causing the fluid to act directly upon these masses.

The author uses an instrument (Fig. 38), consisting of a German silver tube about 2—2½ mm. thick and 7 cm. long. It is perfectly straight in its middle portion, and, in order to accommodate it to the tympanic cavity, it is bent at one end, almost at a right angle, but only to such an extent that its beak is scarcely more than one mm. in length. At the outer end the tube is curved in the opposite direction at an obtuse angle, and is thickened at this extremity in order to allow an india-rubber tube to be fastened over it, by means of which it is connected with a syringe, the most suitable being the so-called English india-rubber syringe. It is important that this india-rubber tube should be as thin and light as possible, so that the instrument may be moved about freely. Toynbee first suggested the employment of such a tube, but Schwartze seems to lay claim to the invention, although the present writer had previously shown its advantage.[1] In his recently published book, Schwartze[2] somewhat acrimoniously refers to the writer's statement, namely, that 'on account of its size and shape, it was barely possible to introduce the instrument (Schwartze's) while the ear was under illumination with the reflecting mirror.' Fig. 39 represents the thinner of the instruments designated as flexible 'antrum-tubes' (*Antrumröhren*), the same size as in Schwartze's book. A comparison with the instrument shown in Fig. 38 will justify the cogency of the above statement in the mind of any one aware of the very limited space and the difficulty of manipulation in the ear.

The tympanic tube is generally introduced through a speculum while the ear (right) is illuminated by means of the head-mirror.

---

[1] *Zeitschrift für Ohrenheilkunde*, vol. viii. p. 28.
[2] *Die Chirurgischen Krankheiten des Ohres*, p. 325.

The auricle and speculum are held with the left hand, while the tube is introduced with the right. The hand which holds the tube lies against the head of the patient, in order to be able to follow it, in the event of movement, without altering the position of the tube; with the other hand the syringe is discharged, or this is done by an assistant. By turning the tube the current can be directed toward all parts of the tympanic cavity. The returning fluid is caught in a vessel held by the patient below the ear. The operation is continued until the returning stream is free from any exudation products. The sensitiveness of the tympanic membrane or its remains, and of the walls of the tympanum, varies greatly. In some cases complete anæsthesia exists, while in others the slightest touch is disagreeable or painful. In the latter cases, or when the sound-conducting apparatus has been preserved, and the tube requires to be introduced through a small perforation, tearing, dragging, and pain may be entirely avoided if the instrument be inserted carefully and be securely kept in position during syringing. The tube is finally withdrawn, in the same direction given it when introduced. It is sometimes impossible to perform this operation in the case of very timid persons, because they cannot keep sufficiently still. In such cases preparatory instillations of a solution of cocaine must be made, or it may be necessary to administer chloroform.

In any case this treatment must be carried out with the greatest care and with a steady hand. The tympanic tube can only be used without injury to the patient by those who have that degree of dexterity and practice necessary in all manipulations in the treatment of the ear. Before commencing this operation the condition and sensitiveness of the parts involved should be accurately ascertained by means of the probe. The pressure exerted in this operation of syringing must be carefully graduated. Slight pressure should be used at first, so that only a weak current of fluid enters into the tympanic cavity. When the patient bears this well, and it causes no giddiness, dull feeling, or headache, the pressure may be gradually and carefully increased. Almost without exception, the author has found that patients tolerate a strong current of fluid without discomfort, and he has succeeded in removing with ease and safety the exudation products which had accumulated in the tympanum and its recesses. In the numerous cases in which he has performed the syringing as described above, he has been frequently astonished at the immense accumulations which were removed. In most cases a permanent cure of the otorrhœa was effected, while in the others syringing had to be repeated, after shorter or longer intervals, in order to remove the masses which had formed anew. In one patient he found in the membrana tympani, anteriorly and superiorly, only a small orifice, scarcely admitting the tympanic tube, the remains of the membrane along with the ossicles having united with the inner wall of the tympanic cavity. He succeeded in passing the hook-shaped probe without obstruction to the posterior part of the tympanum, and by syringing through the small anterior orifice, not only were caseous masses removed from the tympanic cavity, but in the returning fluid a small polypus was found, which probably had its seat in the posterior part of the tympanum, and had been torn off by the current. This caused the disappearance of the symptoms of giddiness, headache, and a dull feeling, which had previously existed.

For the same purpose for which the author has recommended the metallic tympanic tube, Politzer advocated a little tube (*Paukenrörchen*) used by Weber-Liel as a tympanic catheter, which is made like the gum-elastic English urethral catheter, about 1 mm. thick and 7 cm. long. This little tube is very suitable for introducing a current of fluid behind constrictions in the external meatus; being pliable, it is better adapted for this purpose than the rigid tympanic tube. But for removing from the tympanic cavity and its recesses firmly situated and inspissated deposits the little tube is, as a rule, not sufficient. In one case, at least, in which the author had syringed the tympanic cavity with the little tube, he had the opportunity of demonstrating on the cadaver that only a small portion of the deposit had been removed.

If found impossible to remove such deposits by means of the tympanic tube, or, if they accumulate anew, an opening in the mastoid process must be made. Beck, in his Manual, published at Heidelberg and Leipzig in 1827, wrote, even at that time, as follows :—' Trephining the mastoid process is indicated in suppuration or caries in its cells, in order to provide a place of escape for the accumulated matter, to limit the process of destruction, and to promote the separation of carious or necrosed bone.' This operation is especially necessary when the accumulation in the mastoid cannot be reached by means of the tympanic tube, and in the case of swelling in the external meatus and in the tympanic cavity.

Sometimes the cholesteatomatous masses are found firmly adhering together. In such cases they frequently cannot be removed by a stream of fluid, and require first to be softened and loosened. Reactive inflammation often sets in, which either accelerates the separation of the deposits, or is accompanied by more dangerous symptoms, which may terminate fatally. When the diagnosis has been made, that such deposits cannot be removed by the tympanic tube, the mastoid process must be opened externally. In the case of bulging of the posterior wall of the external meatus, the accumulation making its way through the wall from the antrum mastoideum, an incision should be made at the most prominent point. The removal of the accumulated material can then be effected from this spot by the ordinary syringe, the probe, or the tympanic tube.

In the case of acute symptoms brought on by retention of pus, which it has been found impossible to remove, an opening of the mastoid process must be made, even although the bone is sound externally, when the pain and fever continue, with or without œdematous swelling of the soft covering of the mastoid. Regarding the indications for the performance of this operation, Schwartze places special importance on the bulging of the posterior-superior wall of the meatus.

The Operation of Opening the Mastoid Process.

The most exact knowledge of the anatomical conditions is required, on account of the close proximity of the cranial cavity and of the great blood-vessels. In order to be precise on this point, the author performed this operation a hundred times on the dead subject, and convinced himself of the consequences of the operation by sections made through the temporal bone, horizontal to the axis of the external meatus.[1] Two of the sections (Figs. 28—31) show the

---

[1] Von Langenbeck's *Archiv für Chirurgie*, vol. xxi.

great variation in the extent of the cell-spaces. While in Fig. 28 a wide extent of bone exists between the external meatus, on the one hand, and the middle cranial fossa with the sigmoid groove of the lateral sinus, on the other, this distance is considerably diminished in Fig. 29, in which the middle cranial fossa is also deeply situated. In Figs. 30 and 31, which are horizontal sections through the middle line of the external meatus, the varying extent of the region of operation can also be seen. The dangers of the operation are considerably lessened by the circumstance that in temporal bones with well-marked excavation of the sinus outward, the bone is mostly diploetic or sclerotic, and therefore little liable to disease. This explains why Schwartze considers himself justified by his observations on the living subject in assuming that excavation outwards of the sinus is not found so frequently as anatomical investigations have indicated. Nevertheless the rule which the author has already laid down must be observed, that the opening must not be made higher up than the level of the superior wall of the meatus, and that posteriorly it must approach the posterior wall of the meatus as closely as possible. One must always bear in mind while penetrating deeply into the bone that he may come upon the wall of the sinus or the dura mater. It is therefore of first importance that the field of operation should be constantly carefully examined. Inflammatory processes spread from the mastoid antrum to the surrounding cells, and in many cases accumulation of pus results from obstruction to its escape through the tympanic cavity and the external meatus. Therefore ought we always to open the antrum freely along with the neighbouring cells. As we have seen, the antrum is situated posteriorly, and somewhat superiorly with relation to the inner half of the osseous meatus, from which it is separated by a layer of bone 2—5 mm. thick. The antrum in this position forms a prominence on the surface of the mastoid process, occupying a direction parallel to the axis of the external meatus, and lying in the line of attachment of the auricle. We will therefore reach the antrum and the cells with greatest certainty by perforating in this situation. Schwartze's method of entering the bone a centimetre behind the line of attachment of the auricle is not in accordance with the anatomical conditions, neither in regard to the site of the antrum nor the danger of injuring the sinus. In performing the operation, an incision is made through the skin in the line of attachment of the auricle, or close behind it, at a distance of 3—4 cm., so that the middle point of the incision is on a level with the roof of the external meatus. The bleeding is then controlled, and the surface of the bone is denuded of its periosteum both backward and forward, the lips of the wound being held apart by sharp hooks.

The opening in the bone is made in a forward direction, parallel to the axis of the meatus. The operation is performed by chipping off layers of bone with a grooved chisel, giving the canal the shape of a funnel. It ought not to be made deeper than about 16 mm., as otherwise there is a danger of opening the canal of the facial nerve, or the semicircular canals. After the perforation through the bone has been successfully made, and the antrum opened, a stream of fluid injected into it passes through the external meatus. Frequently it does not pass in this way until a few days after the operation. When granulations or carious spots are met with, they may be removed with the sharp spoon. The perforation in the bone must be kept open for some time, at first by drainage tubes, and afterwards by thin leaden tubes.

If in doubt while operating regarding the correct position of the opening one is making, he will best set himself right by introducing a small blunt rod or a thick probe into the external meatus and pressing it against its roof. In this way the upper limit is ascertained, and an estimate can also be formed of the distance of the artificial opening from the meatus posteriorly. The temporal ridge, which was formerly described as corresponding with the level of the middle cranial fossa, is subject to such variation in its direction that it is of very limited value in ascertaining the position of the artificial opening.

Out of the total number of 2568 patients treated at the writer's Poliklinik during 1883 and 1884, opening of the mastoid process was performed in 22 cases. In 7 of these it was performed in consequence of acute inflammation of the middle ear, in one of which the pus had burst through the surface on the inner aspect of the mastoid process; in 4 a sequestrum had formed; in 9 caries was present; in one polypi existed in the mastoid process, and in the remaining case caseous and cholesteatomatous material was found.

Treatment of Polypi.

Before operating upon polypi, information should be obtained regarding the place of origin of the polypus, also whether it is pedunculated or sessile. This is best done by moving the probe round the polypus, and pressing towards it until resistance is met with (Politzer), but we are by no means always able to form a positive and definite diagnosis.

The removal of polypi is effected with a loop-snare. Formerly an instrument, constructed by Wilde, was employed for this purpose, but a more simple instrument, recommended by Blake, is now in use. The wire, instead of running along the sides of a solid rod, is passed through a tube, at whose end the loop is formed. The tube is fixed by a screw at an obtuse angle to a quadrangular rod, which is furnished with one or two movable rings, to which the ends of the wire are fastened (Fig. 40). The rod has another ring at its end for holding the instrument more conveniently. By moving the two lateral rings towards the terminal ring, the loop formed by the wire at the end of the tube is withdrawn and cuts through the polypus, round which it has been placed.

In Blake's snare the tube is closed at its end, and is furnished with two orifices for the wire. In the instrument represented in Fig. 40, the tube is open, and flattened at its end, so that the two branches of the loop lie in the two angles thus formed. (The same instrument, furnished with other tubular pieces for fixing to the rod, can be used for operating upon nasal polypi and adenoid vegetations in the naso-pharynx.) The tube being open, the loop can be completely withdrawn into it, so that even polypi of greater consistence than usual are entirely cut through, while with Blake's instrument this is frequently not quite possible, and the remaining portion of the polypus requires to be torn or twisted off.

The very thinnest flexible iron wire is used, such as gardeners employ for binding up flowers, or thin silver wire. The loop is made corresponding to the size of the polypus. It is most convenient to give the loop a roundish shape over a speculum, and

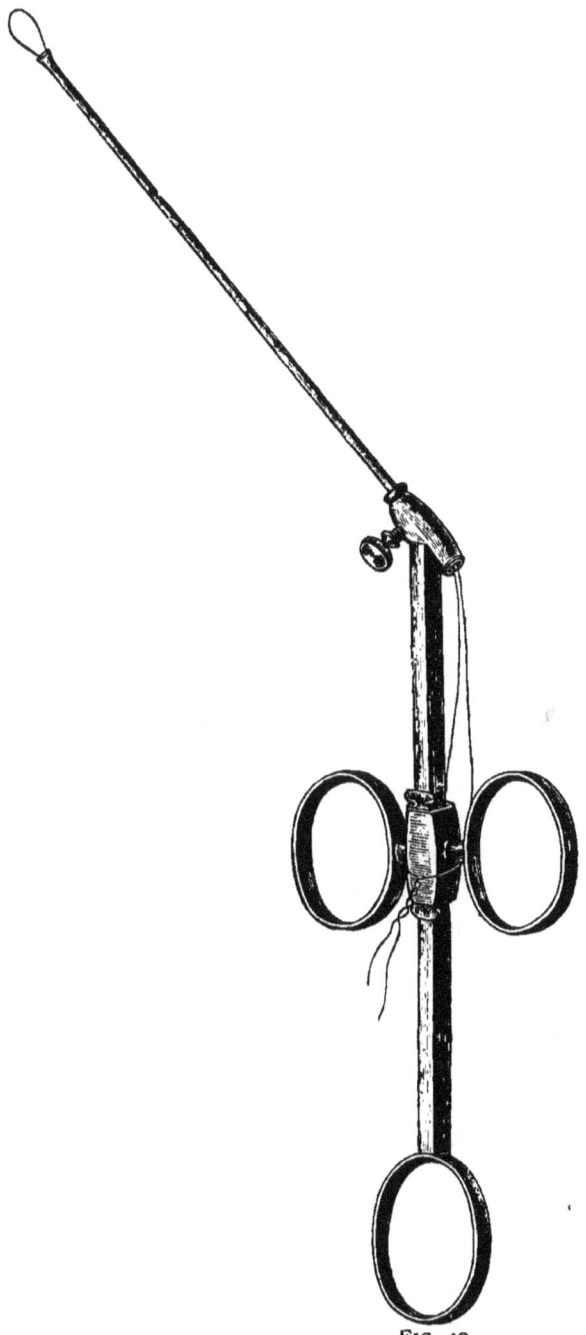

FIG. 40.

then to bend it somewhat on the flat. When the place of attachment of the polypus is ascertained, we place the tube of the snare towards the corresponding side of the meatus. The loop is now passed over the polypus, pressed downwards as much as possible, and then withdrawn. As a rule, we do not succeed in removing the whole mass at the first attempt. After stopping the slight hæmorrhage by means of a cotton plug, the loop of the snare is reintroduced several times if necessary in order to remove what remains. Easy as this operation is in the case of polypi situated at the outer part of a wide meatus, it is very difficult when the meatus is narrow, and the polypi are seated very deeply in it or in the tympanic cavity. But even in such cases these growths can be reached by means of a snare with a thin tube, and under good illumination. If this fail, caustics must be employed. The hæmorrhage after using the snare is almost without exception very trifling, and only in exceedingly rare cases do we require to resort to the tampon.

The galvano-caustic snare is only required in cases of very fibrous polypi. The removal of polypi can be effected more simply and easily by means of the cold wire, the danger of injuring the external meatus with the hot wire being avoided. The galvano-cautery has recently been very highly recommended by Moos and Steinbrügge for the removal of the remains of polypi.

For the purpose of removing small polypi, or what remains after operating with the snare, the curette (Fig. 33) proves most effective.

The caustics in use are liquor ferri perchloridi, argenti nitras, and acidum chromicum. The first named is mildest, and may be employed in the case of very soft polypi and granulations. Chromic acid is the most reliable remedy for destroying fibrous polypi and their remaining stumps; liquefied upon a probe, it must be applied with care, as severe inflammation may be produced by touching the surrounding healthy parts. Its application is therefore only admissible when the probe is handled with precision.

Politzer recommends a very convenient remedy, spiritus rectificatissimus, which often proves effectual in removing polypi. By using it continuously for a length of time, it is possible to remove even firm fibrous polypi. According to Politzer, the spirit should be poured into the ear three times daily by means of a teaspoon, and allowed to remain for 10—15 minutes. This method is to be recommended in all cases where we cannot reach the place of origin of the polypus. It is particularly valuable in the case of patients who are afraid of operation, and in children, in whom the removal of polypi cannot be effected without administering chloroform.

Treatment of the Pathological Processes affecting the Bone.

(a) *Sclerosis.*—We have seen that sclerosis of the mastoid process which accompanies chronic purulent inflammation of the middle ear is sometimes exceedingly painful. In all such cases the pain has been permanently removed by opening the mastoid by means of the chisel, even although no communication was made with the antrum mastoideum. The performance of this operation should therefore be regarded as justifiable under these circumstances.

The author has obtained no good result from painting with tincture of iodine, nor from the use of the various ointments. Only by narcotics, especially hydrate of chloral, can the pain be temporarily relieved.

(b) *Caries and Necrosis.*—When caries or necrosis can be diagnosed, we must, first of all, provide for careful cleansing and disinfection of the parts affected by syringing with a 1—2 per cent. solution of carbolic acid, and thus endeavour to promote a cure. In addition, it is of material importance to remove anomalous conditions of the constitution generally associated with this disease, by means of cod-liver oil, iron, salt-water baths, etc. Irritant applications, cauterisation, etc., are to be avoided, as thereby acute inflammation may arise, the extension of which we may be unable to control. Extension of the carious process to the outer surface of the mastoid is indicated either by a fistulous opening in the skin or by swelling and accumulation of pus over the bone, which must be laid bare by free incision. In this situation regular cleansing is carried out. When a communication exists between the antrum mastoideum and the tympanum, the fluid passes from the fistulous opening through the tympanic cavity, making its exit at the external meatus. When the syringe is used regularly, and the general health is simultaneously improved, a cure will follow. The continuance of a discharge of a very bad odour gives rise to the suspicion that purulent deposits still exist in the interior of the mastoid process, or that sequestra or granulations have formed. The sinus must then be freely opened up again, and enlarged by means of the sharp spoon or chisel. Granulations, carious bone, or sequestra which have formed in the mastoid can thus be removed by the sharp spoon. During the operation the anatomical conditions which we have described at page 125 must be borne in mind. In the same manner as when opening the mastoid process, when its surface is healthy, the field of operation must be laid bare by freely incising the soft parts and separating the edges of the wound with sharp hooks.

In the cases described by Bezold, in which the purulent process extended to the inner aspect of the surface of the mastoid, the opening should not be made on a level with the external meatus, but at the inferior part of the mastoid, the bone being perforated in its whole thickness in order to reach the pus behind. In a case of this kind in which the author operated it was only necessary to extend the fistulous opening in the bone in order to effect a cure.

We have already seen that small sequestra are sometimes spontaneously expelled through the external meatus. In other cases they can be removed by the syringe, the hook-shaped probe, or the small sharp hook, the methods being the same as those for removing foreign bodies from the meatus which we have described. It need scarcely be pointed out that all these manipulations must be performed with the utmost care. In order to proceed with the operation quietly and surely, it is necessary to give the patient chloroform. In cases of the formation of a large sequestrum, the posterior wall of the meatus may require to be removed, in order to obtain sufficient room for its extraction. Sometimes when necrosis takes place in the region of the mastoid process, it is possible to remove a sequestrum lying superficially after making an incision through the soft covering of the bone. In other cases the cortical layer must be removed by means of the chisel or sharp spoon, in order to reach the more deeply situated sequestrum. The outer opening should be made as large as possible, so that the sequestrum may be entirely exposed. After its removal the wound should be kept open by thick drainage-tubes for some time. This method of keeping the wound open and under inspection facilitates the removal of other sequestra after they separate.

In order to stop the hæmorrhage from the large vessels, which is sometimes associated with carious processes, the first proceeding is plugging the external meatus with tampons, used either with or without the solution of perchloride of iron. When great hæmorrhage takes place from the carotid, the tampon is washed away unless firmly wedged into the meatus. In such cases the blood finds its way through the Eustachian tube into the mouth and nose. Compression of the carotid at the neck will only stop the bleeding so long as it is kept up. If found impossible to stop the hæmorrhage, the common carotid must be ligatured, notwithstanding the unfavourable prognosis.

Treatment of other Complications.

In the case of complications involving the interior of the cranial cavity, as when the presence of a cerebral abscess is suspected, all bodily exertion, and everything inducing congestion in the head, must be very carefully avoided. When inflammatory symptoms arise from irritation due to the abscess, they should be relieved by the application of ice-bags, by blood-letting in the region of the temporal bone or of the mastoid process, and the bowels should be carefully regulated by purgatives. Meningitis, phlebitis of the sinus, or thrombosis should be treated in the same way. Schede brought about a cure in the case of an abscess in the temporal lobe by opening it from the outside. While chiselling open the mastoid process, Zaufal came upon a deposit of ichorous pus, situated deeply, accompanied by partial destruction of the floor of the sigmoid groove and of the wall of the sinus. Through this gap the sinus was syringed with a 2 per cent. solution of carbolic acid, but death occurred in 14 days in consequence of an affection of the lungs. While treating the complications, the original disease must not be neglected : the tympanic cavity and its recesses must be regularly cleansed and disinfected. In order to relieve the severe pain, hydrate of chloral or morphia cannot be dispensed with in most cases.

CHRONIC INFLAMMATION OF THE MIDDLE EAR
WITHOUT EXUDATION.

(SYNONYM: *Sclerosis of the Tympanic Cavity.*)

This disease is caused by pathological processes, which lead to thickening and rigidity of the mucous membrane covering the vibrating parts of the organ of hearing, and to the development of membranous bands and adhesions between the ossicula and the walls of the tympanum.

Chronic inflammation without exudation, or 'dry catarrh of the middle ear,' as Von Tröltsch calls it, may be divided into two forms, but intermediate forms are frequently met with.

The first is the *hyperplastic form*, produced by hyperæmic swelling. It can generally be ascertained that a naso-pharyngeal catarrh existed before or at the onset of the disease. The simultaneous swelling of the Eustachian tube may have disappeared after the naso-pharyngeal catarrh has subsided, or it may still exist. The inflammatory swelling with which the mucous membrane of the naso-pharynx, the Eustachian tubes, and the tympanic cavity were at the same time affected, may eventually be limited only to the tympanum. At the beginning of the affection, exudation may have taken place into the tympanum, the exudation becoming absorbed, but the alteration of the mucous membrane remaining. As in all chronic inflammation, new growth of connective tissue and vessels takes place. Membranous bands of connective tissue are developed, binding the ossicula to the walls of the tympanum. In this way it is frequently observed in the dead subject that the malleus and incus are fixed by fibrous bands to both sides of the upper part of the tympanic cavity. In some cases these bands only extend to one side, and are attached either to the malleus or the incus. Frequently the mucous membrane of the fenestra ovalis is thickened, as also that of the ossicula and of the membrana tympani. All these changes more or less impair the vibratory power of the sound-conducting structures.

The disease occurs in persons who are subject to chronic catarrh, as also in individuals of a scrofulous constitution; the plethoric habit often causes the persistence of chronic inflammatory processes. People whose occupation exposes them to frequent changes of temperature and of weather also suffer from this affection. It is more frequent in damp regions, at the coast and in the North, than in the dry climate of the South.

The second form of dry inflammation of the middle ear, namely, *sclerosis proper* of the mucous membrane of the tympanum, originates either in hyperæmic swelling followed by retrograde metamorphosis, or more frequently, without any such process, develops from interstitial condensation. The mucous membrane becomes exceedingly rigid, and may contain calcareous deposits. Ossification takes place, by which the different parts of the sound-conducting apparatus become firmly anchylosed, osseous tissue frequently forming, especially at the fenestra ovalis, so that the annular ligament of the foot-plate of the stapes becomes fixed (synostosis). In addition, the fenestra rotunda may become ossified, or anchylosis may affect the articulations of the ossicula. In all these cases the mucous membrane of the tympanum assumes a paler colour, is free from swelling, and is perfectly dry.

This form of disease is chiefly met with in people of a delicate constitution, of a nervous temperament, and the rheumatic or gouty diathesis, and particularly in those hereditarily predisposed. In almost one-third of the cases of sclerosis similar affections can be traced in other members of the family.

The disease occurs nearly without exception on both sides. Its course varies much. On the one hand, it either develops very slowly and insidiously, the patient noticing accidentally that he is dull of hearing, years perhaps elapsing before the dulness reaches a high degree, or the affection makes rapid progress in a short time. On the other hand, the symptoms may remain stationary after the disease has developed to a certain extent, and even in such a case an acute exacerbation may take place.

The two chief symptoms of both forms of dry inflammation of the middle ear are dulness of hearing and subjective sounds. The latter symptom may precede the former, or the reverse, and in some cases the subjective sounds are absent. The defective hearing and the tinnitus are generally out of proportion to each other, the degree of disparity varying considerably. According to the acoustic importance of the parts of the sound-conducting apparatus affected, the dulness of hearing will be greater or less. If the deafness increase very rapidly, the prognosis with regard to its further development is unfavourable; but with only slow progress, it may be inferred that the pathological change may also proceed slowly or may cease altogether. Patients affected with sclerosis of the mucous membrane of the tympanum often hear better in surrounding loud noises (Paracusis Willisiana).

After sclerotic inflammation has existed for a long time, symptoms often set in from which it may be concluded that the labyrinth has also been affected. This is especially the case in sclerosis proper if the vestibular fenestræ have become implicated. As these symptoms sometimes exist from the onset of the affection on the part of the middle ear as well as of the labyrinth, it must be assumed, as Politzer in particular points out, that trophic disturbances occur in both of these parts. By testing with the tuning-fork we obtain information with regard to the extent the labyrinth is involved.

According to the statements of patients, the character of subjective sounds varies greatly, being described as humming, buzzing, singing, whistling, bell-ringing, knocking, etc. The noises are perceived in the interior of the head, in the ear, and outside the ear, but we are not entitled to draw any conclusion regarding the disease itself from their description. Sometimes various sounds exist simultaneously, and are distinctly defined by the patient; in many cases it is possible by treatment to remove one of the sounds. These subjective sounds are continuous and uniform; sometimes they change for a time, or the patient is at intervals perfectly free from them. In cases of continuous sounds the prognosis is unfavourable; in those that change it is favourable.

It is of special importance for diagnosis and prognosis to ascertain whether the dulness of hearing and subjective noises can be influenced by our methods of examination. We have to make out whether by positive or negative air-pressure in the external meatus, or by the air-douche, an improvement in the hearing or the noises can be effected. If we find that such improvement does take place, we may assume that the inflammatory changes are still in a tractable condition, and we may reckon upon the success of the treatment.

Patients frequently complain of a feeling of dulness, heaviness, and fulness in the head and the ear, which may be associated with giddiness. Sometimes dull stinging pain is complained of, which generally recurs with the slightest colds. Unpleasant sensations are often felt in the external meatus, such as dryness, tension, and itching, inducing the patient to seek relief by scratching.

Only in that form of the disease first described can we make a tolerably reliable diagnosis from the local appearances. From the injected appearance of the membrana tympani, the radiating arrangement of the vessels being plainly visible, and the hyperæmic condition especially marked at the short process and the handle of the malleus, an extensive hyperæmia of the mucous membrane of the tympanum may be inferred, if it can be ascertained that no idiopathic affection of the membrana tympani is present. When the membrane is opaque and of a whitish colour, as if thickened, it may be concluded that a similar change is going on throughout the extent of the mucous membrane of the tympanum. The membrane may be indrawn by obstruction in the Eustachian tube, which condition of the tube may have formerly existed or still exists. If after the air-douche, or after using Siegle's speculum, the membrane along with the malleus still remains in its abnormal position, we may conclude that adhesions and anchyloses exist, producing permanent fixture of the membrane and ossicles.

In the second form of dry inflammation the membrana tympani is as a rule normal. In many cases it is exceedingly pale, the outline of the malleus is very sharply defined, and the membrane presents no deviation from its normal position.

By means of the air-douche we obtain information regarding the condition of the Eustachian tubes. While in the case of the hyperplastic form, with simultaneous obstruction of the Eustachian tube, the auscultation sound is generally very fine and weak and sometimes interrupted, we hear in the sclerotic form an expansive, full current of air striking sharply against the tympanic membrane.

The prognosis in both forms of this affection is as a rule unfavourable. In many cases it is impossible even by early treatment to arrest the increasing dulness of hearing; in others it can be made stationary for a longer or shorter time by treatment. A comparatively favourable prognosis may be given when the symptoms can be affected by the air-douche.

Treatment.—For both of these forms of chronic inflamamtion of the middle ear the air-douche is the most important remedy. In cases of swelling and hyperæmia, it promotes absorption, restores the sound-conducting structures to their normal condition, and stretches or ruptures any adhesions which may have formed. This mechanical treatment is assisted by injections into the middle ear. Amongst the great number of remedies employed in the first-mentioned form of the inflammation, the most effective are astringent solutions, such as sulphate of zinc (0.5—1 per cent.), in order to remove any existing inflammatory condition. In both forms of the affection, iodide of potassium in solution (2—4 per cent.) may be used to promote absorption of the inflammatory products. For the purely dry form of inflammation, the so-called sclerosis of the tympanic mucous membrane, Politzer recommends bicarbonate of soda (1—2 per cent.) As such solutions readily become mouldy, the author employs, instead of the bicarbonate of soda, a solution of borax (sodæ bibor. 0·3, glycerin. 5, aq. destill. 15). This treatment, by soaking through the rigid structures, is believed to bring about a loosening of them and an improvement of their vibratory power, but no doubt the simultaneous employment of the air-douche is the chief cause of the success of these injections. Wreden recommended injections of a solution of chloral hydrate (1—2 per cent). Injections of acetic acid or caustic potash, and solutions of other irritating substances, formerly so much in use, may effect a temporary improvement, but afterwards the increase of the deafness will be the more rapid.

Catarrhs of the naso-pharynx or of the mucous membrane of the Eustachian tubes must receive the necessary treatment. In many cases it is possible to effect an improvement in the hearing by treating these catarrhs after the local treatment of the ear has proved unsuccessful.

Sometimes steam conducted into the middle ear produces a good effect, and although immediately after this treatment the symptoms are aggravated, an improvement will soon follow. Vapour of chloride of ammonium which has been in use for a long time is now rarely employed. In cases of noises in the ear, chloroform vapour, or, according to Burckhardt-Merian, vapour of the iodide of ethyl may be used with advantage.

Catheterism may be performed daily. When it is combined with injection, it is best to employ each on alternate days (Politzer). This treatment is not to be continued for longer than 3—4 weeks, and should only be resumed again after a long interval. It should not be continued if an increasing improvement in the hearing or in the subjective noises cannot be effected by it. Treatment continued too long sometimes aggravates the disease even after improvement has taken place. The air-douche is inadmissible if followed by increased dulness of hearing.

In cases of plethora abdominalis, the waters of Karlsbad or Marienbad have often a beneficial effect when accompanied by appropriate diet. In cases of heart disease, Oertel's method of treatment is recommended, which consists in diminishing the volume of blood to be circulated, by increasing the excretions, and limiting the supply of fluids, and in stimulating the heart by muscular exercise, such as mountain-climbing.[1] Patients of a scrofulous constitution should take salt-water baths. In sclerosis proper, especially if associated with annoying tinnitus, patients will find most benefit from residing in high altitudes.

Although in many cases the prospect of improving the hearing is but small, even as we cannot decline to help a phthisical patient for whom there is little chance of recovery, so ought we not to abandon a patient annoyed by his ear affection, but must at least endeavour to relieve him as much as possible. In many cases we are unable to improve the hearing, but the tinnitus and other symptoms complained of may be alleviated.

Rarefaction of air in the external meatus, a remedy often employed by the old aural surgeons, sometimes produces a beneficial effect upon the tinnitus, but more rarely upon the hearing. The air may be rarefied by a strong india-rubber bag or by other special appliance. Delstanche has recently recommended an instrument by means of which a high degree of rarefaction of air can be obtained. But the effect of rarefaction is mostly temporary. The following

[1] Ziemssen's *Handbuch der Allgemeinen Therapie*, vol. iv., Leipzig, 1884.

internal remedies have sometimes a good effect on subjective noises, namely, bromide of potassium (2—4 grammes daily), atropine (0.002 gm.), liquor arsenicalis Fowleri (2—10 gtt.), also quinine (0·1—1 gramme) or salicylic acid (1—2 grammes) daily. The constant current should also be tried (p. 69).

In the case of sclerosis, Lucae endeavoured to improve the mobility of the sound-conducting apparatus by mechanical treatment of the ossicular chain itself. The instrument employed for this purpose consists of a steel pin furnished with a small pelotte or ball, and resting upon a spiral spring fitted into a handle. This 'spring-pressure probe' is placed upon the short process of the malleus, and then piston-like movements are made.

For improving the hearing in cases of obstruction to the conduction of sound, Politzer recommended a small instrument, by means of which the vibrations of the cartilaginous structure of the auricle are conveyed to the ear. It consists of an elastic sound-conductor, made most conveniently of a drainage tube of the thinnest kind, one end of which is slit up, forming at one side a small plate, which is made to lie upon the membrana tympani. The outer end of the tube is connected with an india-rubber membrane, $1—1\frac{1}{2}$ cm. in diameter, which lies in the hollow of the concha.

If no benefit can be obtained by the above modes of treatment, operations must be resorted to. In the case of great tension and thickening of the membrana tympani, incisions may be made, or the galvano-cautery may be employed to effect paracentesis. The folds of the membrana tympani extending from the short process of the malleus should be cut when they are markedly stretched. In the case of retraction of the membrane and shortening of the tendon of the tensor tympani, tenotomy of that muscle, first performed in the living subject by Weber-Liel, may be resorted to. But as we have already observed, the changes in chronic inflammation of the middle ear are not confined to these parts, and as anchyloses and adhesions may take place throughout the whole extent of the sound-conducting apparatus, so these operations are only successful in exceptional cases. Two cases have been reported in which a post-mortem examination was made after tenotomy during life. In the one case anchylosis of the stapes in the fenestra ovalis was found (Voltolini), and in the other abnormal conditions in the labyrinth (Lucae). Kessel proposed and carried out the removal of the ossicles, afterwards contriving to increase the mobility of the foot-plate of the stapes, an operation more rational and better supported by our knowledge of the pathologico-anatomical conditions. According to Kessel, this operation is indicated as soon as the apparatus of the middle ear has suspended its functions, the bone-conduction being retained for tones of eight octaves and also in cases of very troublesome subjective noises.

The author has repeatedly performed disarticulation of the malleus, and has at least confirmed the experience of Kessel that no harm is done by the operation. In one of the author's cases it diminished considerably the exceedingly troublesome tinnitus, for which all previous treatment had been in vain, and also improved the hearing for more than a year. Only in the case of subjective noises can permanent success be achieved by this operation. Contriving to improve the mobility of the foot-plate of the stapes is proscribed by the nature of the anatomical conditions.

NERVOUS EARACHE.

(SYNONYM: *Otalgia nervosa.*)

By nervous earache we understand that pain which occurs without any traceable inflammation. Whether it arises in connection with the branches of the trigeminal or of the glosso-pharyngeal nerve cannot be determined. The pain is either continuous, or, more frequently, intermittent, and in the latter case it generally sets in during the evening or at night. Most frequently nervous otalgia arises in a reflex manner from carious disease of the molar teeth, as a rule, of the lower jaw. On the other hand Moos observed a case of supra-dental neuralgia preceding purulent inflammation of the middle ear. A healthy tooth had been extracted without giving relief. The toothache disappeared after incision of the membrana tympani in its posterior-superior quadrant, where it was bulging, thereby making an opening for a copious discharge of pus. Otalgia is also due to ulcerative processes in the pharynx or larynx, and to operations on these parts. Earache is particularly common in ulcerative destruction of the epiglottis. Vidal noted pain in the ears of a lady, lasting for several hours, after excision of the tonsils. Sometimes this affection depends upon malarious infection, but in many cases the etiology cannot be given.

Treatment.—Earache arising from carious teeth is, of course, cured by their extraction, but in some cases quinine does much good, even when malarious origin cannot be traced, and in a few cases the author has also obtained success with salicylic acid. In addition, iodide of potassium, chloroform vapour, oil of turpentine, and nitrite of amyl have been employed.

HÆMORRHAGE INTO THE TYMPANUM.

Hæmorrhage into the tympanic cavity not only occurs in the case of polypi or of injury, but also in great venous engorgement, in severe vomiting, and in whooping-cough. Such hæmorrhage, when no perforation of the tympanic membrane exists, causes sudden and great dulness of hearing and pain, a sensation of pressure in the ear, and tinnitus. When the membrana tympani is perforated at the same time, the quantity of blood discharged from the ear is generally slight.

A lady whom the author treated for purulent inflammation of the middle ear with perforation of Shrapnell's membrane had a discharge of blood from the ear every time she was sea-sick. The coagulated blood had to be removed by means of the tympanic tube. Benni[1] observed hæmorrhage from both ears during menstruation, the ears being healthy; but after severe pain, occurring suddenly, copious bleeding took place from both ears, and on examination the membranes were found to be perforated.

Treatment consists in the removal of the effused blood by means of Politzer's method after paracentesis of the membrane, if not perforated previously; the ear should also be syringed with an antiseptic fluid. If the hæmorrhage be followed by inflammatory symptoms, cold should be applied in the form of compresses.

[1] Bericht über den 2. internationalen otolog. Congress in Mailand, *Zeitschrift für Ohrenheilkunde*, vol. ix. p. 407.

CHAPTER IX.

DISEASES OF THE INTERNAL EAR.

ANATOMICAL.

THE osseous labyrinth is formed of exceedingly dense bone, as hard as ivory, and is enclosed in the more porous substance of the petrous bone. It contains the cavities designated as the *vestibule*, the *cochlea*, and the *semicircular canals*, in which is situated the membranous labyrinth, bathed inside as well as outside by the labyrinthine fluid, the endo-lymph, and the peri-lymph respectively.

The vestibule forms an oval cavity divided into two parts by a

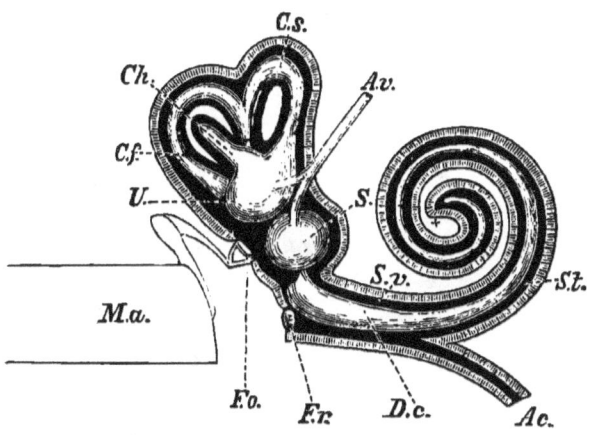

FIG. 41.

perpendicular ledge, *crista vestibuli*, extending along the internal wall, namely, the *recessus sphericus* or *fovea hemispherica* (*sacculi*) in front, and the *recessus ellipticus* or *fovea hemi-elliptica* (*utriculi*) behind. The external wall of the vestibule separates it from the tympanic cavity, and in this wall is situated the *fenestra ovalis* (*F.o.* Fig. 41), in which the foot-plate of the stapes is fastened by means of the annular ligament. In the internal wall of the vestibule are small orifices (*maculæ*), through which the branches of the vestibular nerve enter. The three semicircular canals, which are all situated at right angles to each other, communicate with the posterior part of the vestibule by five apertures. We distinguish the semicircular canals as follows—a horizontal (external) *C.h.*, and two vertical, the frontal (superior) *C.f.*, and the sagittal (posterior) *C.s.* These different canals commence with a dilated lumen, the ampulla; their extremities are of the actual width of the canal, and the two vertical canals have a common termination. Anteriorly the

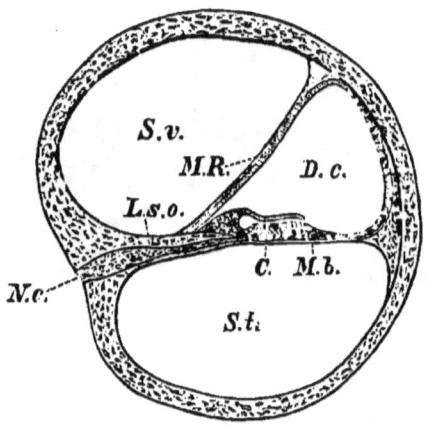

FIG. 42.

vestibule merges into the cochlea, the apex of which is directed outward. The cochlea makes two turns and a half around a central pillar (*modiolus*), which lies horizontally. From the modiolus the so-called spiral lamina, also consisting of bone (*L.s.o.* in Fig. 42, representing a vertical section through one of the windings of the cochlea), projects into the lumen of the cochlea, and is continued to the opposite wall by means of the *lamina spiralis membranacea*, also called the *membrana basilaris* (*M.b.*). The windings of the cochlea are thus divided into two parallel canals. The superior canal commencing at the vestibule is named the *scala vestibuli* (*S.v.*); the inferior, communicating with the tympanum through the *fenestra rotunda*, is named the *scala tympani* (*S.t.*). The two canals communicate with each other through a small opening, the *helicotrema*.

Corresponding with the division of the osseous vestibule, the membranous portion is divided into two small sacs, namely the *sacculus* in front (*S.*, Fig. 41) and the *utriculus* (*U*) behind. Upon the delicate walls of these small sacs, which are connected with each other by a small canal extending to the *aquæductus vestibuli* (*A.v.*), the nerves are spread. Crystals termed *otoliths* adhere to the inner surface of the membranous structures. Posteriorly extend the membranous semicircular canals bathed by the perilymph, and assuming a form corresponding to their osseous enclosure. Besides the membrana basilaris, already mentioned, another membranous structure, called *Reissner's membrane* (*M.R.*), extends from the osseous lamina spiralis to the wall of the cochlea. A third canal is thereby formed between these two membranes, termed the *ductus cochlearis* (*D.c.*), which contains the sound-perceiving organ. A free communication exists between this canal and the sacculus of the vestibule by means of the *canalis reuniens*, which is filled with endolymph. The *aquæductus cochleæ* (*A.c.*) extends from the scala tympani, close in front of the fenestra rotunda, to the jugular fossa, and forms a connection between the perilymph of the labyrinth and the peripheric fluid. The endolymph finds an outlet through the arachnoidal sheath of the auditory nerve into the subarachnoidal space, as well as through the *aquæductus vestibuli* to the posterior surface of the *eminentia pyramidalis* (*crista vestibuli*), which ends blindly in a sac covered by the dura mater.

Corti's arches (*C*), many thousands in number, are situated parallel, and consist each of two small rods or fibres, an inner and an outer, lying upon the *membrana basilaris* in the *ductus cochlearis*. On either side of these rods lie the inner and outer hair-cells. The membrana basilaris, upon which Corti's organ is situated, increases in width from the base to the apex of the cochlea, and upon it, between the rods and the cells, the extremities of the nerve-fibres are extended.

At the extremity of the external meatus the *auditory nerve* divides into the *vestibular and cochlear nerves*. The former supplies the vestibule and the semicircular canals, while the latter is distributed in a radiating manner through the cochlea in the lamina spiralis ossea, forming in that situation a ganglionic plexus from which the nerve terminals extend on the membrana basilaris.

Physiological.

The vibrations of sound are transmitted to the labyrinthine fluid by the sound-conducting apparatus in the middle ear, through the medium of the stapes, which is movably inserted into the fenestra ovalis by means of the annular ligament. Only through the agency of the elastic membrane of the fenestra rotunda can the labyrinthine fluid, confined in its dense osseous capsule, accommodate itself to the variations of pressure produced by the movements of the foot-plate of the stapes. On account of the very narrow lumen of the helicotrema, this cannot take place without the membrana basilaris with the structures upon it being set in motion.

The functional importance of the different parts of the labyrinth has not yet been clearly defined. According to Helmholtz, it seems probable that the vestibule and ampullæ serve for the perception of non-periodic vibrations (noises), the cochlea for that of periodic vibrations (tones). Helmholtz also pointed out that probably in the cochlea the parts near the fenestra rotunda respond to high tones and those near the cupola to low tones. Helmholtz's view, that Corti's arches should be regarded as perceptive organs for the different tones (on account of Hasse's discovery that birds do not possess Corti's organ), had to be modified to the view that the varying length and tension of the membrana basilaris in connection with the capillary cells must be considered as the chief factors in the perception of the different tones, and that by this means the vibrations of sound are analysed and transformed into nerve-stimuli.

Helmholtz's theory of tone-perception in the cochlea was confirmed by Moos and Steinbrügge by pathologico-histological investigation. They found in a case of defective perception of high tones atrophy of the nervous elements of the lowest turn of the cochlea. Baginsky tested the accuracy of Helmholtz's theory by experiments on animals.

The semicircular canals appear to have nothing to do with hearing. According to the experiments hitherto made, they stand more in relation to the equilibration of the body.

The transmission of variations in air-pressure from the external meatus and the tympanum to the labyrinth has been somewhat exactly defined by Politzer's interesting experiments. He inserted hermetically into the superior semicircular canal a small manometrical tube filled with a solution of carmine, and in this way ascertained that when air was condensed in the external meatus as well as in the tympanum (from the Eustachian tube), the fluid in the manometer rose, while it sank in the case of rarefaction of air in both parts. These experiments were subsequently confirmed and elaborated further by Helmholtz, Lucae, and Bezold. According to Bezold, the excursive capacity of the membrane of the fenestra rotunda is five times as great as that of the annular ligament.

While it was formerly assumed that an increase of the labyrinthine pressure occurs when the membrana tympani and the footplate of the stapes are drawn inward, physiological experiments point to the fact that, in the case of rarefaction of air in the middle ear, such as we observe when the Eustachian tube is impermeable, a decrease in the intra-labyrinthine pressure is produced. As the labyrinthine fluid is in communication with the cranial cavity by means of the aquæducts and the arachnoid sheath of the auditory nerve, the view is quite tenable that pressure-changes in the labyrinth can only exist temporarily. Only in the event of the places of outflow of the labyrinthine fluid being affected by pathological changes can it be possible for a permanent alteration to take place in the pressure in the labyrinth.

GENERAL REMARKS ON DISEASE OF THE INTERNAL EAR.

Having in previous chapters treated of the diseases of the sound-conducting structures, we now turn to the affections of the apparatus of perception, the labyrinth, and the auditory nerve in its course and centre in the brain.

As the labyrinth is contained in an exceedingly dense osseous capsule, and obtains its nutrition almost exclusively through the internal auditory artery from the basilar artery, and hence from a vascular origin quite different from the middle ear, it is therefore, with regard to its diseases, somewhat independent of the other parts of the organ of hearing. The implication of the labyrinth, sometimes occurring in severe acute and chronic inflammation of the middle ear, can be explained partly by the capillary vascular communication between the middle ear and labyrinth which was demonstrated by Politzer, and partly also by trophic disturbances affecting both structures. Taking into consideration the position of the different parts of the nervous apparatus of the ear, especially of the labyrinth, being inaccessible to direct examination, it is not remarkable that the diagnosis of nervous deafness was not accurate in former times. Even now, with all the means of examination we have, much still remains to be wished for. When the apparatus of perception is alone affected, the diagnosis is easier. In the case of a completely normal condition of the parts to which we have access, and a decided difference between the bone- and air-conduction, we may conclude that the disease has its seat in the sound-perceiving portion of the organ of hearing, especially when cerebral symptoms co-exist. In the case of simultaneous disease of the sound conducting and perceiving structures, we are unable to form a decided opinion regarding the degree in which the one or the other is affected by the existing disease.

HYPERÆMIA OF THE LABYRINTH.

Hyperæmia of the labyrinth occurs with all those diseases which lead to hyperæmia of the head in general, and especially of the brain, such as the serious exanthemata, typhus, and scarlet fever; in vascular engorgement from the most varied causes, and also in active congestion. The more independent hyperæmia of the labyrinth, which occurs with or without cerebral hyperæmia, is of greater importance to us. The principal symptoms are tinnitus, giddiness, a dull feeling in the head, and impaired hearing. While the hyperæmia lasts, marked injection of the vessels may be observed at the handle of the malleus, which subsides again as the symptoms disappear. We must assume that in these cases we have to deal with vaso-motor disturbance, namely, decreased tonicity of the vessels, due to the diminished influence of the sympathetic in producing contraction. Secondary hyperæmia occurs in the course of acute and chronic inflammation of the middle ear.

From hyperæmia of the labyrinth arise the hearing disturbances observed during the administration of various medicines, especially quinine and salicylic acid, namely, very troublesome tinnitus, with more or less dulness of hearing. These symptoms either last only a few hours or several days, and subside almost without exception quite spontaneously. That they are caused by hyperæmia of the labyrinth was demonstrated by the experiments of Roosa and Kirchner,[1] who, after large doses of quinine and salicylic acid, found hyperæmia and ecchymosis of the tympanic membrane, the tympanum, and labyrinth. The rare cases in which hearing disturbances become permanent may be assumed to have originated from extravasation of blood into the labyrinth.

Treatment.—Appropriate treatment must be employed to remedy defects in the general circulation when the hyperæmia has arisen from that cause. Such treatment must be carried out according to the condition and the constitution of the patients, and upon principles applying to the individual cases. Woakes, for instance, points out that cases of tinnitus which he attributed to hyperæmia of the labyrinth were sometimes cured by Karlsbad salts. It is also frequently possible to obtain in these cases good results from the electric treatment of the sympathetic in the neck with the constant or induced current.

ANÆMIA OF THE LABYRINTH.

In anæmic patients, and all whose strength has been greatly reduced by severe illness, tinnitus and dulness of hearing often occur. Both symptoms disappear when the anæmia is cured and the general health is improved. Besides the administration of preparations of iron, a residence in high altitudes is decidedly

[1] Sitzungsberichte der Würzburger physik.-med. Gesellschaft, 1881.

beneficial. It is well known that fainting fits are sometimes accompanied by tinnitus and dulness of hearing.

While it has not unfrequently been observed that blindness has been caused by acute anæmia, the only similar case with relation to the ear has been communicated by Urbantschitsch,[1] in which, after profuse bleeding from the nose, total deafness on both sides set in, which became permanent. The necropsy showed no changes from the normal state either in the labyrinth or the brain. Abercrombie speaks of a very debilitated patient, who was deaf in an upright position, but who heard well when he lay down or bent forward to such an extent that he became red in the face.

HÆMORRHAGE INTO THE LABYRINTH.

Extravasation of blood or its residue in greater or less quantity has been observed in the labyrinth on post-mortem examination, in cases of acute as well as chronic inflammation. Observations on the living subject also warrant the conclusion that such effusion into the labyrinth sometimes takes place. If slight, the symptoms are very insignificant, while extensive extravasation is characterised by the sudden occurrence of great dulness of hearing or total deafness. Most frequently great extravasation into the labyrinth is of traumatic origin, especially in the case of fracture of the petrous bone, the deafness being generally total, and the tinnitus and giddiness very troublesome. After absorption, the symptoms may abate to a great extent, but dulness of hearing generally remains. Without doubt, the total deafness, which sometimes occurs suddenly and becomes permanent, must be ascribed to hæmorrhage into the labyrinth. In the case of a deaf and dumb boy, the author found that such total deafness had set in suddenly during a paroxysm of whooping-cough. We shall afterwards discuss the extravasation of blood, which is supposed to be the cause of Menière's disease. Let us only note here that on post-mortem examination it has frequently been found (Moos, Politzer, Lucae) that the labyrinth, including the semicircular canals, has been filled with blood without any disturbance of equilibration during life.

Moos, in particular, in the case of chronic processes following

[1] *Archiv für Ohrenheilkunde*, vol. xvi. p. 185.

upon inflammation of the middle ear, repeatedly found deposits of pigment in various parts of the labyrinth. He also proved by the most careful microscopic examinations that the defective hearing occurring in hæmorrhagic pachymeningitis is likewise due to hæmorrhage into the labyrinth.

Moos[1] summarises the results of his investigations as follows:— 'The defective hearing in cases of hæmorrhagic pachymeningitis originates from extravasation by diapedesis into the labyrinth, which accompanies meningeal hæmorrhage, repeated attacks of which may lead to total abolition of the sense. This result is owing to atrophic and degenerative processes in the labyrinth, the course of the auditory nerve as well as its terminations being especially affected thereby. In the production of such processes, disorders of the circulation and of nutrition are chiefly concerned.'

ACUTE INFLAMMATION OF THE LABYRINTH.

Hitherto only a few cases of idiopathic acute inflammation of the labyrinth have been definitely ascertained by post-mortem examination, while those of traumatic origin, or as an accompanying symptom of other diseases, especially of meningitis, sporadic as well as epidemic, often come under observation. In one case Politzer[2] made an exact investigation on the dead subject. The case was that of a deaf and dumb boy of 13, who at the age of $2\frac{1}{2}$ years had suffered from fever with convulsive seizures, followed by otorrhœa in both ears of brief duration. It was found that both tympanic membranes, as well as the mucous covering of both tympanic cavities, were normal, that the stapes was immovable, the niche of the fenestra rotunda filled with an osseous mass, the cochlea and the semicircular canals entirely occupied with newly formed bone, and the vestibule much contracted. The vestibular and cochlear branches of the auditory nerve were intact. According to Politzer, this was a case of acute purulent inflammation of the labyrinth, the pus having probably made its way through the fenestra rotunda into the tympanic cavity, and thence outwards, after which the osseous formation had taken

---

[1] *Zeitschrift für Ohrenheilkunde*, vol. ix. p. 97.   [2] *Ibid.* p. 389.

place in the labyrinth. In a similar case Moos and Steinbrügge [1] found, in addition to many other changes, new formation of connective tissue and bone proceeding from the periosteum, in consequence of which partial obliteration of the lumen of the cochlea in the first convolution had taken place, along with rigidity of the lamina spiralis membranacea. Schwartze has recorded a case of the affection occurring in an adult, which set in with pain in the head and ear, giddiness, unsteady gait, loud subjective noises, dulness of hearing, and frequent vomiting, to which symptoms were soon added those of purulent meningitis. The post-mortem examination showed purulent inflammation of the labyrinth and meninges, no intercommunication being traceable. Whether the labyrinthine inflammation was the primary disease, as assumed by Schwartze, must remain doubtful.

Voltolini believes that, in the case of children, deafness occurring very suddenly and accompanied by meningeal symptoms is due to acute inflammation of the membranous labyrinth. 'Otitis labyrinthica' of Voltolini only lasts a few days, and after the disappearance of the meningitic symptoms total and incurable deafness in every case remains on both sides, along with giddiness and staggering, which only disappear in the course of weeks or months. Even if the above case described by Politzer demonstrated the occurrence of this kind of acute inflammation of the labyrinth, it nevertheless seems to be more probable that in most of such cases simple basal meningitis is present. The course of meningitis is often very rapid :—A well-developed child, previously quite strong, suffers from weak health from about the time of teething until its third year, when suddenly it becomes feverish, and convulsions, delirium, and drowsiness set in ; these symptoms subside as rapidly as they appear, and idiocy, aphasia, or deaf-mutism remains. In other cases the abortive forms of epidemic cerebro-spinal meningitis appear. According to the author's investigations in the deaf and dumb institutions of Berlin, an affection of such brief duration as that of Voltolini's otitis labyrinthica occurs only in isolated cases. As a rule, it lasts much longer, and the convalescence is slow after the disappearance of the meningitic symptoms.

[1] *Zeitschrift für Ohrenheilkunde*, vol. xii. p. 96.

In cases of purulent inflammation of the meninges, deafness is more rarely owing to implication of the auditory nerve, either in its course or its central tracts, than to extension of inflammation to the labyrinth. This is demonstrated by the fact that, although on post-mortem examination the auditory nerve is often found imbedded in pus, not even the slightest deafness had been noticed during the course of the illness; besides, facial paralysis is rarely observed accompanying deafness. Disease of the labyrinth must be superadded before deafness is produced. In several cases post-mortem examination has shown that deafness has resulted from epidemic cerebro-spinal meningitis.

Out of a total of 43 cases of cerebro-spinal meningitis observed by Moos,[1] deafness occurred in 11 during the first 3 days; in 17 between the 3d and 10th day; and in 15, between 14 days and 4 months. The early occurrence of deafness is, according to Moos, most probably due to purulent or hæmorrhagic inflammation of the labyrinth, developing simultaneously with the meningeal affection.

When the defective hearing occurs later, we must assume that the inflammation has proceeded along the sheath of the auditory nerve and thence into the labyrinth—a so-called 'neuritis descendens,' with its consequences.

Moreover, the inflammation may also extend to the labyrinth through the aquæducts. From what he found on post-mortem examination, Lucae believes that it may also extend through vascular cords of tissue from the dura mater to the cancellous tissue which surrounds the capsule of the labyrinth. From a large number of post-mortem examinations (Merkel, Heller, Knapp) the purulent character of the inflammation of the labyrinth has been ascertained.

The prognosis of the deafness, which is absolute in almost all cases, and occurs on both sides, is exceedingly unfavourable. Moos has related a case in which he succeeded in effecting considerable improvement by the constant current.

After the meningitis has run its course, disturbances in the equilibration remain noticeable from the unsteady gait of the patient, probably due to disease of the semicircular canals.

[1] *Ueber Meningitis cerebrospinalis epidemica*, p. 14. Heidelberg, 1881.

Cerebro-spinal meningitis, which in 1864-65 prevailed in various parts of Germany, was of particular severity in Western Prussia, in Pomerania, and Posen, and added greatly to the number of deaf-mutes in these provinces. According to Wilhelmi's statistics regarding deaf-mutes in Pomerania, there were in that province, out of 1637 deaf and dumb persons, 278 from cerebro-spinal meningitis. Great epidemics of this disease also occurred in Germany during 1870-71 and in 1878. Even this year several slight epidemics have been reported.

The fact that inflammation of the middle ear is often associated with that of the labyrinth has been established by post-mortem examination. While Moos in particular has traced cellular infiltration of the membranous labyrinth even in the case of slight inflammation, others have observed purulent accumulation in the labyrinth due to severe inflammation of the middle ear.

Direct extension of purulent inflammation from the middle ear to the labyrinth may take place, but only in very rare cases, by destruction of the membranes of the round or oval window, as also by destruction of the labyrinthine wall. With regard to the separation of the osseous labyrinth in the form of a sequestrum, see page 170.

Treatment.—In acute inflammation the antiphlogistic remedies are used, namely, application of cold, blood-letting, preparations of iodine and mercury, and purgatives. If no success attend this treatment, pilocarpine should be tried, which was first recommended by Politzer at the Otological Congress at Milan in 1880. In some cases of long standing it is still possible to effect an improvement by means of this 'sweating treatment' continued for 2 to 3 weeks. According to Politzer, 2—8 drops of a 2 per cent. solution of hydrochlorate of pilocarpine should be daily injected subcutaneously. In the case of many patients the effect is powerful with small doses of 0·005 to 0·01 gramme of this drug, while in others doses of 0·02 gramme are required. Profuse perspiration and salivation take place in the course of 5—45 minutes after the injection. Treatment by pilocarpine is contra-indicated in cases of weak conditions of the heart.

CHRONIC INFLAMMATORY AND DEGENERATIVE PROCESSES IN THE LABYRINTH.

Chronic inflammatory processes of the labyrinth occur either independently or in connection with disease of the middle ear. Examination of the labyrinth has shown a series of changes which must be regarded as arising from chronic inflammation. Those changes affect all parts of the labyrinth, and appear as hyperplastic as well as degenerative processes, namely, thickening of the membranous labyrinth from hyperæmic swelling, new formation of connective tissue, cellular infiltration, fatty, fibroid, or amyloid degeneration, atrophy, increased vascularity, calcareous or pigmentary deposition, and changes in the labyrinthine fluid. In a case of atrophy of the nerve structures in the first turn of the cochlea, most carefully examined by Moos and Steinbrügge,[1] the mobility of the stapes in the fenestra ovalis was impaired. They leave it undecided whether this atrophy is to be considered as caused by inactivity, or by a permanent increase in the intra-labyrinthine pressure.

The important points in the differential diagnosis between disease of the labyrinth, and that of the sound-conducting apparatus have been already discussed at page 33.

Treatment.—The labyrinth is accessible to treatment only to a slight extent. In most cases we have to limit it to derivative measures, vesication, painting with tincture of iodine, embrocation with iodine or iodoform ointment upon the region of the mastoid process, as also to general treatment, and the treatment of dyscrasiæ. In addition pilocarpine may be tried.

MENIÈRE'S COMPLEX OF SYMPTOMS.

Upon the basis of several cases which came under his observation, in one of which a post-mortem examination was made, Menière defined a form of disease which is named after him. The symptoms of Menière's disease are unsteady gait, excessive giddiness, movements of rotation, vomiting, faintness, dulness of hearing, and tinnitus. In the case which Menière examined post-mortem, he found hæmorrhagic effusion into the semicircular canals. On

[1] *Zeitschrift für Ohrenheilkunde*, vol. x. p. 1.

account of the correspondence of the symptoms observed in this case with those which Flourens noticed in animals on making a section through the semicircular canals, Menière assigns to these structures his complex of symptoms.

Although there can be no doubt that this group of symptoms may occur in affections of the semicircular canals, it must nevertheless be pointed out that the same symptoms may also be produced by affections of the tympanic cavity, on the one hand, and of the auditory nerve and its central tracts on the other. The observations recorded at page 57 lead us to assume that Menière's symptoms originate from stimuli acting from the ear upon the cerebral centres, from which the disturbances in the equilibration, the dyspeptic, and the other nervous symptoms arise. Hughlings Jackson believes that any weakness of health constitutes a factor in the production of aural vertigo, and that the more the power of resistance of the nervous system is lowered, the latter becomes more susceptible to stimuli acting from the ear.

Menière's complex of symptoms may therefore be caused by—
1. Stimuli from the middle ear.
2. Diseases of the labyrinth.
3. Pathological processes in the brain.

1. Symptoms of vertigo may arise from the presence of plugs of cerumen or foreign bodies in the external meatus. Accumulations of exudation products or polypi in the tympanum may also give rise to these symptoms. Sometimes alterations of pressure in the tympanic cavity, due to interference with the ventilation in the case of disease of the Eustachian tubes, suffice to produce vertigo.

2. Sometimes Menière's symptoms are acute, when the disease is described as 'the apoplectic form.' In the slighter cases there is only a temporary feeling of giddiness, with nausea and vomiting. In severe cases the patient suddenly falls to the ground, with or without loss of consciousness. He regains consciousness after a short time, but he suffers from impaired hearing, loud subjective noises, vertigo, unsteady gait, nausea, and vomiting. The disease occurs mostly in strong adults, and, as a rule, only on one side. Sometimes the patient has been dull of hearing before the first attack. After the attack the dulness of hearing increases, and either returns after-

wards to its former condition, or the aggravation becomes permanent. The hearing in a healthy ear may be permanently abolished by the first attack. On the other hand, a greater or less degree of dulness of hearing may set in and disappear again. Either the patient is attacked only once, or the attacks recur at longer or shorter intervals, until finally, if not from the very first, the deafness is complete. In most cases the attack commences with intense tinnitus or aggravation of the subjective noises.

With regard to the seat of the pathological processes which give rise to these symptoms, opinions are much divided, a cerebral or labyrinthine origin or only a defect of innervation being severally assumed.

In a case in which Menière's symptoms were apoplectiform, the writer observed the simultaneous formation of a blood-cyst in the external meatus while the tympanum was in a normal condition. It is therefore probable that, as in the external meatus, rupture of blood-vessels had also taken place in the labyrinth, true Menière's disease being thus caused by extravasation of blood into the labyrinth. Extravasation of blood into the labyrinth also occurs without any symptoms of vertigo. The occurrence or non-occurrence of these symptoms seems to depend on the circumstance whether stimulation or paralysis of the nerves involved has taken place (Moos).

Menière's symptoms are often observed in children, along with those of meningitis, and also in such as have suffered from actual meningitis. On the disappearance of the meningitic symptoms, after existing for a longer or shorter time, deafness and unsteady gait remain. We have already described this disease under acute inflammation of the labyrinth (see page 216). Regarding Menière's symptoms in the case of syphilis and after injury, see pages 225 and 234.

3. Oscar Wolf reports an interesting case in which Menière's group of symptoms was caused by a cerebral tumour.[1] The disease commenced with subjective sounds and dulness of hearing, soon followed by attacks of giddiness, nausea, and vomiting. In the course of two years the symptoms gradually increased in intensity, and symptoms of cerebral disease set in, namely, dilatation of the

[1] *Zeitschrift für Ohrenheilkunde*, vol. viii. p. 380.

pupils, violent headache, psychical derangement, facial paralysis, and lesions in the region supplied by the hypoglossal nerve; death occurred after paralysis of the soft palate and pulmonary symptoms. On post-mortem examination a tumour as large as a cherry was found in the *tonsilla (amygdala) cerebelli*, which had pressed upon the origin of the auditory nerve. A second tumour was found in the cortex of the cerebrum with inflammatory infiltration of the meninges; probably this was a case of gummata.

Treatment.—Disease of the tympanic cavity must receive suitable treatment when it is the cause of the symptoms.

For attacks of the apoplectic form, Charcot recommended the administration of sulphate of quinine in a dose of 0·3—1·0 gramme daily, to be continued for a month. Then 14 days are to elapse, and the same treatment is to be resumed. It is specially important that the general health should be improved and that the nervous system should be invigorated by carefully promoting hardiness of constitution, as by cold-water baths. For the symptoms which remain after the attacks, such as tinnitus and vertigo, bromide or iodide of potassium, as well as the constant current, may be employed with advantage. In cases in which it can be inferred that exudation has taken place suddenly into the labyrinth, Politzer obtained good results from pilocarpine.

CONCUSSION OF THE LABYRINTH.

Concussion of the labyrinth is caused by the action of violence upon the surface of the cranium, as from a fall, knock, or blow, or upon the orifice of the external meatus, but especially by the action of loud sounds. The nerve terminations are affected by the sudden increase of the intra-labyrinthine pressure, which may give rise to permanent or temporary suspension of the sense of hearing. In severe cases not only simple concussion occurs, but also more or less extensive hæmorrhage.

Cases are observed in artillerymen where permanent deafness sets in immediately after the action of loud sounds. In an interesting case reported by Brunner,[1] all tone perception was lost after the

[1] *Zeitschrift für Ohrenheilkunde*, vol. ix. p. 142.

discharge of a rifle in the immediate neighbourhood of the patient. 'The lady heard the keys of the piano rattle, but did not perceive the tones at all.' Some time afterwards she was able to distinguish the tones again. In slighter cases the effect on the hearing is such that everything is heard with a different sound, especially the patient's own voice. Sometimes a double sound (Wolf) is heard with high tones, and in other cases the tones and noises have a rattling or resounding accompaniment. Besides, there is frequently great sensitiveness to the action of sound. In addition, loud subjective sounds set in, such as ringing or singing of a very high pitch. These symptoms may be aggravated by vertigo, headache, and nervous excitement, which do not appear immediately after the injury, but in a few days, and may therefore be attributed to reactive inflammation in the labyrinth. The symptoms of vertigo are sometimes of a distinct character. Hughlings Jackson, for instance, describes a case in which, after the discharge of a cannon, vertigo, deafness, and unsteady gait took place. Since that time the patient suffered from dulness of hearing in the right ear, with subjective sounds, and inclined to the left in walking. The patient always pushed a companion to the left while arm-in-arm with him, and his wife had often to draw his attention to the fact that he was walking towards the left.

In the case of concussion of the labyrinth, the bone-conduction is either greatly reduced or suspended. This fact is useful in making the diagnosis, whether the defective hearing arises from a labyrinthine affection or from a lesion in the middle ear. Politzer in particular pointed out that in traumatic rupture of the membrana tympani, the bone-conduction should be tested, as thereby we are able to ascertain whether the labyrinth is implicated. In the case of artillerymen, dulness of hearing along with subjective noises of a singing character is a frequent complaint. The one circumstance that the dulness is as a rule worse after shooting-practice points to the fact that it is caused by frequently repeated concussions of the labyrinth.

Although functional defects mostly become permanent in severe cases, recovery may take place even after total deafness, so that the prognosis should not always be unfavourable.

Treatment must be limited chiefly to the exclusion of all detrimental influences. Everything likely to produce congestion in the diseased organ should be avoided, and the patient kept very quiet. The influence of loud sounds must be excluded as much as possible, and the meatuses kept well plugged. In order to prevent reactive inflammation, blood-letting, cold compresses, and purgatives may be employed, and all irritating remedies are strictly to be avoided. In the later stages remedies promoting absorption, especially the preparations of iodine, may be used.

SYPHILIS OF THE LABYRINTH.

Apart from the diseases of the external meatus and of the tympanic cavity due to secondary syphilis, this affection also produces disease of the labyrinth.

Hutchinson first pointed out that hereditary syphilis caused deafness. He expressed the view that this deafness was produced by disease of the nervous apparatus, as in 21 cases examined by him, the external and middle ear were in a normal condition. According to Hinton, the affection occurs at the age of puberty, the dulness of hearing becoming rapidly very marked, and having its origin in the nervous structures ; the tuning-fork is not heard, and the dulness of hearing is very great, without any trace of actual disease of the tympanum. Hinton believed that in the poorer classes the affection is more severe, and is less amenable to treatment, while in the better classes the symptoms are less marked, and the treatment is followed by better results. It is remarkable that German authors have written very little with regard to this disease. Von Tröltsch remarks that especially in cases of dulness of hearing in children of syphilitic parents, the perception of sound through the cranial bones is very often affected to an extent out of proportion to the defective perception of speech. The author has observed total deafness in the case of a girl of 6, and also in that of a girl of 8 years, which had set in suddenly in the former and gradually in the latter, both cases being traceable to hereditary syphilis.

Hereditary syphilitic disease of the labyrinth is frequently associated with catarrh of the middle ear. Moreover, parenchymatous keratitis is often accompanied by the labyrinthine affection, the latter sometimes preceding the former. Hutchinson found dulness of hearing in 15 out of 102 cases of syphilitic keratitis. The rapid development of the labyrinthine affection takes place with Menière's symptoms, nausea, giddiness, vomiting, unsteady gait, and headache. According to Knapp, tinnitus may be absent.

The prognosis of hereditary syphilitic affection of the labyrinth is unfavourable. In isolated cases a cure is effected by early and rational antisyphilitic treatment, but unfortunately it is often impossible to improve the generally weak constitution of the patient. Hinton obtained no benefit from preparations of mercury and iodine, but iodine vapour passed into the tympanum seems to have been found effectual by him. Knapp, on the other hand, completely cured a patient by means of calomel and iodide of potassium. Zeissl, in a treatise 'On Lues (Syphilis) hereditaria tarda' (*Wiener Klinik*, part vii. 1885), recommends for recent cases the inunction cure, with simultaneous doses of Zittmann's decoction (decoct. sarsæ co. Ger. Ph.), and for non-progressive cases the preparations of iodine, especially iodide of iron.

The time of appearance of the labyrinthine affection in acquired syphilis varies very much. Sometimes it sets in during the late period of the secondary stage, and sometimes in the tertiary stage. The disease may run an insidious course, and commence with the symptoms of non-purulent chronic inflammation of the middle ear, with or without a simultaneous affection of the pharynx. The tinnitus and slight dulness of hearing which existed from the beginning may increase more or less rapidly. In other cases a high degree of deafness sets in rapidly, almost suddenly, accompanied by Menière's symptoms.

In the case of one of the writer's patients, specific irido-choroiditis developed before the labyrinthine affection; the latter commenced with such extreme symptoms that the patient was in a very sad condition. Suddenly he suffered from a feeling of intoxication, giddiness, pressure, and heaviness in the head, aggravated by nausea and frequent vomiting, troublesome tinnitus, and dulness of hearing. He was so unsteady in his gait that he was unable to walk alone.

By taking iodide of potassium, 2 grammes daily, all the symptoms disappeared rapidly.

Testing the bone-conduction is of importance in the diagnosis of syphilitic disease of the labyrinth. Politzer points out that dulness of hearing of sudden onset, the examination of the tympanum giving a negative result, and the perception through the cranial bones being abolished, may with probability be diagnosed as syphilitic. In the case of every acute or chronic affection of the hearing, where no disease of any consequence can be ascertained in the tympanic cavity, but where bone-conduction is lost, we are led to suspect that the affection is based upon a specific origin. But it must be borne in mind that in old age, even with normal hearing, the bone-conduction is sometimes abolished.

Moos made a microscopic examination in a case of acquired syphilis. The infection had taken place seven years before death. The symptoms of the ear affection were intolerable tinnitus, attacks of vertigo, and very great dulness of hearing. The external meatus and tympanum were normal, and on post-mortem examination periostitis was observed in the vestibule, immobility of the footplate of the stapes, and cellular infiltration of the labyrinth. In a case which was minutely examined by Politzer, he found dense infiltration of the spiral canal of the modiolus (Rosenthal's canal), partly with numerous round cells, and partly with larger bodies, globular, oval, or angular in shape.

Treatment.—While it is possible either to cure or to arrest by early treatment the slighter forms of disease of the labyrinth, due to acquired syphilis, which make slow progress with gradually increasing dulness of hearing, the more severe forms in which extremely defective hearing occurs rapidly are more difficult to treat, those cases especially in which the affection has remained stationary for a considerable time being hopeless.

In cases of acquired syphilis we employ, according to the stage of the disease at which the labyrinthine affection occurs, either mercury or iodide of potassium. As the affection generally develops only in the later stages of syphilis, the latter remedy is most frequently used.

Simultaneous affections of the tympanum should be treated chiefly by the air-douche, all irritant measures being avoided.

The author examined two patients, the one being totally deaf, and the other very dull of hearing, with abolition of perception through the cranial bones, who asserted that the deafness and great dulness of hearing respectively were due to electric treatment. The dulness had been previously only slight, but they said it had distinctly increased immediately after that treatment. A third patient ascribed her deafness to the operations of paracentesis of the membrana tympani and section of the tendon of the tensor tympani.

DEAFNESS IN LEUKÆMIA.

Gottstein, Politzer, and Blau have reported cases in which leukæmic patients were affected with sudden deafness, after more or less extreme vertigo, nausea, and vomiting, accompanied by intolerable subjective noises.

Politzer on post-mortem examination of the labyrinth found the scala tympani of the cochlea occupied by new growth of connective tissue, intersected by a trabecular osseous new formation, the lamina spiralis ossea et membranacea being thereby displaced at several points. Similar changes were found in the vestibule, but to the greatest extent in the semicircular canals. The necropsy showed that exudation of a leukæmic nature had occurred, being quite recent at one place, which had given rise to inflammation, with the production of connective and osseous tissue.

DEAFNESS IN CASES OF MUMPS.

As in leukæmia, deafness also occurs very rapidly in cases of mumps accompanied by Menière's symptoms, either on one or both sides. No cerebral symptoms are observed, and neither fever nor other inflammatory symptoms are present. The deafness is complete.

Knapp believes that, as in the case of orchitis, which sometimes occurs along with mumps, we have to deal with a metastatic process. Lemoine and Lannois, on the other hand, who have observed the simultaneous occurrence of parotitis and the labyrinthine affection, are of opinion that the disease is due to localisation of a general affection in different parts of the body.

The prognosis is exceedingly unfavourable, as up to the present time no case has been reported in which improvement was possible.

On post-mortem examination Toynbee found in a patient who had become deaf from mumps great changes in the labyrinth.

DISEASES OF THE AUDITORY NERVE.

Inflammation affecting the auditory nerve proceeds either from the meninges or from the labyrinth. Sometimes hæmorrhage takes place into the neurilemma with simultaneous affection of the neighbouring parts.

Of greatest importance is *atrophy* of the nerve, produced in a mechanical manner by pressure of tumours or inflammatory products upon its stem. Atrophy may also arise from disease of the nerve-centre or its peripheral expansion.

Accompanying atrophy *fatty degeneration* is often found, along with the deposit of amyloid bodies.

Böttcher and Moos found *calcareous deposits* in the auditory nerve. In general marasmus, in anchylosis of the stapes, and in cancer Politzer found *amyloid degeneration* in the spiral canal of the modiolus.

Of *neoplasms* affecting the auditory nerve, several cases of sarcoma, neuroma, fibroma, and gumma have been described. By the presence of a tumour the nerve may be drawn aside. In a case reported by Virchow a psammoma extending from the dura mater into the internal auditory meatus caused paralysis of the facial and auditory nerves.

OTHER DISEASES AFFECTING THE NERVOUS STRUCTURES.

In addition to the diseases of the nervous structures already described, there is another series of affections, the nature of which has still to be made clear, and which must be regarded partly as *reflex neuroses*, partly as *vaso-motor disturbances*.

Scanzoni[1] observed temporary deafness simultaneously with general vascular irritability and an eruption of urticaria over the

[1] Gynäkologische Fragmente, *Würzburger med. Zeitschrift*, vol. i.

whole body after the application of leeches to the region of the vagina. At the menstrual period, in cases of abortion, or in confinements, often temporary or permanent dulness of hearing or deafness may set in.

Politzer[1] describes a rare form of defective hearing as *angeioneurotic paralysis* of the auditory nerve, which is characterised by sudden pallor of the face, followed immediately by nausea, vertigo, tinnitus, and dulness of hearing. In a case observed by him such symptoms occurred daily, and a cure was effected by applying galvanism to the sympathetic in the neck.

An interesting case of *alternating dulness of hearing* has been reported by Urbantschitsch.[2] The alternations occupied a term of ten days. Within such period the hearing in one ear decreased from a certain maximum of acuteness to nil, while simultaneously in the other ear the hearing increased from nil to that maximum. It must remain doubtful how far the explanation given by Urbantschitsch is correct, who assumes the cause as a change of tension in the tensor tympani muscle.

DEAFNESS IN HYSTERIA.

Partial or total deafness is a symptom rarely observed in hysteria. Hysterical dulness of hearing either occurs independently or along with paresis of other parts, especially as an accompanying symptom of hysterical hemi-anæsthesia. With the latter is also associated anæsthesia of the membrana tympani and the middle ear. When the deafness is not complete, sound-conduction through the bones is more impaired than that through the air.

In the same manner as Bourcq, Charcot, and others effected a transference of sensibility from one side to the other by means of metals, Zaufal, Urbantschitsch, and Walton proved that a transference of hearing can also be made. In the same degree as the hearing decreases in the one ear, it increases in the other.

The higher tones are first transferred, and then the lower. In the case reported by Urbantschitsch[3] the deafness passed over to the side which was previously hyperæsthetic on approximating a

[1] *Lehrbuch der Ohrenheilkunde*, p. 832.   [2] *Wiener med. Presse.*
[3] *Archiv für Ohrenheilkunde*, vol. xvi. p. 171.

horse-shoe magnet to the mastoid process. The high tones were always transferred first, and then the low tones. A return to the previous condition took place in about six minutes in the reverse order. Zaufal succeeded in removing hysterical deafness by frequent application of gold coins. In two cases Uspensky effected a cure by galvanising the sympathetic.

OTITIS INTERMITTENS.

Intermittent disease of the ear arising from malarious infection was first described by Weber-Liel,[1] and has since been repeatedly confirmed. It was regarded by Weber-Liel as a vaso-motor neurosis. The symptoms, which almost always set in towards evening or during the night, consist of neuralgic pains, dulness of hearing, and noises in the ear. The membrana tympani and the tympanum are remarkedly hyperæmic, and a muco-purulent exudation takes place. The attacks generally occur according to the quotidian type, but the tertian form is also observed. The disease may last for weeks or months. Sometimes the neuralgic symptoms are the most prominent. Voltolini reports a case of *otalgia intermittens* where the most severe earache occurred every night, and which disappeared on the first day after the administration of quinine in doses of 0·05 gramme every hour.

Treatment.—The treatment of otitis intermittens consists in administering quinine in the manner usually adopted in malarious infection.

DISEASE OF THE CEREBRAL TRACTS OF THE AUDITORY NERVE AND CENTRE.

In tracing the auditory nerve in a centripetal direction we have first to point out that its course in the brain as well as its central origin is not yet thoroughly known.

The root-fibres extend in the medulla oblongata (1) into the anterior auditory nucleus (Meynert), which lies in the pons; (2) into the inner, and (3) the outer auditory nucleus on the floor of the fourth ventricle.

---

[1] *Monatsschrift für Ohrenheilkunde*, etc., No. 11, 1871 : *ibid.* No. 5, 1878.

Fibres in the medulla oblongata from the auditory nuclei extend (1) upon the tract of the pedunculus cerebelli to the cerebellum of the same and of the opposite side, and end in the *nucleus monticuli* (roof-nucleus) of the cerebellum ; (2) upon the tract of the pedunculus cerebri through the internal capsule to the temporal lobe. The latter tract crosses the median line below the corpora quadrigemina, above the pons. But, according to Wernicke, it has not yet been proved that the continuation of the auditory nerve to the temporal lobe always crosses completely. (3) There is also a decussation in the brain, between the temporal lobe on the one side and the cerebellum on the other.

According to the experimental investigations of Ferrier and Munk, the seat of the hearing-centre is to be sought for in the temporal lobe. Munk distinguishes between 'psychological' and 'cortical deafness' (Rindentaubheit). The former occurs in animals when a superficial part of the cortical substance of the temporal lobe is removed. The dog no longer understands the words which he had learned, such as, 'Pst,' 'Come,' 'Paw,' etc.; but he still hears, and at every noise he points his ears. When a large portion of the surface of the brain is removed, cortical deafness sets in, the dog taking no more notice of any sounds.

Based upon observations on the living subject and subsequent post-mortem examination, Wernicke first expressed the opinion that the centre of the perception of sound has its seat in the first temporal convolution. The symptoms caused by injury of the first temporal convolution are designated as 'sensory aphasia' (Wernicke) or 'word-deafness.' Patients thus affected are able to express themselves by means of speech and writing, but they do not understand spoken words. Sounds are perceived by them, but they are unable to form an idea from what they hear. The pathological processes which give rise to this affection are atrophy, hæmorrhage, and softening.

Neuro-pathologists have hitherto given but little attention to defects of hearing caused by cerebral disease, so that from the cases which are presently known, although they have been carefully examined, no conclusions of any great value can be deduced. In the small number of cases of disease of the auditory nuclei which have hitherto come under observation, the existence of deafness has not yet been definitely traced. It is especially remarkable that deafness has very rarely been observed in bulbar paralysis. When the nucleus of the roof of the cerebellum is injured, the ear of the same side is said to be duller than the other. The symptoms characteristic of tumours in the cerebellum are occipital neuralgia, defective co-ordination, unsteady gait, and restricted movement. Hutin observed in the case of a tumour of the temporal lobe completely crossed deafness, and Vetter also observed it in a lesion of the internal capsule.[1] But in both cases the ears were not examined.

At the place of decussation of the crura cerebri, in the neighbourhood of the corpora quadrigemina, the nuclei of the motor oculi and of the trigeminus are situated; so that in affections occurring in this region defects of hearing are associated with strabismus and double vision, with xerosis of the cornea, neuralgia of the trigeminus, and paralysis of the masseter muscles.

Aphasia is caused by disease of the third frontal convolution, adjacent to the anterior convolution of the temporal lobe. When, therefore, a disease is localised in this region on the left side, sensory aphasia is sometimes combined with aphasia proper, that is, with inability to speak. In a case reported by Westphal,[2] in which the left temporal lobe was almost totally destroyed, no aphasia or dulness of hearing existed, so that the results of the experiments on animals are very much open to question.

Apoplexy is rarely accompanied by defects of hearing—only occurring sometimes in the case of unilateral hæmorrhage in the pons. Aneurism of the arteries, especially of the basilar, does not as a rule produce defects of hearing. Griesinger states that several patients who suffered from it complained of pulsation in the occiput.

Cerebral tumours much more frequently produce defects of vision than of hearing. Tumours at the base of the cranium, which press or drag upon the auditory nerve, are most frequently the cause

---

[1] Moos, 'Zur Genese der Gehörsstörungen bei Gehirntumoren, III. Otol. Congress, Basel, 1884; *Comptes Rendus*, p. 22.
[2] *Berlin, Klin. Wochenschrift*, No. 49, 1884.

of defects of hearing. As, according to Huguenin, inflammation of the meninges develops during the presence of a tumour in the brain, causing in its turn *neuritis descendens olfactoria, optica et acustica*, the disturbances of these various senses are but of little importance in making a diagnosis with regard to the locality of the tumour.

Ladame found auditory defects 7 times in 77 cases of tumours in the cerebellum; 7 in 26 cases in the pons; 5 in 13 in the middle cranial fossa; 2 in 14 in the pituitary region; 3 in 27 in the middle lobe; 6 in 52 cases of multiple tumours. In 5 cases there were only defects of hearing, no other organ of sense being implicated. Total deafness existed in 17 cases, in one of them only temporarily. The other hearing defects were in 9 cases simply dulness; in 6, tinnitus; and in 2, hallucinations. In one case the tinnitus lasted for seven years, and for a long time was the only symptom, and in another case it was the only disturbance of the organs of sense throughout the illness (Moos).

CHAPTER X.

TRAUMATIC LESIONS, NEOPLASMS, AND MALFORMATIONS.

TRAUMATIC LESIONS.

On account of its protected situation, lesions of the external meatus are somewhat rare. They may be occasioned by the entrance of sharp or blunt articles. By violence acting upon the lower jaw, as by a fall or a blow upon the chin, the anterior wall of the meatus, which forms part of the glenoid fossa, may be fractured, producing hæmorrhage from the ear. In rare cases the articular process of the lower jaw is wedged into the external meatus. The osseous portion of the external meatus is generally implicated in cases of fracture of the temporal bone.

Rupture of the membrana tympani, already described under diseases of that membrane, constitutes the most frequent kind of injury to the ear. At page 114 the writer has described two cases of perforation of the membrana tympani by means of knitting-needles, probably with injury of the labyrinth, in which Menière's symptoms of a very extreme character were observed. Another case was recently reported by Schwartze, in which after an injury with a knitting needle a discharge of cerebro-spinal fluid took place, which lasted for eight days, and was so copious that a continuous dripping ensued. Symptoms of cerebral irritation were also manifested, which continued for four weeks. It remains doubtful whether this was a case of lesion of the labyrinthine wall, or of perforation of the tegmen tympani with laceration of the dura mater.

Bezold[1] has recently reported a most interesting case of injury

[1] *Berlin. Klin. Wochenschrift*, No. 40, 1883.

of the ear from stabbing. The knife, which was driven in at right angles to the surface of the cranium, made its way through the tragus and the orifice of the external meatus to the anterior surface of the tympanic plate, penetrated deeply between the anterior wall of the meatus and the articular process of the lower jaw, and injured the internal carotid artery and the Eustachian tube.

Fractures of the base of the skull very frequently involve the ear, as they extend to the temporal bone, and either implicate the labyrinth or still more frequently the tympanic cavity.

According to its development, the temporal bone is composed of three parts. Even in the adult traces exist of this original division. The temporal bone consists of (*a*) the *pars squamosa*, (*b*) *p. petrosa* (the pyramidal portion), and (*c*) the *p. tympanica*. The two former join at the petro-squamosal suture, which extends in the longitudinal direction of the tympanic cavity, through its roof, and through the roof of the antrum mastoideum to the parietal bone. From thence the suture runs in a vertical direction, but somewhat forward, above the mastoid process, and returns to the upper part of the tympanic cavity, above the posterior wall of the osseous meatus. These two parts are joined in front and below by the pars tympanica, which forms the anterior half of the osseous meatus, and takes part in the construction of the fissure of Glaser, and of the musculo-tubal canal.

Two kinds of fracture of the temporal bone are to be distinguished—(1) fracture actually in the lines of suture formed by the development of the bone (diastasis); (2) transverse fracture of the temporal bone, extending through the meatus auditorius internus, and through the vestibule of the labyrinth. The former runs frequently from the apex of the pyramid to the hiatus Fallopii, and through the tegmen tympani. Generally the lines of fracture extend through the osseous meatus in two directions—from its upper and inner extremity to the posterior and anterior walls of the meatus, outward and downward. In these cases the membrana tympani is either not injured at all or only in its upper part. With diastases, as well as with transverse fractures, the facial canal may be implicated. Transverse fractures of the temporal bone are generally caused by force acting upon the occiput, while fractures in the line of the long axis of the pyramid are due to force applied to the lateral surface of the cranium.

There may be no hæmorrhage from the ear even in the case of extensive fractures, while, on the other hand, it may occur in slight cases, and either originate in the external meatus or in the tympanum, the membrana tympani being ruptured. In the latter case the severe hæmorrhage which sometimes occurs proceeds from the middle meningeal artery.

If after an injury a discharge take place of serous watery fluid, sometimes copious in amount, we may conclude that this fluid is *liquor cerebro-spinalis*, and that we have to deal with an opening in the cranium along with rupture of the dura mater. According to the investigations of Schwalbe, it appears probable that in cases of fracture through the labyrinth, cerebro-spinal fluid may also be discharged by way of the internal auditory meatus.

The prognosis of fracture of the base of the skull is mostly very unfavourable, but cases of very severe and extensive injuries are reported to have recovered. When the labyrinth has been implicated by the fracture deafness is total. Hæmorrhage into the tympanum causes considerable dulness of hearing, which passes away on absorption of the effused blood. As a rule, vertigo and noises in the ear remain for a considerable time.

Politzer[1] describes a transverse fracture, which is interesting on account of the meningitis which followed at a later stage. A strong man suddenly fainted, and fell backward upon the ground, hardened by frost. When he regained consciousness after the lapse of several hours, total deafness set in on both sides, with impaired power of speech, pain in the occiput, vomiting, tinnitus, vertigo, and a dull feeling in the head. On examination six weeks afterwards, he was totally deaf, and no changes were observed in the tympanic membrane, tympanum, or Eustachian tubes; neither was there any trace of injury of the cranium. While walking, his gait was so unsteady that it resembled that of an intoxicated person. In the seventh week after the fall, meningitis appeared, under which the patient rapidly sank. The post-mortem examination showed fissures of the petrous bones on both sides, which extended from behind into

[1] *Archiv für Ohrenheilkunde*, vol. ii. p. 88.

the vestibules. The labyrinth was filled with pus, which had passed thence through the internal meatus to the base of the cranium, giving rise to purulent meningitis in that situation.

Treatment.—When the injury implicates the external meatus or the membrana tympani, any fluid blood which may be present should be soaked up with wadding, and the meatus closed by antiseptic dressing, consisting of a cotton tampon steeped in carbolic oil, the whole ear being covered with antiseptic cotton-wool. Sometimes a tampon of cotton wadding in the external meatus is necessary in order to stop the bleeding. All manipulations likely to give rise to irritation, even syringing of the meatus, must be avoided during the first few days after the injury. Only when the cerebral symptoms allow of it, careful syringing with antiseptic fluid may be attempted. When the acute symptoms have yielded to the treatment usually adopted in fracture of the base of the cranium, consisting of antiphlogistic measures, restricted diet, and rest, an improvement of the hearing and of the other symptoms may be brought about by careful employment of the air-douche, in the case of hæmorrhage into the tympanum and an inflammatory condition of the mucous membrane.

NEOPLASMS.

To the rare affections of the organ of hearing belong the malignant growths, carcinoma, enchondroma, and sarcoma. They either grow from the external ear or the tympanum, and lead to destruction of the neighbouring parts of the temporal bone, of the parotid gland, and of the skin. They extend to the interior of the cranial cavity and produce death by pressure upon or implication of the brain.

When the growth originates in the tympanum the membrana tympani is first destroyed, swelling shows itself at the bottom of the meatus, which may readily be mistaken for a polypus, and if removed a new growth rapidly appears. While an ordinary polypus has a smooth, uniform surface and shape, the new growth frequently presents an ulcerated surface. The larger the growth and the earlier destruction and swelling of the surrounding parts appear, the more is the diagnosis confirmed. The pain accompanying the development of the growth is, as a rule, very severe. Carcinoma is observed most frequently; enchondroma and sarcoma rarely.

The author had the opportunity of observing in the case of a boy, $3\frac{1}{2}$ years of age, the development of a soft, round-celled sarcoma, which caused death in seven months. The new growth first appeared as a polypus-like swelling, springing from the tympanum, which rapidly increased in size until it became a tumour as large as a goose egg, projecting from the side of the head. Death ensued, with severe cerebral symptoms. On post-mortem examination it was found that a portion of the temporal bone had been destroyed. A dense mass, $1\frac{1}{2}$ cm. thick, lay upon the inner surface of the cranium in the region of the temporal bone, the dura mater being intact.

Treatment.—As operative interference is regarded as hopeless, the treatment is chiefly confined to alleviating the pain.

MALFORMATIONS.

Malformations are found in all the various parts of the organ of hearing, but those of the external ear, namely the auricle and the external meatus, are most frequently observed. They are caused by arrest of development at an early stage of fœtal life or by a deviation from the normal process of growth. From numerous post-mortem examinations, Hyrtl draws the conclusions (1) that the development of the external sphere of the organ of hearing depends by no means upon that of the middle and internal ear; (2) that the general law of symmetrical formation of all double parts does not apply in pathological processes, and that one ear may exhibit quite different anomalies of formation from the other.

Only a few cases of *supernumerary external ears* have been observed, their situation being usually in front of the normal ear, whose form they assume on a smaller scale. Of more frequent occurrence are the shapeless *auricular appendages*, consisting of cartilage or skin, which are also situated in front of the tragus.

The entire *absence of the auricle* is rarely observed. As a rule, some traces of it exist in the shape of cartilaginous formations or cutaneous appendages. The writer has observed a small flap of skin hanging down from the situation of the auricle, the external meatus being normal. In another case the meatus was closed, and in place of the auricle there was only the tragus, forming a small thorn-shaped process. Not unfrequently a *stunted auricle*, or the *absence of some parts*, or its *abnormal position*, is noted. *Closure of the external meatus* is frequently associated with anomalies of development of the auricle. The closure is either membranous or osseous, and its site is either in the outer or in the more deeply situated parts of the meatus. In such cases the cartilaginous part of the meatus may be present or absent. When the membranous closure is confined to the outer part of the meatus, the membrana tympani may be quite normal. Cases have been observed in which conversation was well understood although a membranous closure existed on both sides, from which the inference can be drawn that the more internal parts were normal. Moos[1] observed a case of osseous closure of the external meatus on both sides, with unilateral malformation of the auricle. Speech was heard at a distance of several metres. Rau operated upon a membranous closure in a boy by excising a circular piece of the structure close to the osseous walls with a cataract knife. After a gelatinous substance had been removed from the meatus by syringing with tepid water, the boy heard at once very distinctly. A long time after the operation the opening became very narrow and finally closed altogether. Several cases have been reported in which this operation has been successful in the case of deaf-mutes. As a rule, however, closure of the external meatus is complicated with defects in the tympanic cavity, offering but little hope of success from operative interference.

Sometimes a barely noticeable anomaly of development is observed close in front of the external ear, consisting of a small depression or a blind fistulous canal, which was first described by Heusinger as *fistula auris congenitalis*, and which, according to Urbantschitsch,[2] is to be regarded as the remains of the first branchial cleft. This anomaly is generally situated about 1 cm. above the tragus, and a little in front of it. Sometimes a cream-like secretion is discharged from the fistula. Urbantschitsch repeatedly observed this malformation as hereditary. In the family of one of the writer's patients both grandparents exhibited this anomaly, along with the

---

[1] *Zeitschrift für Ohrenheilkunde*, vol. x. p. 20.
Monatsschrift für Ohrenheilkunde, No. 7, 1877.

father of the patient and his father's two brothers, as also five brothers and sisters of the patient.

Malformation of the tympanum and of the labyrinth is more rarely observed. The tympanic cavity may be entirely absent, and an osseous mass substituted for it. Its various parts may be abnormally developed, especially the ossicula, which may exhibit the most varied abnormalities, or may be entirely wanting. Contraction and absence of the labyrinthine fenestræ have been repeatedly observed. Complete absence of the labyrinth has also been noted, but the absence or the defective development of some of its parts, the semicircular canals, and the cochlea is more frequently observed. It cannot always be ascertained whether these defects depend upon early inflammatory processes or upon anomalies of development. Sometimes these malformations are combined with defective development of the upper and lower jaw, as well as the palate bones.

Malformations of the tympanum are due to early interruption of development in the region of the first branchial arch. The development of the labyrinth takes place, independently of the middle ear, from the labyrinthine vesicle, for which reason malformations of the labyrinth exist generally by themselves and independent of those of the middle ear.

CHAPTER XI.

DEAF-MUTISM.

DEAFNESS existing from birth or acquired in early childhood is followed by dumbness. When the child does not hear its mother's voice, it is unable to imitate and understand it. A child without the sense of hearing remains dumb, and those children who during their infancy lose their hearing also lose the speech they may have acquired.

The statistics contained in the writer's monograph on *Deaf-mutism and the Education of the Deaf and Dumb* show that amongst 246,000,000, there are 191,000 deaf-mutes, which gives an average proportion of 7·77 in every 10,000 individuals. The proportion is lowest in the Netherlands, being 3·35. In Belgium it is almost as low as 4·39. The proportion in the following countries is below the average, namely Great Britain, 5·74; Denmark, 6·20; France, 6·26; Spain, 6·96; Italy, 7·31, as also in the United States of North America. The following are above the average proportion: Germany, 9·66; Austria, 9·66; Hungary, 13·43; Sweden, 10·23, and Norway 9·22. The proportion is highest in Switzerland, namely 24·5 in every 10,000 inhabitants, and, among non-European countries, in the Argentine Republic. The statistics of the different countries all point to the fact that deaf-mutism is more frequently observed in mountainous regions than in the flat countries, and that in Europe it is of extraordinary frequency in the Alpine districts. In the mountainous regions of Austria the proportion in 10,000 is as follows: Salzburg, 27·8 Styria, 20; Carinthia, 44·1; while the average proportion for Austria is only 9·7. The proportions are similar in Italy and in France. In the latter the high figures not only apply to the regions of the Alps, but also to the Cevennes and Pyrenees, where deaf-mutism is more prevalent.

In Germany the north-east Provinces of Prussia contribute very large numbers to the total of deaf-mutes, namely East and West Prussia, 18·2 (census of 1st December 1880); Posen, 15·4; Pomerania, 12·7 in every 10,000 inhabitants. This seems to contradict the experience met with in other countries, that deaf-mutism occurs more frequently in mountainous districts than in the lowlands. But as the large number of deaf-mutes in these Provinces is due to the epidemic of cerebro-spinal meningitis in 1864-65, we may leave them out of account; otherwise, the proportion in Germany is the same as that in other countries. The proportion in the mountainous regions of South Germany is as follows, namely Baden, 12·2; Würtemberg and Alsace-Lorraine, 11·1; Bavaria, 9—being higher than the proportion of the lowlands in the north; Hamburg and Bremen, 4 and 6·4; Brunswick, 6; Oldenburg, 6·9. In the western Provinces of Prussia it is as follows: Westphalia, 7·4; Hanover, 7·8; Rhenish Prussia and Saxony, 7·6; Schleswig-Holstein, 5·9.

In all countries the number of male deaf-mutes is considerably larger than that of female: while, for instance, in Prussia in 1871 the proportion of the whole male sex to the female was 100—103·4, there were only 85·1 female deaf-mutes to 100 male. Both in regard to congenital and acquired deaf-mutism the male sex proponderates. Deaf-mutism is most frequently met with among the Jews; thus in Prussia (1880), amongst the Protestants, there were 9·89 deaf-mutes in 10,000; amongst Catholics, 10·39; and amongst Jews, 14·38, and a still larger proportion of Jews was noted in Bavaria.

Considerable disagreement exists in the statements regarding the frequency of congenital as compared with acquired deaf-mutism. Schmaltz in former years found, amongst 5425 deaf-mutes, 3665 who had been born deaf, and 1760 who had acquired deafness; but the author's more recent statistics[1] showed that amongst 4547 deaf-mutes, the disease was congenital in 2041 and acquired in 2378. We may therefore assume that in somewhat less than half the number of deaf-mutes the defect is from birth, while in the remaining half it has been acquired through disease.

The explanation of the disagreement between the different statistics is, that, owing to epidemic or endemic conditions, either congenital or acquired deaf-mutism preponderates.

[1] *Taubstummheit und Taubstummenbildung*, p. 52: Stuttgart, 1880.

The chief causes of congenital deaf-mutism are hereditary transmission and the influence of consanguinity of the parents. With regard to heredity, we distinguish between direct and indirect transmission, as well as multiple occurrence in one family. Formerly direct transmission was regarded as doubtful. According to the writer's statistics there were amongst 8037 deaf-mutes seventeen married couples, both being deaf-mutes, who had twenty-eight children with perfect senses. There were also 276 couples, of whom one—either the husband or the wife—was a deaf-mute. These had 419 children with perfect senses, and only eleven deaf and dumb children. In the course of the writer's investigations in the two schools for deaf-mutes in Berlin, two couples were found, all four being deaf-mute. In the case of the one pair, both were deaf-mute since birth, and they had four deaf and dumb girls and one boy with perfect senses. The other couple had three deaf-mute children, both parents having acquired deafness through disease. The statistics as compiled by the author show that in 6834 deaf-mutes there were 430 cases of indirect heredity—that is, 6·8 per cent. Even in the case of congenital deafness in several children of a family, without deaf-mutism in the other members of the family and the parents, we must assume the transmission of a predisposition from the parents to the children. According to various statistics, it has been found that in 100 families with deaf-mute children, there were 85·4 with only one deaf-mute child, 9·3 with two, 3·8 with three, and 1·1 with four. More than four deaf-mute children, and up to eight, were only found in 0·4 per cent. of the families. Cases of acquired deaf-mutism occur almost without exception only singly in each family.

Consanguinity of the parents plays an important part in regard to congenital deafness, although many have disputed this. While French investigators—Boudin and others—stated that the percentage of deaf-mutes arising from such marriages was 25—28, more recent and more extensive investigations have shown that the frequency is not nearly so great. According to the writer's statistical tables, 451 in 8404 deaf-mutes were born of consanguineous marriages, or 5·4 per cent.; the percentage born deaf was 8·1. As the number of consanguineous marriages does not exceed 1—2 per cent. in

France, as well as in Prussia, it has been placed beyond doubt that these marriages favour the occurrence of deaf-mutism. The author met with an interesting example of the influence of consanguineous marriages in one of the Berlin schools for the deaf and dumb. A deaf-mute child had other five deaf-mute brothers and sisters, and although no case of deaf-mutism had occurred in former generations of the family, it was found that the parents, as well as the grand-parents and the great-grand-parents, had been cousins. Thus the pernicious influence of consanguinity did not show itself until after the third marriage, when deaf-mutism appeared in such a dreadful manner.

The opinion has been frequently expressed that the occurrence of deaf-mutism is promoted by unfavourable social conditions. Unhealthy and damp dwellings, insufficient nourishment, and severe physical exertion of the parents, have been regarded as favouring the occurrence of the defect in children. Although these cannot be held as causes of deaf-mutism, it has been demonstrated, especially by Schmaltz,[1] who with the greatest care collected statistics with regard to deaf-mutism in the kingdom of Saxony, that, as a general rule, the defect is somewhat commoner amongst those classes who are poorest, and whose children are neglected. All statistics bear out the fact that acquired as well as congenital deaf-mutism is of somewhat more frequent occurrence in the country than in towns.

When deafness arises from disease, the child loses the speech which it has acquired. This is almost without exception the case with children up to seven years of age; but instances of loss of speech have been observed even when deafness did not occur until the age of fourteen and fifteen. The diseases giving rise to acquired deaf-mutism consist chiefly of inflammation of the meninges, namely simple basal meningitis and epidemic cerebro-spinal meningitis. Huguenin[2] points out that there are no decided marks of distinction between these two diseases due to the possibility of the occurrence of protracted epidemic meningitis, which fact renders it difficult to class the sporadic cases with the one or the other. Almost one-half of the cases of acquired deafness are due to

---

[1] *Die Taubstummen in Königreich Sashsen*, Leipzig, 1884.
[2] *Handbuch der Krankheiten des Nervensystems*, 2d edition, part I., p. 592.

cerebral affections (930 in 1989). Deafness is also caused by typhus and scarlet fever (260 and 205 in 1989). But it seems that the majority of cases of typhus must be attributed to inflammation of the meninges. Diphtheritic inflammation, due to extension of pharyngeal diphtheritis to the ear, should also be mentioned. More rarely deafness is caused by independent ear diseases, by injuries to the head, and other affections. In a recent meritorious work Bircher[1] maintains that it is incorrect to distinguish between congenital and acquired deaf-mutism, and is of opinion that it should be divided into the sporadic and the endemic forms. According to statistics, the extent of deaf-mutism in Switzerland is of an endemic nature, deaf-mutism and goitre being on a complete parallel in this respect. Bircher shows that this condition is related to the geological formation of the soil, that it is only met with upon the marine deposits of the trias and tertiary period, and that primitive mountainous regions, sediments of the quaternary sea, and freshwater deposits are free from it. Based upon extensive investigations in Swiss deaf and dumb institutions, Bircher assumes that in Switzerland sporadic deaf-mutism prevails at the rate of about 20 per cent. and endemic deaf-mutism at the rate of about 80 per cent. He believes that, under the influence of endemic pathological conditions, changes in the cerebral centres of hearing and speech are produced *in utero*. Endemic deaf-mutism, therefore, may exist from birth, or only occur during infancy. In districts where endemic deaf-mutism prevails, the defect of speech frequently predominates over that of hearing, so that it is assumed that the absence of speech is based upon primary defects of the centre of speech. It must remain a matter of doubt in the meantime whether we should record as a cause of endemic deaf-mutism the micro-organisms which Bircher found in the wells of districts where goitre prevailed, and which are absent from the wells of those places free from that disease. Having no special data with regard to the occurrence of deaf-mutism in mountainous regions, the author has pointed out in his monograph on *Deaf-mutism* the desirability of collecting exact statistics of such districts. To Bircher belongs the credit of explaining the remarkable frequency of deaf-mutism in Alpine countries.

---

[1] *Der endemische Kropf und seine Berziehungen zur Taubstummheit und zum Kretinismus*, Basle, 1883.

His investigations indicate the great frequency in these countries of a special kind of deaf-mutism, unknown in the lowlands, or, at least, only very rarely seen. With regard to Saxony, Schmaltz was unable to ascertain that terrestrial conditions had any influence upon the occurrence of deaf-mutism.

Unfortunately, very erroneous opinions still exist with regard to deaf-mutes. Judging from the descriptions frequently given, we should expect to find in the institutions a collection of sickly, badly developed, and stupid creatures, while we actually meet with healthy, bright children, who by their appearance cannot be distinguished from those with perfect senses. People were of opinion that scrofula and pulmonary diseases were very prevalent among deaf-mutes, but this is really the case only to a very limited degree. Deaf-mutes are also reproached with being lazy, cruel, greedy, passionate, etc., peculiarities which do not belong to deaf-mutes on account of their infirmity, but which can always be attributed to defective education.

In the case of many deaf-mutes the power of hearing is not altogether absent. Many hear to such an extent that they are able to repeat words spoken close to the ear. A considerable number of them also learn to speak single words in their homes, but are unable to master language completely. The statistics which have hitherto been collected show that more than one-half (60·2 per cent.) of the total number of deaf-mutes are entirely devoid of the sense of hearing. The fourth part of them are able to perceive sounds (24·2 per cent.); 11·3 per cent. hear vowels, and 4·3 per cent. hear words. The chief point of distinction with regard to the hearing-power of those born deaf and those who have acquired deafness, is, that of the latter the number of the totally deaf is far larger (68·4 per cent.) than that of the former (42·2 per cent.).

The anatomical conditions underlying deaf-mutism are still but little known, notwithstanding the considerable number of reports of post-mortem examinations, amounting to sixty-seven, which the author in his monograph has collected from various sources. In this respect much yet remains to be made clear. It is desirable that in all autopsies of deaf-mutes a careful examination of the organ of hearing should be made, and that the cause to which the infirmity was ascribed during life should be ascertained.

The reports of post-mortem examination show entire absence of the labyrinth in four cases, absence of the auditory nerve in one, and abnormal course of the nerve in one. Frequently changes have been found in the labyrinth, which must be regarded as the effects of inflammation, osseous deposits, degeneration, atrophy.[1] A large number of the reports in our possession have reference to the tympanic cavity. Moos gives most careful records of two cases of anchylosis of the ossicula and ossification at the labyrinthine fenestræ, and Gellé describes a similar case, all three being cases of congenital deaf-mutism. The most varied forms of alteration and destruction affecting the middle ear have been noted, but we have only a few reports recording changes in the brain. Rüdinger found in the brains of deaf-mutes a defective development of the surface of the third frontal convolution.

The curability of congenital deaf-mutism is only to be entertained in very rare cases where the deafness is not absolute and the defect is based upon changes in the middle ear. Two cases are recorded in which the hearing was established by the removal of a membranous closure of the external meatus. But no other cases are known in which treatment has been in any way successful. In the case of a girl who had been totally deaf since birth, the writer ascertained that the hearing was established spontaneously to such an extent that she was able to repeat words spoken close to the ear.

In acquired deafness an attempt at cure is out of the question in all cases in which deafness has resulted from disease of the brain and its membranes, as also from purulent destructive inflammation. When a purulent discharge exists it must be treated. In many cases also an improvement in the hearing may be effected by removing inflammatory processes. Deafness or dulness of hearing associated with naso-pharyngeal catarrh, generally along with exudation, may be made to yield to treatment.

But it is of the greatest importance that the treatment of these affections be not delayed until the defect has existed for a number of years. Rational treatment must at once be instituted, as soon as

---

[1] Compare Politzer's reports and those of Moos and Steinbrügge, p. 202.

the affection makes its appearance. Particularly in the case of independent purulent inflammation of the middle ear, or in inflammation due to scarlet fever, inadequate treatment is often the cause of deafness in children. 'As long as practitioners, otherwise thoroughly qualified, conscientiously availing themselves of auscultation and percussion in any doubtful case of bronchial catarrh, do not hesitate to treat, regardless of censure, every "ear-patient" who comes into their hands with instillations of oil and the like; as long as otherwise thoroughly experienced surgeons speak of "otorrhœa" in scarlet fever, and of "harmless catarrhs of the external meatus;" as long as the question whether it is desirable to hand over the "ear-patients" in large hospitals to trained specialists, is not only merely ventilated in medical circles, but even negatived—in one word, as long as the majority of general practitioners pay so little attention to the aural branch of surgery, so long can we scarcely expect an improvement in the field of hygiene' (Schmaltz). In the case of a child becoming deaf after acquiring speech, we must first of all endeavour to preserve the speech. It should be induced to speak much and correctly, and should be educated in a school for the deaf and dumb. Sending the child to such a school ought not to be delayed until its speech has been completely lost.

A deaf-mute, unable to acquire speech, is thereby excluded to a great extent from communication with his associates. His mental development is most seriously impeded, as he is not capable of receiving impressions of what is happening around him by means of hearing and speech, and thus he cannot share in the knowledge of his hearing fellows.

The great purpose of the founder of the instruction of deaf-mutes was to show the way by which it is possible to teach them to speak, and thereby to save them from mental neglect, and make them useful members of society. During the second half of the sixteenth century the Spanish priest, Pedro Ponce, discovered that deaf-mutes could be taught to speak. Although, in the opinion of his contemporaries, Ponce did excellent work with reference to the instruction of deaf-mutes, and a book also appeared after his death, *On the Art of teaching Deaf-mutes to Speak*, yet only isolated attempts at their instruction were made for a long time, until the year 1778, when, at the request of the Saxon Elector of that time, Heinicke removed with his pupils from Eppendorf near Hamburg to Leipzig, and there founded the first institution for the deaf and dumb. In the same year a school for deaf-mutes in Paris, which had hitherto been maintained by the Abbé de l'Epée, received a subsidy from the State, and in that city also was the foundation laid for the public instruction of the deaf and dumb.

The French and German institutions have been distinguished from each other by the fact that the education in the former has been conducted chiefly by means of the language of signs, while articulate speech has been taught in Germany.

The French deaf-mute, who has only acquired the artificial sign-language, in which the various letters are represented by certain positions of the fingers, is obliged to confine his intercourse to those afflicted like himself, and, except in writing, he can only make himself intelligible to and understand in some measure those of his fellows, blest with all their senses, who have learned his mode of communication. The German deaf-mute can communicate with his more fortunate brethren by speaking to them and understanding what they say. The advantages of the German method of instruction are so overwhelming that recently a beginning has been made in France to introduce it into the institutions in that country.

The instruction of deaf-mutes is conducted either 'intern,' at deaf and dumb institutions, or 'extern,' at schools. Large institutions are of least benefit, as their inmates have little opportunity of intercourse with people in possession of speech, and of putting into practice what they have acquired by instruction. It is different with pupils in day-schools, as the school and the family act complementary to each other.

The results obtained in the instruction of deaf-mutes vary greatly. They depend upon their intellectual capacity, upon the hearing-power which may still remain, and upon their previous ability to speak, also upon the manner of instruction as well as its duration. Considerable variation is observed in the results obtained in the different deaf and dumb schools. The number of those who learn to speak so well that one believes he is conversing with a person in possession of all his senses is very small. At the present stage of the education of deaf-mutes it may, on the whole, be assumed that one-third of their number can be trained with such success that they can converse with everybody. The speech of another third is somewhat less distinct, so that it is not understood by all, and the deaf-mute requires to resort sometimes to the aid of the sign-language. The speech of the remaining third becomes so indistinct after leaving the institution that it cannot be understood. Such deaf-mutes forget it altogether, and communicate with their fellows only by means of the sign-language or writing. In the Deaf and Dumb Association of Berlin, the author made the acquaintance of a joiner, who had been taught in a German institution, and had afterwards resided for several years in Paris, where, by means of writing and reading, he had completely mastered the French language.

The countries in which provision has been made for the instruction of all deaf-mutes are the United States of North America and most of the States of the German Empire.

During the last few years the education of the deaf and dumb has made most satisfactory progress in Prussia. While in 1875 it contained only 37 institutions, with 2351 pupils, the number of institutions in 1882 amounted to 52, with 3792 pupils.[1] In the Prussian schools for the deaf and dumb, 3991 children were under instruction in 1884. In Bavaria only about one-half, in Austria one-fourth, and in Switzerland one-fifth of the total number of deaf-mute children of school-age are under instruction.

It is highly desirable that in all Germany, as well as in every other country, all these unfortunate deaf-mute children should receive the benefit of an education which would rescue them from a state of mental neglect.

[1] *Zeitschrift des K. Pr. Statist. Bureau's*, 1883.

THERAPEUTIC FORMULÆ.

Arranged in the order in which they occur in the Text.

SOLUTIONS FOR CLEANSING THE EAR, page 19.

Common salt in water, 1—2 per cent.
Bicarbonate of soda in water, 1—2 per cent.
Sulphate of soda in water, 5 per cent.
Boracic acid, teaspoonful in 3 ounces of water.
Salicylic acid, in alcohol, 10 per cent. Teaspoonful of the solution in 3 ounces of water.
Carbolic acid in alcohol, 50 per cent. Teaspoonful of the solution in 3 ounces of water.
Corrosive sublimate in alcohol, 1 per cent. Teaspoonful of the solution in 3 ounces of water.

GENERAL REMEDIES, page 67.

(*a*) Local—
    Liquor ferri perchloridi.
    Sulphuric acid.
    Boracic acid.
    Nitrate of silver.
    Chromic acid.

(*b*) Constitutional—
    Preparations of Iodine.
    Preparations of Iron.
    Quinine.
    Cod-liver oil.
    Saline baths.
    Sulphur baths.
    Mineral waters.

Blood-letting, page 68.
Galvanism, p. 69.

ECZEMA, page 78.

(*a*) Local—
    Solutions :—
      Carbolic acid in olive oil, 1—2 per cent.
      Salicylic acid in olive oil, 1—2 per cent.
      Ol. picis liquidæ and oil or alcohol, equal parts.

    Powders :—
      Starch.
      Oxide of zinc.
      Salicylic acid.
      Alum.

    Ointments :—
      Salicylic acid and vaseline, 2—5 per cent.
      Hebra's ointment (ungt. diachyli alb.).
      Spirit of soap (spir. saponatus alkalinus).
      Soap ointment (sapo viridis).

    Caustic :—
      Nitrate of silver.

(*b*) Constitutional :—
    Fowler's solution, 2—6 drops daily.

ANOMALIES OF SECRETION, page 84.

(*a*) Diminished secretion of cerumen.
    Glycerine, applied with camel-hair brush.
    Vaseline, applied with camel-hair brush.
    Electric current (constant).

ANOMALIES OF SECRETION—*continued*.

(b) Increased secretion of cerumen, p. 86.
Instillation of solution of bicarbonate of soda in water, 1—2 per cent.
Instillation of soap and water.
Syringing with tepid water.

INFLAMMATION OF EXTERNAL MEATUS, page 91.
Blood-letting :—
4 to 6 leeches in front of tragus.
Ear-baths :—
Warm water.
Warm salt water.
Warm oil.
Warm moist sponges.
Ice-bags.

Embrocations :—
Blue mercurial ointment and vaseline, equal parts.
Carbolic acid and olive oil, 1—2 per cent.
Solutions for cleansing :—
Corrosive sublimate, 1 in 1000.
Absolute alcohol.
Insufflation :—
Finely powdered boracic acid.
Caustics :—
Nitrate of silver.
Chromic acid.

DESQUAMATIVE INFLAMMATION OF EXTERNAL MEATUS, page 94.
Instillations :—
Salicylic acid in oil, 2 per cent. (subsequent syringing with alkaline solution).
Corrosive sublimate in water, 1 in 300—500.

FUNGUS IN THE EXTERNAL MEATUS, page 96.
Instillations :—
Pure alcohol.
Salicylic acid in alcohol, 2—4 per cent.

HERPES AURICULARIS, page 97.
Ointment :—
Extract of belladonna and vaseline, 10 per cent.
Sedative :—
Hydrate of chloral.

SYPHILIS OF THE EXTERNAL MEATUS, page 98.
Precipitate ointment.
Application of solution of corrosive sublimate.
Powdering with calomel.
Cauterisation.

REMOVAL OF FOREIGN BODIES, page 101.
Instillations :—
Water.
Oil.
Glycerine.
Alcohol.
Petroleum and oil.
Turpentine.
Syringing with tepid water or oil.
Instruments, page 102.
Agglutinative method, page 103.
Suction, page 103.
Galvano-cautery, page 104.

CLOSURE AND CONTRACTION OF THE EXTERNAL MEATUS, page 105.
Laminaria tents.
Sponge tents.
Leaden tubes.

INFLAMMATION OF THE MEMBRANA TYMPANI, page 111.
(a) Acute—
Instillations :—
Warm water or oil with tincture of opium.
Solution of cocaine, 6—10 per cent.
Blood-letting.
Purgatives.
Scarification.
Paracentesis.

INFLAMMATION OF THE MEMBRANA TYMPANI—*continued*.
(*b*) Chronic—
  Insufflations :—
    Alum.
    Boracic acid.
  Caustics :—
    Tincture of the perchloride of iron.
    Nitrate of silver.

THE ARTIFICIAL TYMPANIC MEMBRANE, page 117.
Yearsley's Membrane is impregnated with salicylic acid, boracic acid, or thymol, and moistened in glycerine and water, 1 to 4.

ANOMALIES OF TENSION OF THE TYMPANIC MEMBRANE, page 117.
Incision.
Galvano-cautery.
Painting with collodion.

ACUTE CATARRH AND ACUTE PURULENT INFLAMMATION OF MIDDLE EAR, page 135.
(*a*) Local—
  Application of heat and cold :—
    Ice-bags.
    Cold compresses.
    Priessnitz's Compress.
    Instillation of warm water with tincture of opium.
    Instillation of warm oil with tincture of opium.
    Introduction of steam.
  Instillations :—
    Solution of atropine, ½ per cent., 5 drops several times daily.
    Carbolic acid and glycerine, 1 in 5.
    Solution of cocaine, 5—20 per cent.
    Sulphate of zinc, 5—10 per cent.
(*b*) Constitutional—
  Sedatives :—
    Opium or morphia.
    Hydrate of chloral.
    Iodide of potassium in doses of 8 to 15 grains.

ACUTE CATARRH, ETC.—*continued*.
  Purgatives :—
    Compound infusion of senna (Ger. Ph.).
    Castor oil.
    Mineral waters.
(*c*) Various—
    Blood-letting.
    Air-douche.
    Paracentesis.
    Intra-tympanic injection of warm water through Eustachian catheter.
    Wilde's incision.
    Insufflation of boracic acid.
    Induced electric current.

NASO-PHARYNGEAL CATARRH, page 140.
  Gargles :—
    Inhalations by means of Siegle's steam spray.
    Solution of common salt, 1—2 per cent.
    Solution of bicarbonate of soda, 1—2 per cent.
    Solution of chlorate of potash 1—2 per cent.
  Snuff :—
    Finely powdered borax.

DIPHTHERITIC MEMBRANOUS FORMATIONS IN MEATUS, page 141.
  Lotions :—
    Solution of salicylic acid in spirit, 10 per cent. (1—2 teaspoonfuls of this solution in 3 ounces of water for syringing).
    Warm lime-water.
  Insufflation :—
    Salicylic acid.
  Hypodermic injection :—
    Pilocarpine, about $\frac{1}{12}$—$\frac{1}{6}$th grain, once or twice daily.

CONTRACTION AND CLOSURE OF EUSTACHIAN TUBE, page 146.
  Air-douche.
  Injections :—
    Solution of sulphate of zinc in distilled water, ½—1 per cent.

CONTRACTION AND CLOSURE, ETC.—*continued.*
  Injections :—
    Solution of nitrate of silver in distilled water, 1½—5 per cent.
    Solution of iodine in glycerine (Potas. iodid. 3, iod. pur. 0·3, glycer. pur. 10—30).
  Cauterisation with solid nitrate of silver.
  Pigments for pharynx applied with brush :—
    Solution of nitrate of silver, 2—5 per cent.
    Solution of iodine and glycerine.
  Gargles for pharynx :—
    Solution of chlorate of potash, ½—2 per cent.
    Solution of alum ½—2 per cent.
    Solution of tannin ½—2 per cent.
  Cauterants :—
    Galvano-cautery.
    Chromic acid.
  The snare.
  Bougies.
  Induced electric current.

ABNORMAL PATENCY OF THE EUSTACHIAN TUBE, page 151.
  Nasal douche.
  Injections.
  Insufflations.
  Instillation of glycerine into external meatus and firm plugging.
  Closure of Eustachian tube by catheter-like instruments.

NEUROSES OF MUSCLES, page 151.
  Faradic current.

CHRONIC CATARRH OF THE MIDDLE EAR, WITHOUT PERFORATION OF MEMBRANA TYMPANI, page 156.
  Air-douche.
  Perforation of membrane and air-douche.
  Suction through perforation in membrane, or through Eustachian tube.

CHRONIC CATARRH—*continued.*
  Injections through Eustachian tube :—
    Salt solution, 1 per cent.
    Bicarbonate of soda in distilled water, 1 per cent.
    Liquor potassæ in distilled water, 3 in 30.
    Sulphate of zinc in distilled water, ½—1 per cent.

CHRONIC PURULENT INFLAMMATION OF THE MIDDLE EAR, p. 181.
  Syringing with
    Solution of common salt, 1 per cent.
    Solution of sulphate of soda, 1 per cent.
    Solution of carbolic acid, ½—1 per cent.
    Solution of salicylic acid, ½—1 per cent.
    Solution of boracic acid, 2—4 per cent.
  Insufflations :—
    Finely powdered boracic acid.
    Calomel.
    Iodoform.
    Powdered alum.
  Air-douche.
  Meatus air-douche.
  Cleansing with dry tampons of cotton-wool.
  Other antiseptics used :—
    Permanganate of potash.
    Thymol.
    Iodoform.
  Instillations :—
    Nitrate of silver in distilled water, 5—10 per cent.; 10—20 drops instilled daily or every second day for 1-2 minutes. May be neutralised with salt solution.
    Spiritus vini rectificatus. Instilled two to three times daily.
    Carbolic acid in glycerine, 10 per cent.
    Carbolic acid in oil, 10 per cent.
    Corrosive sublimate solution, 1 in 10,000.

CHRONIC PURULENT INFLAMMATION
OF THE MIDDLE EAR—*continued*.
Caustics :—
    Solid nitrate of silver melted on probe.
    Liquor ferri perchloridi.
    Chromic acid.
The galvano-cautery.
Astringent lotions :—
    Solution of sulphate of zinc, ½-8 per cent.
    Solution of sulphate of copper.
    Solution of acetate of lead.
    Solution of acetate of alumina.
    Solution of tannic acid.
Tympanic tubes for exudation deposits and cholesteatomata.
Snares for polypi :—
    Wilde's.
    Blake's.
    Galvano-caustic.
PAIN IN SCLEROSIS OF MASTOID, page 195.
Operation—
    Opening mastoid.
Narcotic—
    Hydrate of chloral.
CARIES AND NECROSIS OF MASTOID, page 195.
Solution for cleansing :—
    Carbolic acid, 1—2 per cent.
Incision over mastoid or other operation.
Tonics :—
    Cod-liver oil.
    Preparations of Iron.
    Salt-water baths.
CHRONIC INFLAMMATION OF MIDDLE EAR WITHOUT EXUDATION, page 202.
    Air-douche.
    Catheterism.
    Intra-tympanic injections :—
        Solution of sulphate of zinc, ½—1 per cent.
        Solution of iodide of potassium, 2—4 per cent.
        Solution of bicarbonate of soda, 1—2 per cent.

CHRONIC INFLAMMATION OF MIDDLE EAR—*continued*.
    Solution of borax (sodæ bibor. 0·3, glycerin. 5, aq. destill. 15).
    Solution of chloral hydrate, 1—2 per cent.
    Steam.
    Vapour of chloride of ammonium.
    Vapour of chloroform.
    Vapour of iodide of ethyl.
TINNITUS, page 203.
    (*a*) Constitutional treatment—
        Bromide of potassium, 30—60 grains daily.
        Atropine, $\frac{1}{30}$—$\frac{1}{20}$ grain daily.
        Fowler's solution, 2—10 drops daily.
        Quinine, 1½—15 grains daily.
        Salicylic acid, 15—30 grains daily.
    (*b*) Mechanical treatment—
        Rarefaction of air in external meatus.
        Lucae's spring pressure probe.
NERVOUS OTALGIA, page 206.
    Quinine.
    Salicylic acid.
    Iodide of potassium.
    Chloroform vapour.
    Oil of turpentine.
    Nitrite of amyl.
HYPERÆMIA OF LABYRINTH, page 213.
    Karlsbad salts.
    Electric current (constant or induced).
ANÆMIA OF LABYRINTH, page 213.
    Preparations of iron.
    Residence in high altitudes.
ACUTE INFLAMMATION OF THE LABYRINTH, page 218.
    Application of cold.
    Blood-letting.
    Preparations of iodine.
         ,,   ,,   mercury.
    Purgatives.
    Solution of hydrochlorate of pilocarpine, 2 per cent. Inject hypodermically 2—8 drops daily.

CHRONIC INFLAMMATION AND DE-
GENERATIVE PROCESSES IN THE
LABYRINTH, page 219.
  Vesication.
  Painting with tincture of iodine.
  Embrocation with iodine or iodoform ointment over mastoid process.
  Pilocarpine subcutaneously.

MENIÈRE'S COMPLEX OF SYMPTOMS, page 222.
  Quinine in doses of 5 to 15 grains daily.
  Cold baths.
  Bromide of potassium.
  Iodide of potassium.
  Electric current (constant).

MENIÈRE'S COMPLEX OF SYMPTOMS —*continued*.
  Pilocarpine subcutaneously.

CONCUSSION OF THE LABYRINTH, page 224.
  Plugging the meatus.
  Blood-letting.
  Cold compresses.
  Purgatives.
  Preparations of iodine.

SYPHILIS OF THE LABYRINTH, page 225.
  Preparations of mercury, iodine, and iron.
  Decoct. Sarsæ Co. (Ger. Ph.).

OTITIS INTERMITTENS, page 230.
  Quinine.

INSTRUMENTS REQUIRED IN THE TREATMENT OF DISEASES OF THE EAR.

Mirror with head-band (Fig. 2, page 10).
Set of three specula (Fig. 1, page 9).
Siegle's pneumatic speculum (page 16).
Syringe, with glass cylinder (Fig. 10, page 18).
India-rubber syringe (Fig. 11, page 19).
Politzer's bent forceps (Fig. 9, page 18).
Probe (Fig. 8, page 17).
India-rubber bag for air-douche with the following nozzles (Figs. 17, 18, 19, page 38)—(1) For catheterism; (2) Olive-shaped; (3) Politzer's.
Silver catheters, four sizes (page 41).
Bougies, ⅔, 1, and 1⅓ mm. thick (page 51).
Auscultation tube (otoscope) (page 47).
Powder insufflator (page 68).
Metal tympanic tube (Fig. 38, page 185).
Furuncle knife (Fig. 23, page 93).
Membrana tympani knife (Fig. 33, page 138). The same handle serves for holding (*a*) The sharp hook; (*b*) The curette; (*c*) The sickle-shaped knife; (*d*) The blunt-pointed bistoury.
Polypus snare (Fig. 40, page 193). The same handle is used with a larger tubular wire holder for operating upon nasal polypi and adenoid growths in the naso-pharynx.
Tuning-forks (pages 26, 29).
Politzer's acoumeter (page 25).

INDEXES.

R

GENERAL INDEX.

ABDUCENS nerve, implication of, in thrombosis, 179.
Abortion, deafness in case of, 229.
Abscess, cerebellar, 175.
—— cerebral, 164, 174, 197.
—— metastatic, 175.
—— of glands, 173.
—— of mastoid, 171.
Accouchements, deafness in, 229.
Acetate of alumina, use of, 184.
—— of lead, use of, 184.
Acoumeter, 25.
Acute affections, blood-letting in, 68.
Adenoid growths in naso-pharynx, 143.
Ætiology of ear diseases, 62, 63.
Air, treatment by rarefaction of, in meatus, 203.
—— bag, Lucae's, 46.
—— —— Politzer's, 37, 38.
—— compressing apparatus, 46.
—— douche, 35, 47, 113, 200, 202.
—— pressure in labyrinth, experiments regarding, 211.
Alcohol, instillation of, 92, 183.
Alternating dulness of hearing, 229.
Alum as an artificial tympanic membrane, 118.
—— insufflation of, in destructive disease of middle ear, 184.
Ammonium, chloride of, in chronic dry catarrh, 202.
Ampullæ, 208.
—— function of, 210.
Amygdala cerebelli, tumour in, 222.
Amyloid degeneration in labyrinth, 219.
—— —— in Rosenthal's canal, 228.
Anæmia, acute, blindness in, 214.
—— of labyrinth, 213.
—— tinnitus in, 54.
—— treatment of, 73.

Anæsthesia in cerebral abscess, 176.
—— of tympanic membrane and tympanum in hysteria, 229.
Anæsthetising the tympanic membrane, 138.
Anastomosis of vessels of ear, 123.
Anatomy, 76, 82, 109, 120, 207, 230.
Anchylosis of stapes, 5, 29, 163, 203, 215, 219, 226.
—— —— type of deafness caused by, 31.
—— of sound-conducting apparatus, 199.
—— of ossicula in case of deaf-mutism, 247.
Aneurism, cause of deafness, 65, 232, 245.
—— tinnitus in, 54.
Annular ligament, 208.
Annulus cartilagineus, 107.
—— tympanicus, 83.
Anomalies of ceruminal secretion, 83.
—— of hearing from concussion, 223.
—— of taste in purulent inflammation, 156, 159, 162.
—— of tension of tympanic membrane, 118.
Antihelix, 76.
Antitragus, 76.
Antrum mastoideum. *See* Mastoid antrum.
—— of Highmore, 42.
—— petrosum, 172.
—— tubes, 186.
Aphasia, cause of, 232.
—— from meningitis, 216.
—— sensory, 231, 232.
Apoplexy, causing deafness, 232.
—— symptoms of, in cerebral abscess, 177.
Aqueducts of labyrinth, discovery of, 6.

Aqueducts of labyrinth, extension of inflammation through, 217.
Aqueductus cochleæ, 209.
—— vestibuli, 209.
Arsenic in treatment of tinnitus, 204.
Artificial leech, Heurteloup's, 69.
—— membranes, 116.
Artillerymen, concussion of labyrinth in, 222.
—— deafness in, 32, 64.
—— tinnitus in, 223.
Ascaris lumbricoides in Eustachian tube, 152.
Aspergillus, description of, 95.
—— frequency of, 63.
Aspirator for exudation, 157.
Assurance, life, in relation to ear diseases, 163.
Astringents, use of, 184, 202.
Atmospheric conduction of sound, 21.
Atropine in treatment of tinnitus, 204.
Audiometer, Hughes', 26.
Audiphone, Colladon's, 75.
—— Rhodes', 75.
Auditory artery, internal, 212.
—— centre, situation of, 231.
—— meatus, external. *See* External meatus.
—— meatus, internal, psammoma in, 228.
—— nerve, abnormality of, 246.
—— —— absence of, 246.
—— —— anatomy of, 230.
—— —— angeio-neurotic paralysis of, 229.
—— —— atrophy of, 215, 228, 231.
—— —— brain diseases affecting, 66.
—— —— calcareous deposition in, 228.
—— —— decussation of, in brain, 231.
—— —— described by Galen, 3.
—— —— diseases of, 228.
—— —— effect of electricity on, 70.
—— —— fatty degeneration of, 228.
—— —— fibroma of, 229.
—— —— gumma of, 229.
—— —— hyperæsthesia of, 58, 70.
—— —— implication of, in purulent meningitis, 217.

Auditory nerve, Menière's symptoms, from affections of, 220.
—— —— sarcoma of, 225.
—— —— terminations of, 210.
Auditory nuclei, 230, 231.
Aural vertigo. *See* Giddiness.
Auricle, abnormality of, 238.
—— absence of, 238.
—— acute inflammation of, 78.
—— anatomy of, 76.
—— aneurismal dilatation of arteries of, 81.
—— atrophy of, from burn, 79.
—— cysts in, 78, 79.
—— detachment of, 103.
—— diseases of, 76.
—— eczema of, 63, 76, 96.
—— erysipelas of, 81.
—— frost-bite of, 81.
—— gouty deposits in, 81.
—— herpes of, 97.
—— neoplasms of, 81.
—— stunted development of, 238.
—— tophi in, 81.
—— tumours of, 78, 81.
—— wounds of, 81.
Auricular appendages, 238.
Auscultation sounds, 47.
—— —— in chronic dry catarrh, 201.
—— —— in presence of exudation, 155.
—— tube, 47.
Autophony, 60, 149.

Bacilli of tubercle in otorrhœal discharge, 180.
Ball-joint for head-mirror, Hartmann's, 11.
Ball syringe, india-rubber, 19.
Barley-corn in Eustachian tube, 152.
Basal meningitis, causing inflammation of labyrinth, 216.
Basilar artery supply to internal ear, 212.
Baths in treatment of ear diseases, 72.
—— salt-water, in treatment of scrofulous conditions, 203.
Beads in external meatus, 98.
Bell-ringing noises in ear, 200.

Bleeding Eustachian tube, instrument for, 51.
—— from nose, a cause of deafness, 214.
Blepharospasm causing tinnitus, 54, 152.
Blindness from acute anæmia, 214.
—— from thrombosis, 179.
Blood, extravasation of, in othæmatoma, 80.
—— —— into the membrana tympani, 112.
—— —— into labyrinth, 213.
Blood-cysts in external meatus, 107, 221.
—— —— in membrana tympani, 112.
Blood-letting, 68.
—— in acute inflammation, 139.
—— in cerebral cases, 197.
—— in myringitis, 111.
—— supply of external meatus, 83.
—— —— of internal ear, 212.
—— —— of membrana tympani, 109.
—— —— of middle ear, 123.
Blood-tumour, 179.
Blows on the ear, effects of, 64, 113.
Blunt-pointed knife for aural operations, 138.
Boilermakers' deafness, 32, 64.
Bone, atrophy of, 165, 169.
—— petrous, fracture of, 214.
—— sclerosis of, 161, 167.
Bone-conduction, experiments in, 21.
—— in concussion of labyrinth, 223.
—— in diagnosis, 4, 21.
—— in exhausted chronic suppuration, 161.
—— in hereditary deafness, 66.
—— in hysteria, 229.
—— in old age, 226.
—— in syphilis, 226.
Boracic acid treatment, 19, 93, 182.
Borax as snuff, 140.
—— solution, 202.
Boring instruments, 102.
Bougies, dangers of use of, 153.
—— Eustachian, 51, 148.
Brain, abscess of, 164, 174, 197.
—— and labyrinth, simultaneous affection of, 66.

Brain cortex, affection of, in purulent meningitis, 177.
—— lesion of internal capsule of, 232.
—— mode of extension of suppuration to, 174.
—— tumour in, 232.
Branchial arch, first, 239.
—— cleft, first, 240.
Bromide of potassium in treatment of tinnitus, 204.
Bugs in external meatus, 98.
Bulbar paralysis, absence of deafness in, 232.
Buzzing sounds in ear, 200.

CALCAREOUS deposits in auditory nerve, 228.
—— —— in labyrinth, 219.
—— —— in membrana tympani, 13, 62, 131, 159, 163, 199.
Calcification of membrana tympani, 13.
Calomel, use of powdered, 184.
Canal of facial nerve, anatomy of, 120.
—— —— first described, 4.
—— —— implication of, 162.
Canalis reuniens, 209.
Capsule for insufflation, 50.
—— internal, of brain, lesion of, 232.
Carbolic acid, in treatment of eczema, 78.
—— —— solution for syringing, 19, 184.
Carbolised glycerine, 139.
Carcinoma of ear, 237.
Cardiac complications, 203.
Caries in otitis externa, 89.
—— of mastoid, 6, 195.
—— of osseous meatus, 107.
—— of petrous bone, 169.
—— of teeth, 65, 205.
—— of temporal bone, 6.
—— of walls of tympanum, 156.
—— superficialis, 169.
Carotid artery, common, ligaturing, 197.
—— —— internal, hæmorrhage from, 197.

GENERAL INDEX.

Carotid artery, implication of, 170.
—— —— position of, 120.
Caseous products, 165.
Catarrh, cause of middle ear disease, 128, 131.
—— of Eustachian tube, 145.
—— of middle ear, acute, 129.
—— —— chronic, 63, 153.
—— —— chronic dry, 198.
—— of naso-pharynx, acute, 140.
—— —— cause of ear disease, 65.
—— —— effect on Eustachian tube, 141.
—— —— evil of neglect of, 66.
—— —— necessity for treatment, 202.
Catgut, use of, for bougies, 51.
Catheter, disinfection of, 45.
—— Eustachian, 41.
—— Frank's method of inserting, 44.
—— injection through, 49, 50.
—— Kramer's method of inserting, 44.
—— Politzer's method of inserting, 44.
—— Weber-Liel's tympanic, 188.
Catheterism, 36, 40, 46.
—— emphysema resulting from, 46.
—— in chronic dry catarrh, 203.
—— obstructions in, 42.
—— of Eustachian tube, first proposed, 6.
—— —— accidents in, 46.
Catholics, proportion of deaf-mutes among, 242.
Caustics, 67, 68, 183, 194, 202.
Cauterets, sulphur baths at, 73.
Cautery, galvano-, use of, 104.
Cavernous sinus, extension of thrombosis to, 179.
—— tumours, 81.
—— —— in ear diseases, 2.
—— —— situation of, 231.
Cerebellar abscess, 175.
Cerebelli tonsilla, tumour in, 222.
Cerebellum, pedunculus of, 231.
—— tumours in, 232.
Cerebral abscess, 174.
—— —— case of cure of, 197.
—— —— from purulent inflammation of middle ear, 164.

Cerebral affections as cause of deaf-mutism, 245.
Cerebral symptoms from otitis externa, 89.
—— —— in acute purulent inflammation of middle ear, 132.
—— tracts of auditory nerve, disease of, 230.
—— tumours as cause of deafness, 232.
—— —— cause of Menière's symptoms, 221.
—— —— tinnitus in case of, 54.
Cerebro-spinal fluid, discharge from ear of, 236.
—— meningitis as cause of deaf-mutism, 216, 242, 244.
—— —— epidemics of, 218.
Cerebrum, tumour in cortex of, 222.
Cerumen, inflammation arising from presence of, 84.
—— inspissated, in Eustachian tube, 153.
—— removal of, 65, 83.
Ceruminal accumulation, earliest treatment of, 1.
—— —— cause of vertigo, 220.
—— glands, description of, 82.
—— plugs, causing giddiness, etc., 57.
—— —— effects of, 84.
—— —— frequency of, 62, 63.
—— —— solutions for softening, 186.
—— secretion, anomalies of, 83.
—— —— diminished, 83.
—— —— increased, 84.
Chalybeate waters in treatment of ear diseases, 73.
Cheeks, erysipelatous swelling of, 179.
Cherry-stones in external meatus, 98.
Children, acute catarrh of tympanum in, 129.
—— acute inflammation of tympanum in, 128, 132.
—— diseases of Eustachian tube in, 141.
—— frequency of ear diseases in, 62, 63.
—— Menière's symptoms in, 221.

GENERAL INDEX.

Chirping sounds in the ear, 53.
Chisel, use of, for removal of exostosis, 106.
Chloral hydrate, injection of solution of, into middle ear, 202.
Chloroform vapour, use of, 203.
Chlorosis, tinnitus in, 54.
Cholesteatomata, 165.
Chorda tympani, description of, 123.
—— —— implication of, 162.
Chromic acid, use of, 68, 184.
Chronic inflammation, electricity in treatment of, 69.
Cicatrices in membrana tympani, 14, 16, 50, 134.
Circulation, disorders of, causing ear disease, 65.
Clamps on tuning-forks, 27.
Cleansing the ear, 17, 181.
Cleft palate, 143.
Clonic spasms of muscles, 151.
Cocaine, 111, 138, 187.
Cochlea, 207, 208.
—— absence of, 240.
—— atrophy of, 34, 210, 219.
—— condition of, in leukæmia, 227.
—— function of, 5, 210.
—— ossification of, 215.
—— sequestrum of, 170.
Cochlear nerve, 210.
Coins, gold, application of, in hysterical deafness, 230.
Cold as cause of ear disease, 63.
—— and heat, application of, 136.
—— baths, treatment by, 72.
—— fluids in syringing, evils of, 20.
Colladon's audiphone, 75.
Collodion in treatment of relaxed membrana tympani, 119.
Complex of symptoms, Menière's, 219.
Concha, 76.
Concussion, effect of, 114.
—— of cranial bones, 113.
—— of labyrinth, 115, 222.
Conduction of sound, 21, 141.
—— atmospheric, 21.
—— bone, 4, 21.
—— cranio-tympanal, 21.
Condylomata in external meatus, 97.
Cone of light, 12.

Consanguinity as cause of deaf-mutism, 243.
Consonants, volume of sound of, 23.
Constipation in purulent meningitis, 178.
Constitutional treatment of ear diseases, 71.
Conta, mode of testing with tuning-forks, 27.
Conversation tubes, 73.
Convulsions in cerebral abscess, 176.
—— in thrombosis of sinuses, 179.
Corium affected by otomycosis, 96.
Cornea, xerosis of, associated with deafness, 232.
Corn-seeds in external meatus, 98.
Corrosive sublimate solution, 19, 184.
Cortical deafness, 231.
Corti's arches, 209.
Cotton, absorbent, 20.
—— holders, 20, 65, 117.
Cotton-wool pellets acting as foreign bodies, 98, 114.
—— —— for artificial membrana tympani, 116.
Cotunnius, fluid of, 207.
Coughing from presence of foreign body, 100.
—— from reflex irritation, 83.
—— rupture of membrana tympani from violent, 113.
Crackling sounds in ear, 55.
Cranial bones, concussion of, 113.
Cranial fossæ, extension of ear disease to, 170.
—— fossa, middle, extension of otitis externa into, 89.
—— —— —— tumours in, 233.
—— —— posterior, implication of, 175.
—— nerves, extension of pus to, 174.
—— sinuses, hæmorrhage from, 170, 178.
—— —— phlebitis of, from cerebral abscess, 175.
Cranio-tympanal conduction, 21.
Crista vestibuli, 207, 209.
Crossed deafness, cases of, 232.
Crura of stapes, 122.
Curette, 137.

DEAF AND DUMB INSTITUTIONS IN BERLIN, investigations in, 216.
Deaf-mutes, defective development of brain of, 247.
—— instruction of, 249.
—— proportion of, in various countries, 241.
Deaf-mutism, 241.
—— acquired, 242, 246.
—— anatomical conditions found in, 246.
—— anchylosis and ossification in case of, 247.
—— congenital, 243.
—— —— proportion of, 242, 246.
—— consanguinity as cause of, 243.
—— curability of, 247.
—— endemic, 245.
—— from cerebro-spinal meningitis, 216, 218, 242.
—— from diphtheritic inflammation, 245.
—— from meningitis, 216.
—— geological conditions in relation to, 245.
—— heredity as cause of, 243.
—— injury, a cause of, 245.
—— intra-uterine causes of, 245.
—— post-mortem examination in case of, 247.
—— sporadic, 245.
Deafness after paroxysm of whooping-cough, 214.
—— cases of temporary, 228.
—— case of, in upright position, 214.
—— chronic progressive, case of, 33.
—— cortical, 231.
—— crossed, cases of, 232.
—— from epidemic cerebro-spinal meningitis, 217.
—— from epistaxis, 214.
—— from purulent inflammation of labyrinth, 214.
—— from tumours in brain, 233.
—— hereditary, 66.
—— —— syphilis as cause of, 224.
—— in fracture of petrous bone, 214.
—— in hysteria, 229.
—— in leukæmia, 227.
—— in mumps, 227.

Deafness, psychological, 231.
—— simulated, testing, 34.
—— to words, 231.
—— types of, 30.
Decayed teeth a cause of ear disease, 65.
Dentaphone, 75.
Diagnosis, chapter on, 8.
—— bone-conduction first employed in, 4.
—— differential, 4.
—— errors in, of acute purulent inflammation of middle ear, 132.
Diapedesis, extravasation by, into labyrinth, 215.
Diastasis, fracture by, 235.
Diathesis, phthisical, 71.
—— scrofulous, 71.
Diphtheritic inflammation of ear, 65, 134, 135, 245.
—— —— treatment of, 141.
Diplacusis, 59.
Diploetic veins in petrous bone, 178.
Diplopia associated with deafness, 232.
Direct light, examination by, 8.
Drainage tubes, 197.
Drill for removing exostosis, 106.
Ductus cochlearis, 209.
Dulness of hearing, alternating, 229.
—— —— from presence of cerumen, 85.
—— —— from tumours in brain, 233.
—— —— in locomotive drivers, 64.
—— —— intensified by electric treatment, 227.
—— —— statistics of, 62.
Dura mater, extension of inflammation from, to labyrinth, 217.
—— —— —— of pus to, 174.
Dysphagia from presence of foreign bodies, 100.

EAR. *See* also External ear, Middle, etc.
—— effects of blows on, 64.
—— influence of affections of nose and naso-pharynx on, 65.
—— noises in the, 52.
Earache, 130.
—— nervous, 205.

Ear-baths, 91.
Ear diseases, ætiology of, 62, 63.
—— —— earliest mention of, 1.
—— —— frequency of, 62.
—— —— precautions in, 64.
—— rings, evil effects from wearing, 77.
—— scoop, 65.
—— speculum first suggested, 3.
Early treatment, importance of, 66.
Earwig in external meatus, 98.
Ecchymosis of membrana tympani from action of drugs, 213.
Eczema of auricle, 63, 76, 78, 96.
—— of external meatus, 76, 77.
Education of deaf and dumb, 248.
Electric apparatus for testing hearing, 26.
Electrical treatment of ear disease, 69, 139, 148, 213, 217.
Embolism from thrombosis, 180.
Eminentia pyramidalis, 123, 209.
Emotion a cause of noises in ear, 152.
Emphysema, cause of ear disease, 65.
—— of skin over mastoid, 126.
—— resulting from catheterism, 46.
Enchondroma, 237.
Encysted tumours, 81.
Endolymph, 207.
Epidermal layer of membrana tympani, 107.
—— plugs, symptoms of, 94.
Epidermis, desquamation of, from syringing, 65.
—— loosening of, 13.
Epiglottis, ulceration of, cause of otalgia, 205.
Epilepsy from presence of foreign bodies, 100.
Epileptic seizures in thrombosis of cerebral sinuses, 180.
Epistaxis a cause of total deafness, case of, 214.
—— plugging in, a cause of inflammation, 132.
Epithelium of tympanic cavity, 121.
Equilibration, disturbance of, 57, 217.
—— function of semicircular canals, 211.

Equilibration, undisturbed, in cases of extravasation of blood, 214.
Erysipelas of auricle, 81.
Erysipelatous swelling of face in thrombosis, 179.
Ethmoid cells, 42.
Ethyl, iodide of, vapour, 203.
Eustachian bougies, 51.
—— catheters, 41.
—— —— disinfection of, 45.
—— —— syphilis inoculated by, 44.
—— prominence, 40.
—— tube, 4, 5.
—— —— abnormal patency of, 60, 149.
—— —— absence of mouth of, 146.
—— —— acute catarrh of, 145.
—— —— atony of muscles of, 143.
—— —— barley-corn in, 152.
—— —— bougieing, 148.
—— —— catarrh of, 202.
—— —— cauterising, 51, 147.
—— —— cicatrices in, 148.
—— —— collapse of mouth of, 143.
—— —— condition of, in cleft palate, 143.
—— —— contraction and closure of, 141.
—— —— description of, 126.
—— —— destruction of, 146.
—— —— dilating, by bleeding, 51.
—— —— diseases of, 141.
—— —— —— causing vertigo, 220.
—— —— —— in children, 63.
—— —— effects of deglutition on, 127.
—— —— folds at mouth of, 41.
—— —— foreign bodies in, 152.
—— —— function of, 126, 127.
—— —— influences of affections of nose and naso-pharynx on, 65.
—— —— injection through, 49, 147.
—— —— length of, 51.
—— —— modes of inserting catheters into, 44.
—— —— obstruction of, 145.
—— —— patency of, 149.
—— —— situation of mouth of, 40.
—— —— tonsils of, 142.
—— —— total closure of, 146.
—— —— transmission of tuberculosis to ear through, 180.

Examination of the ear, 16.
Exanthemata as cause of ear disease, 65, 128, 131.
Exhausting tympanum of exudation, 157.
Exophthalmos from thrombosis, 179.
Exostosis in external meatus, 105.
—— operation on, 106.
External ear, first description of, 5.
—— —— frequency of diseases of, 63.
—— —— inspection of, 8.
—— —— statistics of diseases affecting, 63.
—— —— supernumerary, 238.
External meatus, anatomy of, 82.
—— —— applying remedies through, 67.
—— —— atrophy of walls of, from ceruminal plug, 84.
—— —— beads in, 98.
—— —— blood-cysts in, 107, 221.
—— —— —— with Menière's symptoms, 221.
—— —— caries and necrosis of, 107.
—— —— chronic inflammation of, 90.
—— —— closure of, 77, 104, 238.
—— —— collapse of walls of, 75.
—— —— contraction of, 104.
—— —— cure of deaf-mute by removal of membranous closure in 247.
—— —— desquamative inflammation of, 93.
—— —— diphtheritic inflammation of, 90.
—— —— diseases of, 81.
—— —— dryness of, 83.
—— —— eczema of, 76.
—— —— exostosis in, 105.
—— —— extravasation of blood in, 107.
—— —— foreign bodies in, 98.
—— —— —— in, causing Menière's symptoms, 220.
—— —— fungus in, 95.
—— —— hyperostosis in, 105, 107.
—— —— inflammation of, acute, 86.
—— —— —— of, chronic, 90.
—— —— —— circumscribed, 86.
—— —— —— diffuse, 88.

External meatus, leaden tubes for dilating, 105.
—— —— lesions of, 234.
—— —— methods of dilating, 105.
—— —— nerve-supply of, 83.
—— —— opening posterior wall of, to remove foreign body, 103.
—— —— stenosis of, 9, 173.
—— —— syphilis of, 97.
Exudation-aspirator, Schalle's, 157.
Exudation causing tinnitus, 55.
—— deposits, 164.
Eyelids, erysipelatous swelling of, 179.

FACE, erysipelatous swelling of, in thrombosis, 179.
Facial nerve, 120, 162.
—— paralysis, 162, 170.
—— —— defective hearing in, 59.
—— veins, implication of, in thrombosis, 179.
Fainting-fits, tinnitus in, 214.
—— from syringing, 86.
Faintness from ceruminal plug, 85.
—— from Menière's disease, 219.
Faradic current in ear disease, 69, 139, 148.
Female deaf-mutes, proportion of, 242.
Fenestra ovalis, 120, 199, 204, 208.
—— rotunda, 15, 120, 199, 209, 215.
Fenestræ, anchylosis at, 66.
—— changes at, 163.
—— discovery of, 4.
—— extension of inflammation through, 218.
—— labyrinthine, absence of, 240.
—— —— ossification of, in deaf-mutism, 247.
Fibrous tumours, 81, 166.
Fistula auris congenitalis, 239.
Fistulæ between abscesses and carious bone, 175.
—— from disease of osseous meatus, 107, 108.
Fistulous openings behind ear, 173, 195.
—— —— in caries and necrosis of meatus, 107, 108.
Fomentation, treatment by, 91.
Foramen cæcum, 180.

Forceps, danger of, for removing foreign bodies, 102.
—— Politzer's, 14.
—— use of, for removing cerumen, 85.
Foreign bodies, as cause of inflammation of middle ear, 131.
—— —— of vertigo, 220.
—— —— cotton-wool pellets acting as, 98.
—— —— dangers from, 3, 99, 102.
—— —— early treatment of, 123.
—— —— fatal case of, 100.
—— —— hook for, 137.
—— —— in Eustachian tubes, 152.
—— —— in external meatus, 98.
—— —— removal of, 101, 104.
Forficula auricularis in external meatus, 98.
Formulæ, electrical, 70.
Fossæ, cranial. *See* Cranial fossæ.
Fossa jugular, 121.
—— navicularis, 76.
—— Rosenmüller's, 41.
—— subarcuata, 170.
Fovea hemi-elliptica, 207.
—— hemispherica, 207.
Fowler's solution, 78, 204.
Fracture of base of skull, 235.
—— of cranial bones, 113, 114.
—— of petrous bone, 214.
—— of temporal bone, 114, 235.
Friedrichshall, treatment by mineral wells at, 73.
Frontal convolution, third, defective in deaf-mutes, 247.
Frost-bite of auricle, 81.
Fulness in ear, feeling of, from presence of cerumen, 85.
Fungus in the external meatus, 95.
Furuncle knife, 92.
Furunculosis, 86.
—— treatment of, 92.

GALTON's whistle, 26.
Galvanic hyperæsthesia of auditory nerve, 70.
Galvanism, application of, 69, 229, 230.

Galvano-cautery, for destroying foreign bodies, 104.
—— for paracentesis of tympanic membrana, 204.
—— treatment of anomalies of tension of tympanic membrane by, 119.
—— used as snare, 71.
Gangrene of auricle, 81.
Gargles, 148.
Gastein, treatment by baths at, 72.
General therapeutics of ear, 67.
German military regulations regarding ear disease, 164.
—— system of instruction of deaf-mutes, 249.
Germany, epidemics of cerebro-spinal meningitis in, 218.
Giddiness from acute inflammation of labyrinth, 216.
—— from cerebral abscess, 176.
—— —— ceruminal accumulation, 85.
—— —— ear disease, 57.
—— —— fracture of petrous bone, 214.
—— —— hyperæmia of labyrinth, 212.
—— —— Menière's disease, 219.
—— —— otitis labyrinthica, 216.
—— —— purulent meningitis, 178.
—— —— syringing, 86.
Glands, abscess of, 173.
—— implication of, in otitis externa, 89.
Glandulæ ceruminales, 82.
Glaser, fissure of, 124, 235.
Glass beads in external meatus, 98.
Glosso-pharyngeal nerve, implication of, in thrombosis, 179.
Glottis, œdema of, 172.
Glycerine, use of, 101.
Goitre, cause of deaf-mutism, 245.
—— —— of ear disease, 65.
Gold coins, application of, in hysterical deafness, 230.
Granulation growths, 93, 166, 173.
Growths, adenoid, in naso-pharynx, 143.
—— malignant, 237.

Growths on auricle, 81.
Gumma of auditory nerve, 228.

HÆMATOMA, 79.
Hæmorrhage from cranial sinuses, 178.
—— from internal carotid, 197.
—— from jugular and carotid, 170.
—— in operating on mastoid, mode of controlling, 197.
—— into cerebral abscess, 177.
—— into the labyrinth, 214.
—— into semicircular canals in Menière's disease, 219.
—— into temporal convolution, 231.
—— into the tympanum, 206.
—— meningeal, 215.
Hallucinations from tumours in brain, 233.
—— in purulent meningitis, 176.
—— of hearing, 56.
Hand-mirror, 10.
Hard palate, 41.
Hartmann, artificial membrane, 118.
—— cotton-holder, 20, 65.
—— double ball-joint for head-mirror, 11.
—— electrical apparatus for testing the hearing, 26.
—— experiments in pneumatic cabinet, 127.
—— investigations in Berlin Deaf and Dumb Institutions, 216.
—— manometrical experiments, 128.
—— method of testing simulated deafness, 35.
—— syringe, 18.
—— tympanic tube, 108, 186.
Headache, from presence of foreign bodies, 100.
—— in cerebral abscess, 176.
—— in purulent meningitis, 178.
Head-band for mirror, 10.
Hearing, alternating dulness of, 229.
—— anomalies of, 223.
—— defects of, from cerebral tumours, 232, 233.
Hearing-distance, 22, 24.

Hearing, dulness of. *See* Dulness of hearing.
—— —— intensified by electric treatment, 227.
—— electric formula of, 70.
—— hallucinations of, 56.
—— in perforation of Shrapnell's membrane, 161.
—— melodies, 55.
—— painful, 59.
—— power of, in deaf-mutes, 246.
—— situation of centre of, 231.
—— statistics of dulness of, 62.
—— testing the, 21.
—— transference of, by metals, 229.
—— trumpet, 74.
—— tubes, 73, 75.
Heart disease, a cause of ear disease, 65, 203.
Heat and cold, application of, 136.
Hebra's ointment, 78.
Helicotrema, 209.
Helix, 76.
Hemianæsthesia, hysterical, dulness of hearing in, 229.
Hemicrania, from presence of foreign bodies, 100.
Hereditary predisposition to ear disease, 66.
—— syphilis, as cause of deafness, 224.
Herpes auricularis, 97.
Heurteloup's artificial leech, 69.
Hiatus subarcuatus, 170.
Hissing in the ear, 53.
Hook for foreign bodies, 102, 137.
Hook-shaped probe, 102.
Humming sound in ear, 54, 200.
Hyperacusis, 58.
Hyperæmia, blood-letting in, 68.
—— of the labyrinth, 212.
—— of membrana tympani, 13.
Hyperæsthesia acustica, 59.
—— of auditory nerve, 58.
—— simple galvanic, 70.
Hyperostosis of external meatus, 105.
Hyperplasia of osseous tissue in sclerosis, 168.
Hysteria, acute hearing in, 59.
—— deafness in, 229.

ICE-BAGS, in cerebral cases, 197.
Ice-compresses, application of, 136.
Idiocy, from meningitis, 216.
Innervation, disturbances of, 151.
Incisura intertragica, 76.
Incisuræ Santorini, 82.
Incus, 4, 121, 144.
India-rubber ball syringe, 19.
Infants, muco-purulent exudation in tympana of, 156.
Infectious diseases, their predilection for ear, 135.
Inflammation. *See* External ear, Middle, etc.
—— extension of, to inner surface of apex of mastoid, 171.
—— from foreign bodies, 65.
—— from syringing, 65.
—— purulent, importance of early treatment in, 66.
—— —— type of deafness from, 31.
—— reflex cause of, 65.
—— treatment of, by electricity, 69.
—— —— of, by leeches, 68.
—— of tympanum extending to labyrinth, 218.
—— —— producing pigment in labyrinth, 215.
Injuries of the ear, 234.
Insects in external meatus, 98, 103.
Inspection of the ear, 8.
Inspissated cerumen. *See* Cerumen.
Instillations, 65, 67, 137.
Instruments for removing foreign bodies, 102.
Insufflation capsule, 50.
—— modes of, 68.
Intermittent ear disease, 230.
Internal auditory artery, 212.
—— meatus, psammoma in, 228.
—— capsule of brain, lesion of, 232.
—— carotid artery, implication of, 170.
—— —— position of, 120.
—— ear. *See* Labyrinth, Auditory nerve, etc.
Iodide of ethyl vapour, 203.
—— of potassium, use of, 202, 206.
Irido-choroiditis, syphilitic, 225.
Iris-hook for foreign bodies, 102.

Iron in constitutional treatment of ear disease, 71.
—— perchloride of, as caustic, 184.

JACOBSON'S nerve, 123.
Jugular fossa, 121.
—— sinus, case of dilatation of, 54.
—— vein, internal, thrombosis of, 179.

KARLSBAD salts in labyrinthine hyperæmia, 213.
Keratitis, parenchymatous, 255.
—— syphilitic, 225.
Keratosis obturans, 94.
Knocking sounds in ear, 200.
König's cylinder, 26.

LABYRINTH, absence of, 240, 246.
—— acute inflammation of, 215, 218.
—— air-pressure experiments in, 211.
—— anæmia of, 213.
—— anatomy of, 207.
—— and brain, simultaneous affection of, 66.
—— atrophy of, 215, 219.
—— changes in, in deaf-mutism, 247.
—— chronic inflammation of, 219.
—— concussion of, 114, 222.
—— congestion of, 69.
—— degenerative processes in, 219.
—— deposits of pigment in, 215.
—— development of, 240.
—— extension of inflammation of middle ear to, 218.
—— —— —— to, from dura mater, 217.
—— extravasation of blood into, 213.
—— functions of, 210.
—— general remarks on disease of, 211.
—— hæmorrhage into, 214.
—— hyperæmia of, 212.
—— —— induced current in treatment of, 213.
—— hyperplastic processes in, 219.
—— implication of, in chronic dry catarrh, 200, 204.
—— injury of, 58, 234.
—— malformation of, 239.
—— purulent inflammation of, 215.
—— reactive inflammation of, 223.

Labyrinth, sequestrum of, 170.
—— syphilis of, 224.
—— tinnitus in affections of, 54.
Labyrinthine fenestræ, absence of, 240.
—— —— ossification of, in deaf-mutism, 247.
—— fluid, 207.
—— —— relation of aqueducts to, 7.
Lamina spiralis membranacea, 208.
—— —— —— case of rigidity of, 216.
—— —— ossea, 208.
Laminaria bougies, 51.
—— —— breaking in Eustachian tube, 153.
—— tents, 105.
Larvæ in external meatus, 98, 103.
Larynx, spasm of muscles of, 151.
—— ulceration of, a cause of otalgia, 205.
Lateral sinus, destruction of wall of, 197.
—— —— excavation of, 190.
—— —— extension of disease to, 173, 179.
—— —— —— of otitis externa to, 89.
—— —— relation of, to meatus, 125.
Laudanum, instillation of, 137.
Lead, acetate of, use of, 184.
Leaden tubes for dilating meatus, 105.
Leather hearing-tubes, 74.
Leeches, application of, 68.
Leukæmia, deafness in, 227.
Lenses for speculum, 9.
Lesions of the ear, traumatic, 234.
Levator veli muscle, 127.
Life assurance, eligibility for, in ear disease, 163.
Ligament, annular, 21, 122, 208.
—— —— anchylosis of, 199.
—— of the axis of the malleus, 121.
—— superior, 122.
Liquor Cotunnii, 7, 207.
Lobule, 76.
—— eczema from piercing of, 77.
—— tumours of, 81.
Locomotive drivers, dulness of hearing in, 64.
Longitudinal sinus, extension of thrombosis to, 179.
Loop-snare, for polypi, 192.

MACULÆ of the vestibule, 208.
Magnifying lenses for speculum, 9.
Malformations, 238.
Malignant growths, 81, 237.
Malingering deafness, 34.
Malleus, appearance of, in indrawn membrane, 143.
—— description of, 110, 121.
—— disarticulation of, in treatment of sclerosis, 205.
—— discovery of, 4.
—— extirpation of, 149, 183.
—— foreshortening of, 14, 144.
—— ligament of axis of, 121.
—— superior ligament of, 122.
Mal-nutrition, treatment of, 71.
Malpighian layer of skin affected by otomycosis, 96.
Manometrical experiments on Eustachian tube, 61, 128, 143.
Manubrium mallei, 110, 121.
—— —— position of, in indrawn membrane, 14, 143.
Marasmus, from presence of foreign bodies, 100.
Margo tympanicus, 109.
Massage, treatment of othæmatoma by, 80.
Masseter muscles, contraction simultaneous with tensor tympani, 123.
—— —— paralysis of, associated with deafness, 232.
Mastoid antrum, 120, 124, 172.
—— —— sclerosis of, 161, 167.
—— —— sequestrum in, 160.
—— cells, condensation of, 161.
—— —— periostitis of, 168.
—— —— sclerosis of, 167.
—— —— swelling of mucous membrane of, 168.
Mastoid process, abscess on surface of, 171.
—— —— caries of, treatment of, 195.
—— —— cells of, extension of otitis externa into, 89.
—— —— dehiscences of, 126.
—— —— emphysema of skin over, 126.
—— —— extension of inflammation to inner surface of apex, 171, 196.

GENERAL INDEX. 271

Mastoid process, incision over, Wilde's, 139.
—— —— necrosis of, 172, 195.
—— —— œdema over, 179.
—— —— operation of opening the, 189.
—— —— periostitis of, 171.
—— —— pressure upon, affecting tinnitus, 56.
—— —— sclerosis of, 195.
—— —— sequestrum in, 172, 173.
—— —— trephining the, 6, 140, 188.
—— veins, implication of, in thrombosis, 179.
Measles as cause of ear disease, 65, 128.
Meatus. *See* External meatus.
—— air-douche, 181.
—— psammoma in internal auditory, 228.
Medulla oblongata, root-fibres of auditory nerve in, 230.
Membrana basilaris, 208.
Membrana flaccida Shrapnelli, 12, 109.
—— —— —— perforation of, 160.
—— Reissneri, 209.
—— tympani, adhesions of, 134.
—— —— anæsthesia of, in hysteria, 229.
—— —— anatomy of, 109.
—— —— anomalies of tension of, 118.
—— —— appearance of, in children, 12.
—— —— —— in acute catarrh, 130.
—— —— —— of, in chronic catarrh, 201.
—— —— —— of, in Eustachian tube affections, 143.
—— —— artificial, 116.
—— —— atrophy of, from presence of ceruminal plug, 84.
—— —— bulging of, 14, 130, 137.
—— —— calcareous deposits in, 62, 159.
—— —— calcification of, 13.
—— —— changes in position of, 14.
—— —— chronic inflammation of, 112.

Membrana tympani, cicatrisation of, 14, 16, 50, 134.
—— —— cysts in, in acute catarrh, 130.
—— —— degeneration of, 13.
—— —— description of, 11, 109.
—— —— destruction of, 15.
—— —— —— of, in scarlet fever, 134.
—— —— deviations from normal condition of, 13.
—— —— discoloration of, 13.
—— —— diseases of, 109.
—— —— divisions of, 13.
—— —— ecchymosis of, 213.
—— —— epidermal layer of, 13.
—— —— extravasation of blood in, 112.
—— —— exudation sacs in, 14.
—— —— folds of, 110, 144.
—— —— granular appearance of, 14.
—— —— hyperæmia of, 13, 213.
—— —— hypertrophy of, 13.
—— —— indrawing of, 14, 62, 118, 142, 201.
—— —— infiltration of, 13.
—— —— inflammation of, 110.
—— —— knife, 119, 137, 157.
—— —— loss of substance of, 15.
—— —— miliary tubercles in mucous membrane of, 181.
—— —— mobility of ascertained, 16.
—— —— movements of, 15, 149.
—— —— nerve-supply of, 110.
—— —— normal appearance of, 11.
—— —— opacity of, 13.
—— —— paracentesis of, 6, 7, 137.
—— —— perforation of, 134, 159.
—— —— position of, 11.
—— —— rupture of, 113, 234.
—— —— sclerosis of, 16, 134.
—— —— thickening of, 13.
—— —— treatment by incision of, 204.
—— —— vesicles in, 14.
Menière's complex of symptoms, 219.
Meningeal hæmorrhage, 170, 215.
Meninges, inflammation of, in tumour of the brain, 233.

Meningitis accompanying cerebral abscess, 175.
—— basal, a cause of deaf-mutism, 244.
—— case of transverse fracture with, 236.
—— cerebro-spinal, a cause of deaf-mutism, 242, 244.
—— course of, 216.
—— epidemic cerebro-spinal, 216.
—— from chronic purulent inflammation, 164.
—— in otitis labyrinthica, 216.
—— in tumour of brain, 233.
—— Menière's symptoms with, 221.
—— purulenta, 177.
—— —— a cause of deafness, 217.
—— simple basal, 216.
Menstruation, dulness of hearing at, 229.
—— hæmorrhage into tympanum occurring with, 206.
—— influence of, on ear disease, 66.
Mental disturbances in cerebral abscess, 176.
—— irritability in purulent meningitis, 178.
Mercury, perchloride of, solution, 19.
Metastasis in mumps, 227.
Metastatic abscesses, 175.
Microbes in furunculosis, 87.
Micro-organisms, a cause of deaf-mutism, 245.
Middle Ages, remedies for ear diseases in, 3.
Middle cranial fossa, extension of disease to, 89, 170.
—— —— —— tumours in, 233.
Middle ear, absence of, 239.
—— —— accumulations in, cause of vertigo, 220.
—— —— acute catarrh of, 129.
—— —— acute inflammation of, 128.
—— —— acute purulent inflammation of, 131.
—— —— anæsthesia of, in hysteria, 229.
—— —— anatomy of, 120.
Middle ear, blood-supply of, 123.
—— —— caries in, 156.
—— —— changes in, as cause of deaf-mutism, 247.
—— —— chronic catarrh of, 153.
—— —— —— without exudation, 198.
—— —— purulent inflammation of, 158, 163.
—— —— description of, by Valsalva, 5.
—— —— diphtheritic affections of, 134, 141.
—— —— disease of osseous walls of, 167.
—— —— diseases of, 120.
—— —— dry catarrh of, 198.
—— —— exudation in, 13, 154.
—— —— frequency of diseases of, 63.
—— —— hæmorrhage into, 206.
—— —— heredity in chronic dry catarrh of, 199.
—— —— hyperæmia of, 213.
—— —— hyperplastic form of chronic dry catarrh of, 198.
—— —— inflammation of, extending to labyrinth, 218.
—— —— injections into, 202.
—— —— Menière's symptoms from affections of, 220.
—— —— miliary tubercles in mucous membrane of, 181.
—— —— muco-purulent exudation in, of infants, 156.
—— —— nerve-supply of, 123.
—— —— purulent inflammation of, its neglect a cause of deaf-mutism, 248.
—— —— transmission of tuberculosis, to, 180.
—— —— trophic supply of, 124.
—— lobe of brain, tumours in, 233.
—— meningeal artery, hæmorrhage from, 170.
Military regulations (German) regarding ear disease, 164.
—— service, eligibility for, in ear diseases, 163.
Millers, deafness in, 64.

Mineral waters in treatment of ear diseases, 73.
Mirror, reflecting, 4, 10.
Malarious infection as cause of ear disease, 230.
Mould fungi, 95.
Mouth-plate mirror, 11.
Mumps, deafness in, 227.
Muscles, neuroses of, 151.
—— of ear, intrinsic, discovered, 4.
—— of Eustachian tube, atony of, 143.
—— of larynx, spasm of, 151.
—— of neck, swelling at, 171.
—— of soft palate, paresis of, 145.
Muscular sounds, 54.
—— spasms, causing tinnitus, 55.
Musical instruments used as acoumeters, 25.
Myringitis acuta, 110.
—— chronica, 112.
—— desquamativa, 94.
—— frequency of, 63.
—— treatment of, 111.
Myxomata, 166.

NARROWING of meatus, 104.
Nasal polypi, snare for, 192.
Naso-pharynx, adenoid growths in, 143, 192.
—— catarrh of, 65, 131, 140, 202.
—— influence of affections of, on ear, 65.
Navicular fossa, 76.
Neck, swelling at muscles of, 171.
—— symptoms in, from thrombosis, 179.
Necrosis, 89, 107, 156, 169, 195. *See also* Caries.
Neglect of ear diseases, evil of, 66.
Neoplasms of auditory nerve, 228.
—— of auricle, 81.
—— of ear, 237.
Nerve, auditory. *See* Auditory nerve.
Nerve-supply, 83, 110, 123, 210.
Nervous otalgia, 65, 205.
—— structures, diseases of, 207.
—— —— type of deafness in disease of, 32.
—— symptoms of foreign bodies, 100.
—— tinnitus aurium, 52.

Neuralgia associated with deafness, 232.
—— from carious teeth, 65, 205.
—— from exostosis, 106.
—— of trigeminus, 161.
Neuralgic pains, induced current for, 139.
—— symptoms in otitis intermittens, 230.
Neuritis descendens, 217.
Neuroma of auditory nerve, 228.
Neuroses of muscles, 151.
—— reflex, 228.
Nitrate of silver, use of, 58, 184.
—— in eczema, 78.
Nitrite of amyl for otalgia, 206.
Noise, hearing better in, 59, 100.
Noises in the ear. *See* Tinnitus aurium.
—— loud, causing vertigo, 567.
—— perception of, 210.
Nose, bleeding from, a cause of deafness, 214.
—— blowing the, restoring patency of Eustachian tube, 145.
—— catarrh of, cause of middle ear disease, 131.
—— —— treatment of, 147.
—— clamps, 46.
—— influence of affections of, on ear, 65.
—— pieces for Politzerisation, 38.
—— rupture of cerebral abscess into, 175.
Nostrums for toothache, effect of, on ear, 65.
Nucleus monticuli, 231.
—— —— injury of, 232.
Nystagmus, 58.

OCULO-MOTOR NERVE, implication of, in thrombosis, 179.
Œdema of glottis, 171.
—— of orbits from thrombosis, 179.
—— over mastoid process, 179.
Oil, instillation of, 65, 101, 137.
Ointments, 68, 78.
Old age, bone-conduction in, 226.
Opacity of membrane, 13.
—— —— from acute catarrh, 131.
Opium, instillation of tincture of, 137.

S

Optic nerve, implication of, in thrombosis, 179.
Orbits, œdema of, from thrombosis, 179.
Orchitis in mumps, 227.
Osseous meatus, caries and necrosis of, 107.
—— —— stenosis of, 173.
—— tissue, hyperplasia of, 168.
Ossicula, 121.
—— abnormal development of, 240.
—— absence of, 240.
—— anchylosis of articulations of, 199.
—— —— in case of deaf-mutism, 247.
—— necrosis of, 141.
—— operation of removing, 205.
—— sclerosis of mucous membrane of, 163.
Ostia pharyngea tuba, 127.
Ostitis interna osteoplastica, 168.
—— of mastoid process, 168.
—— ulcerative, 169.
Ostium tympanicum tubæ, 120.
Otalgia intermittens, 230.
—— induced current for, 139.
—— nervosa, 205.
—— reflex cause of, 65.
Otoliths, 209.
Othæmatoma, 79.
—— extravasation of blood in, 80.
—— in the insane, 79.
Otitis externa circumscripta, 63, 86.
—— —— complications of, 89, 90.
—— —— desquamativa, 93.
—— —— diffusa, 63, 88.
—— —— frequency of, 63.
—— —— occurrence of caries in, 89.
—— intermittens, 230.
—— labyrinthica, 216.
—— media acuta, 128.
—— —— catarrhalis acuta, 129.
—— —— —— chronica, 153.
—— —— purulenta acuta, 131.
—— —— —— chronica, 158.
Otomycosis aspergillina, 95.
—— —— frequency of, 63.
—— —— treatment of, 97.
Otophones, 75.
Otorrhœa, 5.
—— cerebralis, 175.

Otorrhœa, chronic, a cause of tuberculosis, 180.
—— constitutional treatment of, 72.
—— prognosis of, 163.
—— purulent, 173.
Otorrhœal discharge, bacillus in, 180.
Otoscope, Toynbee's, 47.

PACHYMENINGITIS HÆMORRHAGICA, 215.
—— —— its connection with othæmatoma, 80.
Painful hearing, 59.
Palate, cleft, condition of Eustachian tube in, 143.
—— hard and soft, 41.
—— soft, action of 127.
—— —— clonic spasm of, 151.
—— —— paresis of muscles of, 145.
Paracentesis in acute purulent inflammation of middle ear, 137.
—— in myringitis, 111.
—— mode of performing, 138.
—— of membrana tympani first performed, 6.
—— —— —— for removal of exudation, 156, 157.
—— —— —— for sclerosis, 204.
Paracusis, 59.
—— Willisii, 59, 100.
Paralysis, angeio-neurotic, of auditory nerve, 229.
—— bulbar, absence of deafness in, 232.
—— facial, 162, 170.
—— from presence of foreign bodies, 100.
—— in cerebral abscess, 176.
—— in purulent meningitis, 178.
—— of masseter muscles associated with deafness, 232.
Parenchymatous keratitis, 224.
Paresis of muscles of soft palate, 145.
—— of soft palate, effect on Eustachian tube, 143.
Parotid gland, implication of, in inflammation of meatus, 89.
—— —— —— of middle ear, 134.
Parotitis, deafness in, 227.
Paukenröhrchen, 188.

Pearl tumours, 165.
Pedunculus cerebelli, auditory fibres in, 231.
Perception of pitch, irregular, 33.
Perchloride of iron, use of, 184.
Perichondritis auriculæ, 78.
Perilymph, 207.
Periosteum of external meatus, 89.
Periostitis of mastoid process, 171.
—— in acute purulent inflammation of middle ear, 134.
—— of mastoid cells, 168.
—— of vestibule in acquired syphilis, 226.
Petrosal sinus, superior, implication of, 179.
Petro-squamosal suture, 235.
Petrous antrum, 172.
—— bone, caries and necrosis of, 169.
—— —— fracture of, 214.
—— —— implication of diploetic veins of, 178.
Pharyngeal diphtheria, extension of, 135.
Pharynx, catarrhs of, cause of middle ear disease, 131.
—— treatment of catarrh of, 147.
—— ulceration of, a cause of otalgia, 205.
Phlebitis, 178.
—— from chronic purulent inflammation, 164.
—— of cranial sinus associated with cerebral abscess, 175.
Phthisical diathesis, treatment of, 71.
Phthisis pulmonalis in relation to ear disease, 180, 183.
Pia mater, infiltration of, in purulent meningitis, 177.
Piano for testing hearing, 25.
Pigmentary deposition in labyrinth, 219.
Pilocarpine in diphtheritic inflammation, 141.
—— in labyrinthine inflammation, 218.
—— in Menière's disease, 222.
Pin-head perforation, 130.
Pitch, irregular perception of, 33.

Pitch of tinnitus, 52, 54.
Pituitary region, tumours in, 233.
Plethora abdominalis, treatment of, 203.
—— cause of ear disease, 65.
Plexus of nerves, tympanic, 123.
Plugging the posterior nares a cause of inflammation of middle ear, 132.
Pneumatic cabinet, Hartmann's experiments in, 127.
—— speculum, Siegle's, 16.
Pockets of Von Tröltsch, 110.
Politzerisation, 36.
Polypi, 166.
—— a cause of vertigo, 220.
—— from furunculosis, 88.
—— in caries and necrosis of meatus, 107.
—— in Eustachian tube, 153.
—— in tympanum, 16.
—— treatment of, 71, 192.
Polypus snare, 192.
Pons Varolii, tumours in, 233.
Posterior cranial fossa, extension of disease to, 170, 173.
Potassium, bromide of, in tinnitus, 204.
—— iodide of, use of, 202, 206.
Poulticing, 91.
Powder-blower, 68, 182.
Powdered alum, 184.
Powders, mode of applying, 68.
Pregnancy as cause of ear disease, 65.
Preventive measures in ear disease, 64.
Priessnitz's compresses, 137.
Probe, examination with, 16.
—— hook-shaped, 102.
—— use of, 85.
Processus brevis mallei, 12, 110, 122.
—— —— —— appearance of, in indrawn membrane, 144.
—— cochlearis, 120.
—— lenticularis, 122.
Progressive deafness, 33.
Promontory, 120.
—— appearance of, in indrawn membrane, 144.
—— shining through membrane, 13.
Prophylaxis of ear diseases, 62, 64.

Psammoma of dura mater, 228.
Psychical phenomena of hearing, 56, 57.
Psychological deafness, 231.
Pulmonary diseases, prevalence of, among infants, 21.
―――― tuberculosis in relation to ear diseases, 180.
Pulse, the, in cerebral abscess, 176.
―――― the, in purulent meningitis, 178.
Pupils, state of, in purulent meningitis, 178.
Pyæmia, 178.
Pyramid, 123.

QUININE, a cause of hyperæmia of labyrinth, 213.
―――― as cause of sounds in ear, 56, 213.
―――― in treatment of ear disease, 71.
―――― ―――― of Menière's disease, 222.
―――― ―――― of otalgia, 206.
―――― ―――― of otitis intermittens, 230.
―――― ―――― of tinnitus, 204.

RÂLES from presence of exudation in tympanum, 154.
―――― heard by otoscope, 40.
Rarefaction, treatment by, in external meatus, 203.
Rattling sound in ear, 55.
Recessus ellipticus, 207.
―――― sphericus, 207.
Reflector for examining the ear, 8.
―――― mode of fixing, to mouth-plate, 11.
Reflex causes of ear disease, 65.
―――― coughing, 83.
―――― neuroses, 228.
―――― origin of otalgia, 205.
―――― psychosis, 57.
―――― symptoms, 83, 85, 100.
―――― vertigo, 58.
―――― vomiting, 83.
Reissner's membrane, 209.
Remedies for ear diseases in Middle Ages, 3.
―――― general, 67, 71.
Resonance and tinnitus, 53.
Resonants, their effect in autophony, 150.

Rhagades in eczema, 77.
Rhinoscopy in diagnosis of closure of Eustachian tube, 146.
Rivinian notch, 109, 121.
Rotation, movements of, in Menière's disease, 219.

SACCULUS vestibuli, 209.
Sal ammoniac vapour, 50.
Salicylic acid a cause of hyperæmia of labyrinth, 213.
―――― ―――― in treatment of diphtheritic inflammation, 141.
―――― ―――― in treatment of eczema, 78.
―――― ―――― ―――― of otalgia, 206.
―――― ―――― ―――― of tinnitus, 204.
―――― ―――― solution for syringing, 19.
Saline baths, 72.
Salpingo-palatine fold, 41.
―――― pharyngeal fold, 41.
Salt-water baths in scrofulous conditions, 203.
Sarcoma of auditory nerve, 228.
―――― of ear, 237.
Scala tympani, 209.
―――― ―――― in leukæmia, 227.
―――― vestibuli, 209.
Scarification in meningitis, 111.
Scarlet fever as cause of aural disease, 65, 128, 131, 134, 245.
Scrofula as cause of ear disease, 65, 128.
―――― prevalence of, among deaf-mutes, 246.
―――― treatment of, 203.
Scrofulous diathesis, predisposition to ear disease in, 128.
―――― ―――― treatment of, 71, 72.
Sea-sickness causing hæmorrhage into tympanum, 206.
Semicircular canals, as place of origin of Menière's disease, 220.
―――― ―――― discovery of, 4.
―――― ―――― experiments on function of, 57, 220.
―――― ―――― extravasation of blood into, 214.
―――― ―――― functions of, 211.
―――― ―――― hæmorrhage into, 219.
―――― ―――― ossification of, 215.

Sensory aphasia, 231.
Septum narium, convexity of, 42, 43.
Sequestra, removal of, 196.
Shrapnell's membrane, 12, 109, 122.
—— —— perforation of, 160, 161, 183.
—— —— rupture of, 114.
Sigmoid fossa, distance of, from meatus, 125.
Sinus, cavernous, extension of thrombosis to, 179.
—— cranial, hæmorrhage from, 170, 178.
—— —— phlebitis of, 175, 178.
—— jugular, dilatation of, 54.
—— lateral, destruction of walls of, 197.
—— —— excavation of, 190.
—— —— extension of disease to, 174, 179.
—— —— —— of otitis externa to, 89.
—— —— relations of, to meatus, 125.
—— longitudinal, extension of thrombosis to, 179.
—— superior petrosal, destruction of walls of, 179.
Simulated deafness, testing, 34.
Singing in the ear, 53.
Small-pox, cause of ear disease, 65, 128.
Smell, sense of, affected by chronic suppuration, 159.
Snare, galvano-caustic, 71, 194.
—— loop, 192.
Sneezing in purulent inflammation of middle ear, 162.
—— restoring permeability of Eustachian tube, 145.
—— rupture of membrana tympani from violent, 113.
Snuff, borax as, in naso-pharyngeal catarrh, 140.
Soda, bicarbonate of, use of, 202.
Soft palate, action of, 127.
—— —— clonic spasm of, 151.
—— —— electrical treatment of muscles of, 148.
Solutions for injection into tympanum, 49.
—— used in syringing, 19.

Sound-conduction, 121.
—— —— through air, 21.
—— —— —— bones, 4, 21.
—— conductor, Politzer's, 204.
Sounds, auscultation, 47.
—— in ear. *See* Tinnitus aurium.
—— loud, causing concussion, 222.
—— —— —— deafness, 64.
—— —— —— vertigo, 57.
—— —— effect of, on ear, 113.
Spasms, muscular, causing tinnitus, 55.
—— of muscles of soft palate, 151.
Spatula-shaped instrument for removing foreign bodies, 102.
—— —— —— handle for, 138.
—— —— probe, 102.
Spectacle-frame for head-mirror, 11.
Speculum, Brunton's, 9.
—— cylindrical cone-shaped, 8.
—— description and use of, 8.
—— first suggested, 3.
—— Kramer's, 8.
—— Siegle's, 9.
—— Wilde's, 9.
Speech, importance of high tones in, 34.
—— testing with, 23.
Sphenoidal sinus, 41.
Spinal accessory nerve, implication of, in thrombosis of jugular vein, 179.
Spiral lamina, 208.
Spirit lotion, use of, 92, 183.
Sponge tents, 105.
Sputum, transmission of tuberculosis to ear by, 180.
Stabbing, case of injury by, 234.
Stapedius, 123.
—— muscle, contraction of, 152.
—— tenotomy of, for tinnitus, 54.
Stapes, anchylosis of, 5, 29, 163, 204, 215, 219, 226.
—— —— of annular ligament of, 199.
—— capitulum of, 15, 122.
—— description of, 121.
—— discovery of, 4.
—— dislocation of, 114.
—— pressure inwards, causing tinnitus, 54.
Staphylococci, 87.
Steam, application of, 65, 137.

Sterno-cleido-mastoid muscle, swelling at, 171.
Strabismus associated with deafness, 232.
Stylo-mastoid artery, hæmorrhage from, 170.
Suction for removing foreign bodies, 103.
—— —— —— exudations from tympanum, 157.
Sulcus tympanicus, 15, 109.
Sulphur baths, treatment by, 73.
Sulphate of copper, use of, 184.
—— of soda solution, 20.
—— of zinc, use of, 184, 202.
Sunlight, examination by, 11.
Suppuration, acute, 131, 158.
—— chronic, 158.
—— mode of extension to brain, 174.
—— of the ears, frequency of, 62.
—— of parotid gland from otitis externa, 89.
Sympathetic affection of opposite ear from foreign body, 101.
—— nerve, application of galvanism to, 69, 229.
—— —— diminished influence of, causing hyperæmia of labyrinth, 213.
—— —— electric treatment of, for hyperæmia of labyrinth, 213.
Symptomatology, 52.
Synostosis of stapes in fenestra ovalis, 199.
Syphilis, 224.
—— affecting labyrinth, 226.
—— as cause of ear disease, 65.
—— effect on Eustachian tube, 143, 146.
—— inoculated by Eustachian catheter, 45.
—— of meatus, 97.
—— treatment of, 225.
Syphilitic irido-choroiditis, case of, 225.
—— keratitis, 225.
Syringes, description of, 18.
—— Pravaz's, 50, 157.
Syringing, cause of giddiness and fainting, 86.
—— directions to be observed in, 18.

Syringing, evil effects of, 65.
—— —— of cold fluids in, 20.
—— for removal of ceruminal plugs, 85.
—— —— —— of foreign bodies, 101.
—— solutions used in, 19.

TASTE, sense of, affected by chronic suppuration, 159, 162.
Teeth, decayed, cause of otalgia, 65.
—— sound-conduction through, 22.
Tegmen tympani, 120.
—— —— extension of suppuration through, 175.
Temperature in cerebral abscess, 176.
—— in purulent meningitis, 178.
Temporal bone, anatomical description of, according to development, 234.
—— —— caries of, 6.
—— —— development of, 235.
—— —— fractures of, 235.
—— lobe of brain, abscess in, 175, 176, 197.
—— —— —— case of tumour in, 232.
—— —— —— situation of centre of hearing in, 231.
Temporary deafness, cases of, 228.
Tenotomy knives, 138.
—— operation of, 204.
Tensor tympani, 122.
—— —— contraction of, causing tinnitus, 55, 151.
—— —— —— of tendon of, 144.
—— —— muscle, 55.
—— —— nerve-supply of, 123.
—— —— spasm of, 151.
—— —— tenotomy of, 204.
—— veli muscle, 55, 127.
Testing simulated deafness, 34.
—— the hearing, 21.
—— —— with acoumeter, 25.
—— —— with speech, 23.
—— —— with tuning-fork, 26.
—— —— with watch, 22.
Therapeutics, general, of ear, 67.
Thrombosis, erysipelatous swelling of face in, 179.
—— from cerebral abscess, 175.
—— from chronic purulent inflammation of middle ear, 164.

Thrombus sebaceus, 84.
Tinnitus aurium, 52.
—— causes of, 52, 152.
—— character of, in chronic dry catarrh, 200.
—— effect of electric current in, 70.
—— first described as a symptom, 5.
—— from muscular spasms, 55.
—— from presence of cerumen, 85.
—— from tumours in brain, 233.
—— in acute inflammation of labyrinth, 216.
——. in anæmia, 213.
—— in artillerymen, 223.
—— in concussion of labyrinth, 223.
—— in fainting fits, 214.
——— in fracture of petrous bone, 214.
—— in hyperæmia of the labyrinth, 212, 213.
—— in Menière's disease, 219.
—— synchronous with pulse, 151.
—— treatment of, 203.
—— —— by electricity, 56, 70, 71.
Tone, perception of, 210.
—— —— —— cases of defective, 222.
——— treatment in tinnitus, 56.
Tonsilla cerebelli, tumour in, 222.
Tonsils of the Eustachian tube, 142.
—— of the pharynx, 142.
Toothache from furunculosis, 88.
—— nostrums for, affecting ear, 65.
Tophi in auricle, 81.
Toynbee's otoscope, 47.
—— tympanic tube, 186.
Trephining, indications for, 189.
—— mastoid first proposed, 6.
—— —— operation of, 188.
—— sclerosed bone, 168.
Trigeminus, 65.
—— implication of, in thrombosis, 179.
—— neuralgia of, 161.
—— —— associated with deafness, 232.
—— pain from pressure upon, by sclerosed mastoid, 168.
Tuba Eustachii, 4.
Tubercle bacilli, 180.
Tuberculosis, 180.
—— as cause of ear disease, 65.

Tumours, cerebral, as cause of deafness, 221, 232, 233.
—— in temporal lobe, case of, 232.
—— of auricle, 78, 81.
—— pearl, 165.
Tuning-forks, graphic statement of tests with, 30.
—— testing with, 26, 29.
Turbinated bodies, 41, 143, 147.
Turpentine, oil of, for otalgia, 206.
Tympanic apparatus, function of, 122.
—— catheter, Weber-Liel's, 188.
—— cavity. *See* Middle ear.
—— membrane. *See* Membrana tympani.
—— part of temporal bone, 235.
—— plexus of nerves, 123.
—— ring, 83.
—— tube, 50, 106, 157.
—— —— Hartmann's, 185.
Tympanophony, 60, 149.
Tympanum. *See* Middle ear.
Types of deafness, according to test with tuning-fork, 31.
Typhoid fever a cause of ear disease, 65, 128, 131.
Typhus fever a cause of deaf-mutism, 245.
—— —— ear in, 135.

ULCERATIVE ostitis, 169.
Umbo, 12, 109.
Utriculus vestibuli, 209.

VAGUS, implication of, in thrombosis of jugular vein, 179.
Valsalvian experiment, 5, 36.
Vapours in treatment of chronic dry catarrh of tympanum, 202.
—— introduced through Eustachian tube, 49.
Vapour of chloroform in tinnitus, 203.
—— —— —— otalgia, 206.
Vascular sounds, 54.
—— supply of internal ear, 212.
Vasomotor defects, electricity in treatment of, 69.
—— disturbances, 213, 228, 230.
Vein in foramen cæcum, 180.
—— internal jugular, 121.

Venous engorgement, hæmorrhage into tympanum from, 206.
—— hæmorrhage, 170.
—— sounds, 54.
Vertebræ, pressure upon cervical, affecting tinnitus, 56.
Vertebral canal, affection of, in purulent meningitis, 177.
Vertigo, auditory. *See* Giddiness.
Vestibular nerve, 210.
Vestibule, the, 207.
—— function of the, 210.
—— periostitis of, 226.
Vision, defects of, from cerebral tumours, 232.
Vomiting, causing hæmorrhage into tympanum, 206.
—— from presence of ceruminal plug, 85.
—— in acute inflammation of labyrinth, 216.
—— in cerebral abscess, 176.
—— in Menière's disease, 219.
—— in purulent meningitis, 178.

Vomiting, reflex, 83.
Vowels, volume of sound of, 23.

WARM BATHS, treatment by, 72.
Watch, testing hearing with, 22.
Whistling sound in ear, 200.
Whooping-cough, causing hæmorrhage into tympanum, 206.
—— —— deafness after paroxysm of, 214.
Wilde's incision, mode of performing, 139.
—— speculum, 9.
Word-deafness, 231.

XEROSIS of cornea associated with deafness, 232.

YAWNING, restoring patency of Eustachian tube, 145.

ZINC, sulphate of, use of, 184, 202.
Zittmann's Decoction, 225.

INDEX OF AUTHORITIES.

ABERCROMBIE, 175, 214.
Abraham, 75.
Abul Kasem, 3.
Albers, 153.
Alexander of Tralles, 3, 103.
Andry, 152.
Apollonius, 1.
Aristotle, 4.

BAGINSKY, 47, 58, 211.
Beck, 188.
Becker, 182.
Bendelack-Hewetson, 139.
Benni, 206.
Berthold, 11, 124.
Bezold, 21, 24, 29, 62, 63, 66, 90, 93, 97, 125, 131, 141, 171, 180, 182, 196, 211, 234.
Bircher, 245.
Blake, 118, 192.
Blau, 90, 227.
Böck, 55, 151.
Boerhaave, 5.
Bonnafont, 46, 111.
Böttcher, 228.
Boudin, 243.
Bourcq, 229.
Bremer, 55, 106, 151.
Brenner, 53, 59, 69, 70.
Brown, 99.
Brugsch, 1.
Brunner, 52, 53, 56, 61, 150, 152, 222.
Brunton, 9.
Buchanan, 83.
Buck, 168.
Buhl, 180.
Burckhardt-Merian, 20, 97, 131, 134, 135, 138, 141, 203.
Bürkner, 63.

Burnett, 160.
Burow, 45.

CAPIVACCIUS, 4.
Celsus, 2
Cerlata, Peter de la, 4.
Charcot, 222, 229.
Cheselden, 7.
Cleland, 6.
Colladon, 75.
Conta, 27.
Cooper, Astley, 7.
Cotugno, 6.
Crampton, 170.
Czermak, 11.

DAUSCHER, 153.
Deleau, 6, 7, 36, 102, 103.
Delstanche, 46, 117, 203.
Dennert, 25, 146.
Du Verney, 5.

ERB, 69, 70, 71.
Erhard, 46, 184.
Eschle, 180.
Eustachius, 4.

FABRICIUS, 156.
Fallopius, 4.
Ferrier, 231.
Field, 106.
Fleischmann, 152.
Flemming, 149.
Flourens, 57, 220.
Frank, 44, 50, 60, 100, 116, 156.
Fränkel, E., 100.

GADESDEN, 3.
Galen, 2, 3.

T

INDEX OF AUTHORITIES.

Galton, 26.
Gellè, 124, 247.
Gerlach, 142.
Goltz, 58.
Gottstein, 54, 94, 141, 152, 184, 227.
Griesinger, 179, 232.
Gruber, 39, 104, 118, 119, 146.
Gudden, 80.
Guyot, 6.

HABERMANN, 54, 181.
Hagen, 53, 69, 184.
Hasse, 210.
Hassenstein, 117.
Haygarth, 86.
Heckscher, 152.
Heidenreich, 46.
Heinicke, 106, 249.
Heller, 217.
Helmholtz, 121, 122, 210, 211.
Hensen, 57.
Hessler, 160, 168, 183.
Heusinger, 239.
Hinton, 47, 118, 153, 157, 224, 225.
Hippocrates, 1, 91.
Hitzig, 152.
Hocker, 103.
Hoffman, 10.
Holmes, 55.
Hughlings-Jackson, 220, 223.
Huguenin, 233, 244.
Hutchinson, 224, 225.
Hutin, 232.
Hyrtl, 238.

INGRASSIAS, 4.
Itard, 6, 7, 25, 36.

JAGO, 149.
Jasser, 6.

KESSEL, 25, 46, 110, 205.
Kiesselbach, 53.
Kirchner, 87, 213.
Knapp, 7, 23, 117, 131, 132, 137, 217, 225, 227.
Knorre, 106.
Köbner, 45.
Koch, 180.
Kölliker, 83.

König, 26.
Köppe, 56.
Kosegarten, 118.
Koyter, 5.
Kramer, 6, 7, 46, 51, 92, 101.

LACHARIÈRE, 97.
Ladame, 233.
Lannois, 227.
Leblanc, 177.
Le Cat, 5.
Leiter, 74.
Lemoine, 227.
Levi, 100.
Lincke, 7, 24, 46.
Lindenbaum, 146.
Löwenberg, 60, 87, 93, 103, 183.
Lucae, 27, 28, 39, 46, 56, 59, 106, 118, 119, 152, 181, 204, 205, 211, 214, 217.
Luschka, 82.

MACH, 22.
MacKeown, 119.
Mayer, 95, 153.
Meissner, 153.
Menière, 184, 219, 220.
Merkel, 217.
Meyer, L., 57, 80.
Meyer, R., 174.
Meynert, 230.
Middeldorpf, 71.
Moldenhauer, 103.
Moos, 7, 34, 35, 54, 64, 90, 100, 106, 107, 110, 141, 161, 162, 166, 167, 179, 194, 205, 210, 214, 215, 216, 217, 218, 219, 221, 226, 228, 232, 233, 239, 247.
Morand, 6.
Morpurgo, 160, 183.
Mosler, 162.
Müller, Joh., 55, 60.
Munk, 231.

NATHAN, 180.

ODENIUS, 170.
Oertel, 203.

PASTEUR, 87.
Paul of Ægina, 3.
Petit, J. L., 6.
Pilcher, 100.
Politzer, 7, 12, 14, 17, 21, 25, 26, 27, 29, 37, 38, 39, 46, 55, 60, 68, 74, 99, 103, 116, 119, 123, 139, 144, 145, 154, 156, 160, 181, 184, 185, 188, 192, 194, 200, 202, 203, 204, 211, 212, 214, 215, 216, 218, 223, 226, 227, 228, 229, 236.
Pomeroy, 46.
Ponce, 248.
Poorten, 150.
Pravaz, 50, 80, 157.
Prout, 23.

RAU, 239.
Reichard, 62.
Rein, 99.
Reynolds, 152.
Rhazes, 3.
Rhodes, 75.
Rinne, 22, 28, 29.
Riolan, 6, 7.
Rokitansky, 175.
Roosa, 213.
Rüdinger, 149.

SABATIER, 100.
Saemann, 51.
Saissy, 51.
Sassonia, 4.
Scanzoni, 228.
Schalle, 153, 157.
Schellhammer, 5.
Schmaltz, 242, 244, 246, 248.
Schmidekam, 57.
Schulte, 162.
Schwalbe, 236.
Schwartze, 7, 51, 56, 85, 111, 151, 153, 154, 157, 181, 183, 186, 189, 190, 216, 234.
Siebenmann, 95, 96.
Siegle, 15, 140.
Semeledei, 11, 153.
Serapion, 3.

Steinbrügge, 34, 166, 167, 194, 210, 216, 219.

TOYNBEE, 7, 47, 85, 117, 118, 129, 176, 186, 228.
Treviranus, 6.
Tröltsch, Von, 7, 9, 10, 46, 56, 62, 91, 92, 113, 121, 143, 148, 170, 175, 180, 198, 224.
Türck, 56.

URBANTSCHITSCH, 57, 112, 145, 148, 153, 162, 214, 229, 239.
Uspensky, 230.

VALSALVA, 5, 6.
Vesalius, 4.
Vetter, 232.
Vidal, 206.
Virchow, 228.
Voltolini, 35, 104, 153, 170, 204, 216, 230.

WAGENHÄUSER, 184.
Walb, 97.
Walton, 229.
Weber, E. H., 22, 28, 29.
Weber-Liel, 50, 92, 157, 183, 188, 204, 230.
Wedel, 86.
Weil, 56, 62, 63.
Wendt, 85, 100, 168.
Wernicke, 231.
Westphal, 232.
Wilde, 7, 9, 163, 192.
Wilhelmi, 218.
William of Saliceto, 3.
Willis, 4, 60.
Woakes, 213.
Wolf, Oscar, 23, 24, 221.
Wolf, Ph. H., 50.
Wolke, 25.
Wreden, 90, 93, 94, 95, 176, 202.

YEARSLEY, 116, 117, 182.

ZAUFAL, 50, 101, 104, 197, 229, 230.
Zeissl, 225.

PRINTED AT THE EDINBURGH UNIVERSITY PRESS,
BY T. AND A. CONSTABLE, PRINTERS TO HER MAJESTY.

www.ingramcontent.com/pod-product-compliance
Lightning Source LLC
Chambersburg PA
CBHW032048230426
43672CB00009B/1514